birthing normally
after a caesarean or two

Emmanuel Bujold

Consultant obstetrician and gynaecologist, and author of VBAC studies:

What a pleasure it is to read about a subject I thought I was tired of! In fact, it's worth taking another look at this topic...

Hélène Vadeboncoeur provides a lovely mixture of scientific data and birth stories, which does justice to the dramatic situation a woman finds herself in when she decides to have a vaginal birth after a previous caesarean.

I sincerely believe that all caregivers and women who need to choose whether or not to arrange a VBAC should read this little gem of a book. Pregnant women will find many answers to questions, as well as a great deal of other necessary information and—most of all—reassurance and comfort if they decide to choose to have a VBAC. Thank you, Hélène, for giving us all this gift—the key to transforming a birth from a trauma into a wonderful experience.

birthing normally
after a caesarean or two

— a guide for pregnant women —

exploring reasons and practicalities for VBAC

Hélène Vadeboncoeur

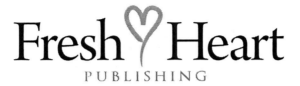

1st British edition with notes and references

First published in Great Britain in 2011 by
FRESH HEART PUBLISHING
a division of Fresh Heart Ltd
PO Box 225, Chester le Street, DH3 9BQ
www.freshheartpublishing.co.uk

© Fresh Heart Publishing 2011

The moral right of Hélène Vadeboncoeur to be identified as the author of this work has been asserted in accordance with the Copyright, Designs and Patents Act 1988.

All rights reserved. No part of this publication may be reproduced, stored in a retrieval system, or transmitted, in any form or by any means, electronic, mechanical, photocopying, recording or otherwise, without the prior permission of the publisher. Nor may this publication be circulated in any form of binding or cover other than that in which it is published and without a similar condition being imposed on the subsequent purchaser.

A CIP catalogue record for this publication is available from the British Library

ISBN: 978 1 906619 15 2

Original French text *Une autre césarienne ou un accouchement naturel?
S'informer pour mieux décider* published by Carte Blanche in Quebec, Canada, with extracts from the 1st edition of the same book, *Une autre césarienne?
Non, merci*, published by Editions Québec/Amérique, Canada
This English edition is an updated, adapted version of the original French texts and includes additional new material
French texts translated and edited by Sylvie Donna
Printed in the UK by Lightning Source UK Ltd
Cover design by Fresh Heart Publishing
Cover photo of Annie Bourgeois and Rafaël Bourgeois Mailloux
Designed and typeset by Fresh Heart Publishing
Set in Franklin Gothic Book, Bookman Old Style and Comic Sans MS

Disclaimer

While the advice and information contained in this book are believed to be accurate and true at the time of going to press, neither the author, nor the translator, nor the editor, nor the publisher can accept any legal responsibility for loss, damage or injury occasioned to any person acting or refraining from action as a result of information contained. The advice is intended as a guideline only and should never be used as a replacement for consultation with midwives, doctors or consultants.

Photo © Regroupement Les Sages-Femmes du Québec, Canada

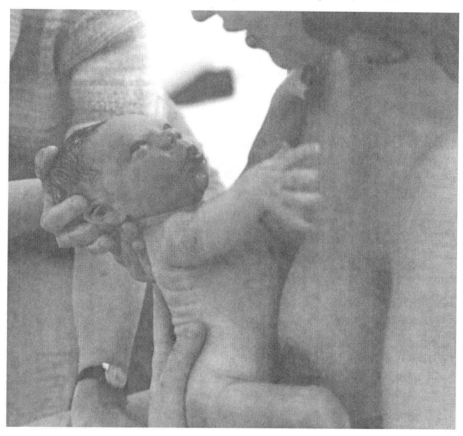

Dedication

- ♥ For my mother, Marie Gaboury, who was one of the first women in Quebec to insist on giving birth without general anaesthesia.
- ♥ For my father, Pierre Vadeboncoeur, from whom I inherited a love of writing.
- ♥ For my children, Nicholas and Isabelle... Without them this book on birth would never have seen the light of day and I would never have become a researcher in perinatalogy.

**Whatever you dream of doing, begin!
There's genius in audacity, power, magic.**
Goethe

Contents

Acknowledgements x

A few words from a professor of midwifery, Mavis Kirkham... xii

... and a few words from a mother, Nina Klose xiv

Introduction 1

Who's this book for? How can it help you? 1

• Birthframe 1: The author's experience—a caesarean followed by a VBAC 2

• Birthframe 2: The author's partner's comments on the two experiences 4

Part 1: To birth or to section, that is the question 7

CHAPTER 1:

The current situation 8

Different viewpoints 8

Rising caesarean rates 8

The trivialisation of the caesarean 9

Reasons for promoting normality, and ways of doing so 14

Changing trends from a historical perspective 15

VBAC rates 16

Changing feelings about pregnancy and birth 18

Changing patterns of information transfer 19

The need for change 20

The significance of recent changes for VBACs 21

Official policies 22

Women started having fewer VBACs... 23

A first consensus development conference on VBAC is organised 24

Reasons why so many caesareans take place and so few VBACs 27

To summarise... 30

• Birthframe 3: Caregivers who were very reluctant to support a VBAC 31

• Birthframe 4: Very different responses from different consultants 33

• Birthframe 5: Preparing properly, but seeing it all from various points of view 35

CHAPTER 2:

The risk element, whatever your decision 38

Risks relating to VBACs for mother and baby 39

Understanding what a rupture really is 39

The level of risk: 0.2% - 0.6% for spontaneous labour 41

Factors which increase the risk of uterine rupture 43

The role of subjectivity when considering a repeat caesarean 48

The real increase in risk... the risk of litigation? 49

Risks associated with caesareans for both mother and baby 52

A comparison of risks associated with caesareans and VBAC 58

The advantage for your baby of letting birth start spontaneously 60

To summarise... 62

• Birthframe 6: A scan which wrongly 'revealed' the baby was too big for a VBAC 66

• Birthframe 7: Being encouraged to have a VBAC, with various conditions... 70

CHAPTER 3:

Persuasive reasons to have a VBAC 71

The need for a decision, whatever people around you think 71

Pros and cons for the baby of either a VBAC or a caesarean 72

How women make a decision 74

Why did you have a caesarean before anyway? 76

Was your caesarean necessary or not? 77

Clear medical indications for a caesarean ('absolute indications') 78

Possible but controversial indications ('relative indications') 78

Myths about problems people believe a caesarean can prevent 82

What are your chances of having a VBAC? 82

What if a woman refuses to have a VBAC? 96

What if you're refused a VBAC? 97

Hospitals which are focused on increasing the VBAC rate 99

To summarise... 102

• Birthframe 8: Persuaded of the reasons, but still unsure... her body decided! 103

• Birthframe 9: A successful VBAC, despite a family history of caesarean birth 104

Some hospitals are focused on increasing the VBAC rate

Part 2: How to prepare for a safe, successful VBAC 112

CHAPTER 4:

Consider the emotional aftermath 113

Consider your own feelings 113

Consider the impact on your family 120

Consider the impact on your partner 120

Possible psychological effects of caesareans on mothers 121

Consider the impact on your baby 122

Let yourself heal 123

To summarise... 128

• Birthframe 10: Dealing with the emotional aftermath 130

• Birthframe 11: Believing it was possible was the biggest barrier to overcome 133

• Birthframe 12: Preparing differently and then deciding to trust the baby 135

• Birthframe 13: Experiencing a new kind of emotional landscape 140

It's important to consider your feelings and the impact of your decision on yourself, your family, your partner and also on your baby

CHAPTER 5:

Create a supportive environment 151

Use the antenatal period wisely 151

Consider finding antenatal classes 153

Prepare physically 155

Prepare mentally 158

Find the right birthplace 164

Find a supportive caregiver 167

Appreciate the benefits of getting the support you need 171

Deal with people around you effectively 174

To summarise... 176

• Birthframe 14: Getting different treatment from different caregivers 177

• Birthframe 15: Resentment because of the way in which decisions were made 179

• Birthframe 16: Having trouble finding support, but getting there in the end 181

• Birthframe 17: Developing increasing confidence in supportive environments 182

CHAPTER 6:

Make wise decisions during labour 188

Things to avoid, ideally 189
Things to do to facilitate a vaginal birth 190
Frequently asked questions about VBAC labour and birth 196
To summarise... 210
• Birthframe 18: Encountering complete lack of support in hospital 212
• Birthframe 19: A twin VBAC with wise care during labour 213
• Birthframe 20: An important glimmer of positivity amongst all the negativity... 214
• Birthframe 21: Learning how to do it normally: a VBAC after two caesareans 216

CHAPTER 7:

Remember the reasons for birthing normally... 218

Current trends and the quest to reclaim vaginal birth 220
Birth as a reflection of values... 223
Why should you want to give birth yourself? 224
But how on earth can you do it? 229
Whatever happens, keep a sense of perspective 231
To summarise... 232
• Birthframe 22: A VBAC after four caesareans and better postnatal recovery 233
• Birthframe 23: Preparing for a VBAC but deciding to have a section after all 234
• Birthframe 24: A VBAC which didn't work out, but she was pleased she'd tried 235
• Birthframe 25: Taking risks or doing the safest thing? Not disturbing labour... 236
• Birthframe 26: Seeing the benefits of antenatal rather than postnatal pain 239
• Birthframe 27: Consequences of unsupportive and supportive environments 242

Why should you want to give birth yourself?

Useful contacts 246
Bibliography 248
Further reading 249
Notes and references 251
Glossary 284
Index 298
About the author 314

Acknowledgements

First, I would like to thank my partner, Steve, for supporting me during the writing of this book—for patiently putting up with tables in the kitchen and living room covered in documents, yet again! I really appreciate the way he lovingly prepared supper almost every evening during his holidays so as to let me work throughout the evenings. His support is particularly remarkable if you take into account that it took me five years to complete my PhD just a few years before. Fortunately, this book didn't take quite as long!

I want to thank all the women who wrote to me after the first French edition of this book came out. I feel honoured that they showed me so much trust and am very encouraged by their accounts of VBACs, particularly since some of these normal births were difficult to arrange. You will be able to read some of these women's accounts in the pages of this book. I am grateful to all the people who allowed me to use their accounts.

I would also like to thank the people who willingly agreed to read chapters of this book, or indeed the whole book. I am particularly grateful to the health professionals, who I interviewed for the first French edition, and also to everyone who helped me with my research. In particular, my thanks go to...

- My mother, Marie Gaboury, who provided feedback on the whole script
- Guy-Paul Gagné, obstetrician/gynaecologist and director of the Quebec programme 'AMPRO' of the Society of Obstetricians/Gynaecologists in Canada
- France Lebrun, head of nursing at the medical centre in Saint-Eustache
- Lise Gosselin, nurse at the Haute-Yamaska community health centre
- Catherine Chouinard, head of the perinatology project at the Quebec association of public health
- Sylvie Thibault, doula and director of 'Mère et Monde' (Mother and the World)
- Josette Charpentier, doula of 25 years' standing
- Célyne Purcell, mother of two children born by caesarean, who gave feedback on the manuscript before trying to have a VBAC, and who allowed me to use a photo of her with her second baby
- Audrey Gendron, who gave me feedback on the manuscript while pregnant with her fourth child
- Jacques Viau, co-owner of the Biosfaire bookshop and good friend, who sadly left this world in August 2009
- Martin Renaud, of the Ministry of Health and Social Security in Quebec, for statistics for Quebec for the last few years
- Annie Bourgeois, who kindly agreed to be photographed with her son for the front cover when she was seven months pregnant—the photo was taken by her father, the photographer Jacques Bourgeois

Acknowledgements xi

- Marie-Josée Aubin and Sebastien Larocque who have allowed me to use the photos which record their first meeting with Tommy on 21 July 2007
- Céline Bianchi, Judith Harvie and Antoinette Geha, who have allowed me to use photos with their birth stories
- My sister, Rachel Vadeboncoeur, for her artwork on page 313—see http://saltspring.tripod.com/rachel/ for more information about her work
- Cheyla Reader, my niece, who—with her youthful enthusiasm—helped me verify the hundreds of references of this book, and my pregnant daughter-in-law, Nathalia Guerrero Velez, who helped with the Index
- Sylvie Donna, the wonderful founder of Fresh Heart Publishing, whose knowledge of French and whose creativity helped make this UK edition a very useful tool for English-speaking pregnant women, their partners and—who knows?—perhaps their health caregivers too

The publisher would also like to thank:

- The contributors of birthframes: Hélène, Steve, Judith, Antoinette, Lorraine, Coleen's husband, Audrey, Marie-Josée and Marie-Josée (two of the contributors happened to have same name), Isabelle, Céline and Célyne (two contributors who *nearly* had the same name), Nina, Estelle, Huguette, Irene, Marie-Claude, Nicole and Raymond, as well as Nicole and Robert, Pierrette, Diane, Shirley, Michelle, Chantale, Françoise, Susie, André and Christine
- The following contributors of birthframes, who also contributed the photographs which appear on pages xii, 65, 69, 110, 111, 129, 138, 139, 245: Antoinette, Marie-Josée, Judith, Céline and Marie-Josée
- *MAMANzine,* Lysane Grégoire from 'Groupe Maman' and the women who wrote Birthframes 6, 9 and 17 (which originally appeared in vol.11, no.1, Sept 2007)
- Regroupement Les Sages-Femmes du Québec, Canada (Quebec Association of Midwives) for graciously allowing the use of the photos on pages v, xiii, xvi, 7, 112, 157, 195, 200, 208, 215, 241, 245 and 310
- The medical/cultural anthropologist, expert on childbirth and midwifery and author, Robbie Davis-Floyd (RE Davis-Floyd), for contributing the beautiful photos which feature on pages 101, 154, 155, 187, 188, 205, 219 and 231 and the original photographers Rachel Yellin, Michelle Welborne, Robbie Davis-Floyd, Noa Mohlabane, Erin Brown, Yeshi Neumann, Elayne Klein and Bliss Dake

If any material has been used accidentally without appropriate acknowledgement, or if any details are incorrect, please contact the publisher with details so that amendments can be made in future editions. Every possible effort has been made to ensure that all details of contributions are correct.

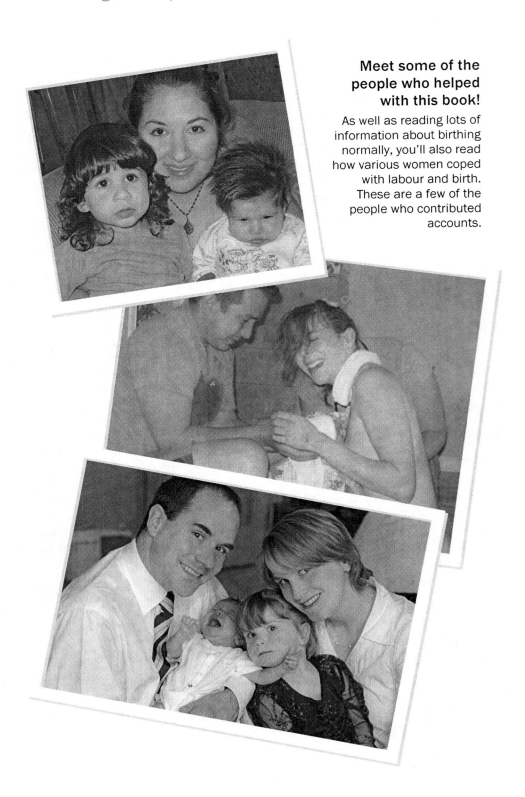

Meet some of the people who helped with this book!

As well as reading lots of information about birthing normally, you'll also read how various women coped with labour and birth. These are a few of the people who contributed accounts.

A few words from a professor of midwifery...

Maternal choice in childbirth has been Department of Health policy since 1993, yet even well into the 21st century so often women feel they have no option but to go along with what their caregivers see as the right way to have their baby, even when that seems right for the organisation rather than the individual woman. This book is the antidote to that situation.

Hélène Vadeboncoeur has written a balanced and highly informative book. She shows how the present pressures towards caesarean section are the product of our social circumstances and are not inevitable, though they may feel like a train had rushed in and taken over. She shows how this situation results from our society's reliance on technology, the shortage of midwives and the 'muzak' of fear which pervades maternity services.

> Hélène shows how the current situation results from our society's reliance on technology, the shortage of midwives and the 'muzak' of fear which pervades maternity services

This book presents a wealth of information, whilst being very user friendly. It is clearly written and thoroughly but unobtrusively referenced. Statistics are presented which clearly illuminate the arguments. Research evidence is well presented. Risks are examined and placed in context with appropriate statistics, and links are made which do not appear in obstetric texts. Overall, the book makes clear that there is not just one obstetric reality, but several, and that these are not necessarily the ones we hear as unavoidable solutions.

Yet there is a limit to what statistics and research can show. Stories tell so much that statistics cannot convey: the variety and nuances of women's experiences and responses to their experience. The great variety of the women's VBAC stories told here is fundamental to the structure of the book.

> There is a big difference between choosing a VBAC and achieving one and the chapters on creating a supportive environment and making wise decisions during labour are immensely helpful

There is a big difference between choosing a VBAC and achieving one and the chapters on creating a supportive environment and making wise decisions during labour are also immensely helpful, as are the useful contacts listed.

This rich resource is full of helpful information and telling experience. I shall be recommending it to women considering VBAC and to my colleagues as a book which can help us change individual women's experience and maternity services for the better.

Mavis Kirkham
Emeritus Professor of Midwifery
Sheffield Hallam University

... and a few words from a VBAC mother

I always grieve after a birth. It feels right to own the sadness of the baby no longer inside me. Loss of my huge and beautiful pregnant self, a time when I was a queen among women. Loss of sleep! It was so much easier having that baby taken care of automatically inside my body! Add to that the losses connected with a caesarean section, and it's nearly too much to bear.

Even now, nearly 12 years later and after two subsequent vaginal births, I still feel tearful when I recall my first birth. I so wanted to give my baby a good birth, to bring him into the world myself, out of my body, to welcome him into my arms. He was born by emergency caesarean. Why?

My mum birthed me and my two brothers vaginally. "Birth is the most powerful experience a woman can have!" she told me, when I was growing up. I felt certain that my body would know what to do, and birth my son instinctively, as she had. I was so looking forward to that transformative experience, to feeling the power of my body bring forth life.

Blessed by my two daughters' natural births two and eight years after my son's, I suppose I have made peace with my own experience of the caesarean. But I still feel sad for my son—it was his loss, too. I believe there is a spiritual significance in how we enter the world, a deep and lasting effect from the experience of those most sensitive moments of the rift from the perfection of the Womb. My mother's joy, fears, strength, the way she held and nursed me, have had a profound effect on me throughout my life. Surely, how I birthed my son affects him, too.

I ask myself whether I am being needlessly hysterical. After all, he was born healthy, he was never separated from us, I nursed him straight away and for over a year. He is a fine, healthy, well-adjusted kid. But wouldn't the start of his independent life have been gentler, better, happier for him if he had entered the world through the birth canal?

What was his experience? A knife entered the amniotic sac first. Then rubber gloves. Then he was pulled out, carefully, feet first. Suctioned. Examined under a heat lamp. I could hear his little mewing cries from the corner of the room while the paediatrician checked him over and wrapped him up.

I am sure it is scary being born. When my second baby, my first daughter, was born, she cried, too, when her face rose to the surface of the birth pool. I held her naked against my skin and she looked into my face in wonder. Soon nursing, she quickly calmed. My son nursed easily too. But I couldn't hold him right away. I was strapped to the gurney, being wheeled from the operating theatre. My husband, dressed up in green scrubs so he could be there for the operation, carried the baby, a tightly wrapped and squalling bundle, down the corridor to our recovery room. I never held him naked to my skin until I brought him home from the hospital a week after his birth.

... and a few words from a VBAC mother

"Any postnatal depression?" the health visitor asked on her final visit.

"I had a caesarean. I feel very upset about it. I cried every day for a month after the birth," I reported, getting weepy again.

"Oh, that's normal. You had a major abdominal operation. You're doing fine," she said, and discharged me.

I helped myself overcome the experience of my son's caesarean birth by planning how I would do it next time. The day after I found I was pregnant a second time, I started hunting for an independent midwife. And I asked myself again and again, Why did I have a caesarean? Perhaps it was my trust in the system. The antenatal classes never warned me: "The system will try to make you into a statistic. You've got to fight!" On the NHS, I never saw the same midwife or doctor twice... I wasn't going near a hospital for this birth. A midwife who knew me might make all the difference.

It takes a lot of work to prepare for a VBAC. There's the rational side— informing yourself about risks and benefits; finding a midwife or doctor who supports you; keeping your body healthy and strong. But the emotional work is even bigger, and even more important. Why did this happen to me? Can I accept this loss, forgive myself for my first failure? Can I get back on the horse? What will it mean for me if I 'can't' give birth vaginally next time either?

The losses we experience are gifts, too. To help myself grow into giving birth on my own, I made lists such as '10 reasons why the caesarean was a gift.' (I was inspired to do this by VBAC campaigner Nancy Wainer-Cohen.) Through this process I realised that I'd experienced something new (major surgery in an operating theatre), and that I'd learnt compassion for others like me whose birth experiences were not as they longed for. Of course, I also knew the fact that my son was born healthy was a gift—and I even felt that my grief was a gift.

I found an independent midwife I loved and trusted. I prepared myself every way I could. And I was lucky. When I laboured with my second child, it hurt like hell. But I was so thrilled that my body was doing what I always knew it could, I hardly noticed. I felt such joy and peace when I had brought her into my arms. The rush of love, the bonding after a natural birth is like holding a lover in your arms after the first time you make love.

I loved my son when he was born, too. But it was a more rational, reasoned connection. "I know he must be mine, because the doctors say so." With my daughter, there was no question at all. It was a physical bond, as overwhelming as desire. I lay awake all night with my newborn daughter sleeping on my chest, skin to skin. "I did it! She's here! She's mine!" I was so excited, I could hardly sleep.

The gift of a good birth is worth dreaming and fighting for with every child. This book can help you heal the inner scars that every caesarean leaves behind. It'll also help you prepare and inform yourself to make a different journey with your next birth.

Nina Klose

xvi   birthing normally after a caesarean or two

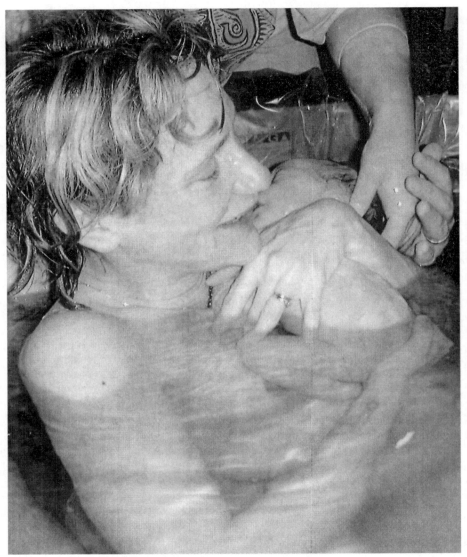

Photo © Regroupement Les Sages-Femmes du Québec, Canada

*A woman hugs her baby, just after it was born... normally, not by caesarean.
This mother experienced her pain before the birth, not afterwards.*

The gift of a good birth is worth dreaming and fighting for
with every child

Introduction

Who's this book for? How can it help you?

If you've had a caesarean before and are thinking about giving birth vaginally next time, this book is for you... as well as for your partner, who will also be concerned about the birth of your next baby. I realise it can be stressful to take responsibility for making choices about birth, and that it can be tempting to want the 'doctor' to decide and take charge of you. However, I think birthing decisions should really be made by women and couples.

It is possible that some of this book will shock you, that emotions about your previous caesarean(s) will resurface for the first time, or that they will re-emerge, even if you think you've put those feelings behind you. Don't let that stop you. As you will see when you read the birth stories in this book (called 'birthframes'), this is perfectly normal. You will also see that letting the emotions generated by a traumatic birth or a non-existent one emerge will actually help you 'heal'.

I hope that after reading this book you will feel more serene and at peace with the choices you have made for your future birth. And if you choose to give birth normally, I hope you find all the help you need to support you in this incredible adventure...

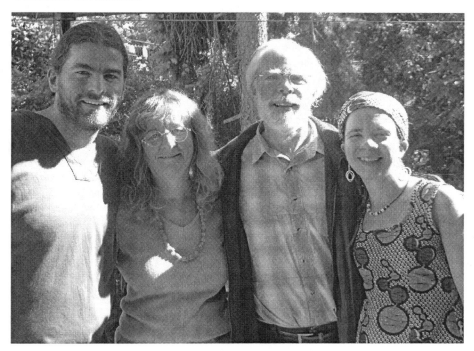

Hélène with her partner, Steve, and their children, Nicholas and Isabelle

Birthframe 1

The author's experience—a caesarean followed by a VBAC

Before I start talking about birth generally, since this is such a personal topic, as the author of this book I think I should start by telling you about my own experience. Giving birth to my children changed my own life and also that of my partner. Things did not go to plan and in 1976 I gave birth to my first baby by caesarean section after 30 hours of labour, which had been induced and augmented. My son was a brow presentation, diagnosed while I was pushing... which meant that his head remained pressed against my pelvic bone. Our consultant did all he could to ensure that my labour didn't end up as a caesarean, but without success. This man, who we had a marvellous relationship with, told us—after I'd suffered a postpartum haemorrhage (PPH) which almost sent me into the next world—that I'd been his 'worst birth in 12 years of practice'. I would have preferred not to have had this honour. And so would my partner. This life event was a brutal shock and signalled our entry into adulthood. Then life went on, painfully at first. In the years that followed I don't remember thinking about my caesarean a great deal. My only concern was to distance myself from the questions which regularly came into my head. It was only when we finally decided to try for another baby, four years later, that the impact of my first birth made itself felt. The day I found out I was pregnant I saw a newspaper headline which read: 'Post-caesarean, women can still birth naturally'. I immediately knew that this was what I wanted, even though the idea had never dawned on me before. I knew that neither my fears nor my doubts would stop me. Nevertheless, in the autumn of 1980 it wasn't easy to find a consultant who would accept me for a vaginal birth after a caesarean (a VBAC). I met two or three who would have accepted me 'if...' one thing, or 'if...' something else. In the end I found one who didn't see any problem in my having a VBAC, at least the first few times we met. But then, in the seventh month of my pregnancy, I had to start looking again because my doctor was becoming more and more nervous. The day before my daughter was born, I went to see a different doctor who hesitantly told me I could have a VBAC as long as my baby didn't weigh more than six and a half pounds at birth—bearing in mind that my first had weighed 7lb 5oz. Nevertheless, he admitted that my pelvis was normal.

That evening I felt intensely discouraged and I said to myself, "OK, that's enough searching. It's now up to the grace of God." For once, I went to bed without having done my antenatal exercises, thinking, "To hell with everything!" I don't know who heard me that night, or whether my daughter in my womb understood the consultant's words, but at 5 o'clock the next morning my waters broke and contractions started; it was exactly one month before my due date. Shaking with nerves and excitement—the first time I hadn't gone into labour spontaneously—my partner and I finally calmed ourselves down and got ourselves to the hospital a few hours later.

> I felt intensely discouraged and I said to myself, "OK, that's enough searching. It's now up to the grace of God."

Labour went well up to the moment when, after 12 minutes of pushing, my doctor—the one who I'd been with for most of my pregnancy—decided that I couldn't push any more... I protested a little but finally accepted that he would extract the baby with forceps, since he insisted: "He's premature and being pressed against the perineum for too long can cause cranial lesions." Even though I wasn't annoyed it was all finally over after 15 hours of labour, accepting this shortcut was an enormous error on my part, which I have long had difficulty forgiving myself for. Later, I realised that this doctor's words had had no scientific basis. In other words, I realised that this doctor had said something scary so as to make me let him use forceps, just as he usually did when he attended a birth.

While I was looking after my children and working over the next few years I tried to accept the feeling that the most important part of birth, for me, had been taken away from me: the part where I would have brought my baby into the world. And while I was preparing the first edition of this book I even came to the point of wanting to get pregnant again, just to get over that feeling. Fortunately, though, I didn't—thanks to my partner, who realised this was not a good reason for having a baby. But all that time, I did think about writing this book... although it took me several years to do so, since I could not feel pleased at having had a VBAC whose outcome had left me feeling so depressed.

The way some women reacted to my initial 8-page article on VBAC (back in 1986) convinced me that I should continue writing, so as to provide information to women and couples who'd previously experienced a caesarean and also to help myself come to terms with my own history. I had no idea what was in store... First of all, after spending many hours in medical libraries, reading birth stories and speaking to open-minded, progressive health care professionals, I found answers to those questions which had come into my head ever since I'd had my caesarean. Each new glimmer of understanding, however small, helped to console me on a very deep level. For example, I discovered that my postpartum haemorrhage (for which nobody had been able to provide an explanation) could have been due to the use of syntocinon (artificial oxytocin)—which I'd had plenty of all through my labour—and not to another uterine 'deficiency'. On the other hand, I also made plenty of discoveries which disturbed me further: I realised that my caesarean—which had been necessary at the point when it was carried out—could have been avoided if things had been managed differently from the beginning of my labour or if I hadn't had an epidural. I could have waited for my labour to begin spontaneously, for example. All of these thoughts evoked a huge flood of emotion, principally made up of sadness and anger. I often had to put my work to one side because I was only capable of continuing with it several weeks later. On many occasions over a long period I dreamt that I would one day be able to push my own baby out into the world. Those three years of research left me convinced that there is not just one obstetric reality, but several, and that these realities are not necessarily the ones we hear as unavoidable solutions. We women need to have our say because we're the people most immediately affected by birth. This is the main point I want to make in this book... And as I finish writing and editing I feel as if I really have given birth a third time. But this time there was no intervention!

Birthframe 2

The author's partner's comments on the two experiences

For our first baby, Hélène and I were ready to have a natural birth. We had attended antenatal classes and had found a super doctor. Hélène had had a beautiful pregnancy and everything looked good. The only thing was that she was overdue.

After three weeks, the consultant told her she needed to be admitted to hospital because her waters had been leaking for a few days. It was a Monday morning. He gave her a test which suggested the slight possibility that an infection was developing. Then he induced labour, using prostaglandin pessaries, followed by a syntocinon drip. At home Hélène had already had some castor oil—which had brought on a few contractions, but not real labour. So Hélène's contractions had started but everything was moving forwards very slowly and quietly. Over the course of several hours, I felt myself going deeper into myself and I felt Hélène going deeper too. There were moments when I felt desperate, not believing that she would ever give birth or that a baby would eventually come out. I felt as if I was in an unreal world. Several times I left the room and even the corridor and headed for the stairwell to cry because of my own sense of impotence. Then I went back in and we continued.

> Several times I left the room and even the corridor and headed for the stairwell to cry because of my own sense of impotence. Then I went back in and we continued.

She was put to sleep for several hours during the night between Monday and Tuesday, so that she could rest. Finally, after about 30 hours of labouring with the constant help of the syntocinon drip—except for when she slept—Hélène started pushing, which didn't achieve much. Then forceps were applied and they almost got stuck. This last intervention made Hélène shout out in pain. Then, when the consultant said he was going to have to perform a caesarean section, I accompanied her into the operating theatre because she was very worked up. There, I stayed right near her until everything was ready. Then our doctor asked me if I wanted to stay. I said: "Why not?" and I sat down behind her. This was how I came to attend the caesarean, with Hélène under general anaesthetic.

At the moment of the operation I felt nothing—I was already beyond that. I was just anxious for it to be over, for us to wake up from this nightmare. I no longer believed we were going to have a baby.

They did the caesarean and during this procedure I saw them fighting to disengage our baby, who was stuck in Hélène's pelvis. A midwife was pushing through Hélène's vagina while the consultant pulled with all his strength at the abdominal incision. He was 6 foot 6 inches tall and shaking while he did that. When they succeeded in getting our baby out, it seemed to me he was dead. He wasn't dead, just knocked out as a result of the general anaesthetic—that's what I learnt afterwards.

Slowly, I came back down to earth and saw my son, who—by that time—was now wide awake. It was as if I was looking at myself; I saw myself in his eyes. This feeling didn't last long but it was beautiful and I still remember it.

A little later, when I was not far from Intensive Care, I heard Hélène talking incoherently. They didn't want me to go in to see her, but I pushed the midwife out of the way and went in anyway. Hélène hadn't yet come to her senses. I told her we'd had a little boy. She didn't believe it. I told her she'd had a 'bad trip' and that it would all soon be over. Then, I put my hand on her dressing, just at the place where her baby bump had been. Then she began to come to her senses. But in the days that followed, and occasionally in the few weeks after that, for a few seconds at a time she would relive those moments when she didn't feel she belonged to herself any more, which made her very afraid. Above all, she was afraid of reliving those moments of her labour and birth.

After that there were other difficulties: she haemorrhaged one week later, then again *two* weeks later, and had to have blood transfusions; I saw her bleeding and watched her life draining out of her. At that time we reassured ourselves that it hadn't all been for nothing and that we should learn something from the experience.

We decided to get married, so as to make more of a commitment towards each other. It was one way of making what had happened meaningful, also a way of finding the strength to keep going through what we were experiencing. We had experienced the illusion of a perfect birth which had come face-to-face with reality. Each successive intervention was like a train which was accelerating, but going nowhere. I had experienced a feeling of impotence like I'd never felt before.

A few years later, we had another baby and this time Hélène wanted to give birth vaginally. I don't know if she wanted to prove she was capable of giving birth to another baby, or if it was a question of wanting a daughter. Both feelings were very much there.

I went along with her desire to have another baby, but what I discovered in the course of our lively antenatal appointments with our midwives—we had some 'secret' midwives as well as our routine care—was that I didn't actually want to have another child. I was afraid of reliving that whole experience, which had left me feeling so empty... because after the caesarean, for more than a year, Hélène had been exhausted, without energy, so everything had been down to me. At the same time, I was starting up a business, so I was embarking on *two* birthing experiences.

When she was a few weeks pregnant Hélène set out to find a hospital or a consultant who would accept her for a VBAC. This was very much *her* project. I was pretty oblivious to it all. I supported her, but she was the one who provided all the impetus. The plan was that when she found a consultant , I would go along with her. I thought it was odd to have to fight so much and do so much research just so as to find someone suitable. And since I'm wary of being rude, when she arrived at the consultant's office with her list of questions and requests, I confess to having been a bit embarrassed. I'm not sure I was very supportive. To me, a VBAC seemed to be a privilege which a consultant might confer on us—so why also insist on 'no drip', etc? Besides, I knew so little. Hélène didn't know much more, but she knew more than I did. Later on, as her pregnancy progressed, we got a lot of support from our secret midwives and it was then that I began to believe that a VBAC really would be possible and to feel that I could support Hélène in this.

When it came to her second birth, Hélène went into labour before her due date. In the early hours of the morning one day, her waters broke and we realised her labour had started. It was exciting, although my main feeling was "I don't want to go to the hospital!" I had the impression that if we were in the hospital we'd be swept along in a process over which we'd have no control. But Hélène didn't want to stay at home. She didn't feel confident enough to stay. Nevertheless, we left it until the late afternoon before we went to the hospital, with a midwife visiting us throughout the day.

In the car the contractions started to get stronger. The midwife had come to meet up with us in the labour ward. Everything was going well: contractions were very strong and the midwife was Hélène's main supporter. I didn't have much idea what I was doing there. But what was going on between the two of them was very beautiful. The midwife was being quite wonderfully supportive and after several hours Hélène was fully dilated, without having taken any medication.

At 10.30pm, she was taken into the delivery suite. Our doctor arrived and he was obviously in a bad mood: not only had we been 'late' in going into hospital (when Hélène was 5cm dilated), the registrar (a woman) had also allowed our own midwife to come into the labour ward, against his wishes. He gave Hélène 'permission' to push. It was beautiful. Everything was going well. She was proud to be pushing. But things didn't progress quickly enough for the consultant and after 12 minutes, on the false pretext that the baby was premature and that it was therefore at risk of brain damage if Hélène pushed for too long, he said he would have to use forceps to get the baby out. He performed an episiotomy—a big one—behaving as if he was conducting an orchestra, clicking and clacking his instruments. I had the impression that with this intervention it was as if he was trying to punish Hélène. Nevertheless, the forceps seemed to be used gently—he didn't pull hard and he proceeded carefully. Our daughter was born and she was put on Hélène's abdomen. As for me, I didn't feel much. I didn't have any great feeling of joy. I didn't feel 'out of it' either. It was as if the presence of the consultant—his attitude—had stopped me from feeling any emotion. Once again, a train had rushed in and taken over. It's when I go into a labour room or delivery suite that I lose all power, that I feel powerless once more—and that was certainly also the case with our birth attendant.

Sometimes I relive the scene, I mentally re-enact the whole thing, saying to the consultant: "No, no, don't perform an episiotomy," or "You must let her push." I wish I'd been more assertive. I didn't know what my rights were, or what it was possible to do. A lot of my weakness was due to a lack of information and that led to my complete lack of assertiveness. I think Hélène resents the fact that I didn't assert myself with enough strength at that moment. Neither her nor I felt fully confident. All along it was as if we were walking on egg shells. This made Hélène want to go into hospital and develop an almost symbiotic relationship with the midwife who accompanied us there. There was a kind of insecurity which made us want to hang on to something and pass on responsibility for what happened. We did not experience this VBAC in peace and harmony, but rather a little out of breath and feeling very weak. It was almost as if we felt that having a VBAC was a sin. I was afraid that the consultant would arrive and pop our bubble—that we would be found out. Perhaps we needed that last month of the pregnancy (which we didn't have) in order to prepare more fully.

Part 1:

To birth or to section, that is the question

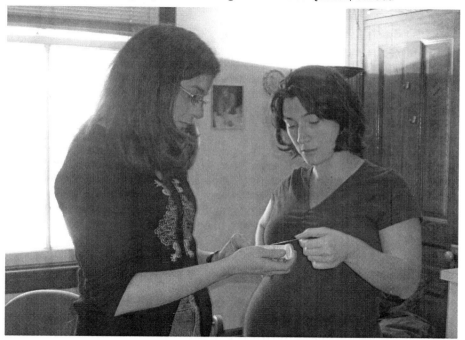

A mother and her midwife consider some test results

What should influence you when you make this decision, which is extremely important for both you and your and baby?

In the first chapter...

- Recent changes in attitudes
- Changing rates of VBAC
- Reasons why so many caesareans take place, and so few VBACs

CHAPTER 1:

The current situation

Different viewpoints

Although vaginal births after caesareans (VBACs) are common and strongly recommended by both women and many professionals, we live in a world which is increasingly considering caesareans the norm—so all that we say about VBAC needs to be considered in this light. However, for decades people have been worrying about rising caesarean rates around the world, and now, early in the new millenium, the caesarean rate is continuing to rise.

Rising caesarean rates

Rates of caesareans vary a great deal in different regions and in different countries around the world and rates also vary between urban and rural areas in the same country, or between the state and the private sector. In 2007 WHO published the results of an enormous international study on caesarean rates.[1] All African countries except two had rates below the recommended level, while in Europe, North America, Latin America and the Caribbean most countries had rates which were above the maximum recommended. In certain regions, for example in Africa, the necessary resources for carrying out caesareans were not available, and in other regions, such as Latin America, where resources were comparatively readily available (compared to the situation in the so-called developed world and developing countries), high average rates were mainly due to the extremely high rates in private clinics. This does not mean that all women in Latin American countries who *needed* a caesarean actually had one, of course...

In Europe, in countries such as Italy and Portugal, caesarean rates are now higher than in the USA and Canada—a situation which has only developed fairly recently. The average age when women have their first baby is higher than it was before (which means that more caesareans are carried out, because complications tend to increase as women age) and lower VBAC rates have resulted in higher caesarean rates. The personal preferences of consultants (i.e. obstetricians) and the way in which they perceive their clients' opinions may also have helped to make the caesarean rate increase.[2] In the USA almost a third of women now have a caesarean (32.8% in 2008, according to the Center for Disease Control), in Canada more than a quarter of women have one, and in the UK 24.6% of women have this kind of surgery. The average caesarean rate in selected hospitals in four countries in South East Asia was 27% in 2008/9, and in China 46% of women now have a caesarean section (but rates can approach 90 to 95% in big cities).[3] In Latin America, according to a WHO survey, published in 2005, the median rate of caesarean was 33%,[4] but—again—there are informal reports of 90-95% in private hospitals. In some parts of Latin America and China, caesarean rates appear to be amongst the highest in the world!

The caesarean rate in different areas of the world from 2003 to 2005

Region of the world	Average caesarean rate	Minimum and maximum caesarean rates in regional areas
Africa	3.5%	1.8%—14.5%
Oceania	14.9%	4.9%—21.6%
Asia	15.9%	5.8%—40.5%*
Europe	19.0%	15.2%—24%
North America	24.3%	22.5%—24.4%
Latin America and the Antilles	29.2%	18.1%—29.3%*

*Note that these upper rates are averages, so aren't as high as in private hospitals. The low rates in government hospitals in the same area bring down the averages.[5]

The figures for the chart on the next page were sourced from the OECD (The Organisation for Economic Co-operation and Development).[6] This chart includes rates from 25 of 30 Organisation for Economic Co-operation and Development member countries in the years 2003-2005. Data on caesareans in other countries was not readily available. In 2005, caesareans accounted for more than 25% of all live births in 12 industrialised countries, including the United States (30%). Nearly 40% of births were by caesarean in Italy and Mexico. The Netherlands had the lowest rate of caesareans (14%), and four of the six lowest rates were in Nordic countries. In the last few years, the situation has not changed substantially, although rates in some countries—notably China and Brazil are said to be as high as 90% or even 95% in urban centres and/or private clinics.

The trivialisation of the caesarean

According to Diony Young, editor of the scientific journal *Birth: Issues in Perinatal Care* in the USA a woman runs an increased risk of having a caesarean if she's too big or too small, too early or too late, too old or too fearful, too tired of being pregnant or too tired of being in labour... if she's having twins, if the baby's breech, if she's previously had a caesarean, or if she's due and so is the weekend, Christmas, Thanksgiving, or New Year's Eve. She says the woman's also at risk if her doctor is in doubt, scared of a lawsuit, too busy, going out of town, or convinced that a caesarean is always safer...[7]

She says there are many pretexts for carrying out a caesarean

birthing normally after a caesarean or two

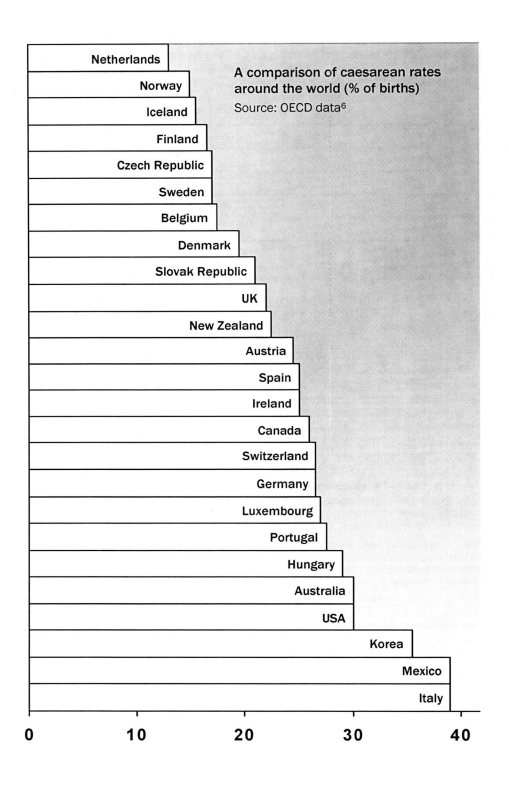

Even in 1984, one doctor (a certain Dr Joey Schulman) said: "It's difficult to believe we've reached the point where 20% to 25% of our offspring have to be delivered by an operation for medical reasons. Would Mother Nature have designed the female body such that 1 in 5 would need to be operated on in order to give birth?"[8]

Would Mother Nature have designed the female body such that 1 in 4 or 5 would need to be operated on in order to give birth?

At a time when caesareans have become more common than ever, the reflections of Diony Young and Dr Schulman are still relevant today. We are living at a time when caesarean surgery has become trivialised. Caesareans are often carried out for reasons other than urgent medical need. Most of the stakeholders I have consulted—consultants, GPs, perinatal nurses, maternity assistants, researchers in perinatology, etc.—agree that many labours are artificially induced and that many caesareans are carried out for the sake of convenience: the hospital's, the doctor's and even for ours, the women concerned. This is obviously the case for repeat caesareans, which—in the majority of cases—are only carried out because that's how the women gave birth previously. However, it's also the case when some caesareans are carried out on first-time mothers... The operations may be carried out not only because either the baby or the mother is in distress, but also because labour is taking 'too long', because the labouring woman has simply had enough, because the consultants are overwhelmed, or because nobody wants to take the risk of disturbing the anaesthetist (who lives a long way away), right in the middle of the night.

One person told me women request caesareans. One nurse, Janelle Marquis, said on hearing this: "It's not necessarily the women who are requesting caesareans the first time they give birth. But they do often arrange a managed labour for themselves—that is to say, they get induced at a time which is convenient to all parties concerned. The consultant has his client come into hospital early in the morning, he gives her prostaglandins and a drip of synthetic oxytocin (synotocinon)—as much as is needed to get her labour going, and he'll also break her waters. Nevertheless, sometimes all this still isn't enough to start off the woman's labour, but since her waters have been broken the consultant feels they shouldn't wait longer than 24 hours before she has the baby, so she ends up having a caesarean." Marlyse, a perinatal nurse, was offered precisely this kind of birth by her consultant, who was a woman. The consultant said: "Listen. You've got two other children... I'll get you going at 38 weeks, on a Monday, so you can find childcare." Stunned, Marlyse replied: "Look... I know what I'm talking about. That way, contractions will hurt more and my labour will end up with a caesarean." After thinking about it, she decided to give birth at home—a decision which, amongst other things, sorted out her childcare problem.

In the magazine *La vie en rose* (special edition, 2005, page 109), the midwife Isabelle Brabant (the author of a well-known French book on birth[9]) explains the contradictions of the recent climate: "Everywhere we hear all this talk about 'women's choice', which is both sudden and highly suspect. Everyone's all too ready to accept that women have the right to choose caesareans on demand or that they may choose to have their menstruation suppressed... Where was 'women's choice' when we were refusing episiotomies (which they gave us all the same)? And where is 'women's choice' when we want to give birth squatting? Everywhere, we also hear so much about risks that it limits us more than it protects us, even when the emphasis is on risks for the baby."

> We hear so much about risks that it limits us more than it protects us, even when the emphasis is on risks for the baby

In the last two decades of the last century women expecting their first baby didn't ask for a caesarean. It is only in the last few years that we have witnessed the phenomenon—little known in the past—where pregnant women request a caesarean even for their first birth because they prefer not to give birth vaginally. Several celebrities such as Britney Spears and Madonna in the US and Elizabeth Hurley in the UK have done the same.[10] But this phenomenon really seems to have grown because of the influence of the media.[11] After all, recent studies reveal that only a very small number of women request a caesarean for non-medical reasons.[12] Nevertheless, in the American survey *Listening To Mothers* only one woman out of 1,600 women interviewed replied that she had had an elective caesarean on demand, for non-medical reasons.[13]

In order to honour women's choices, consultants often agree to carry out caesareans[14] even if the organisations which represent them don't necessarily endorse their decisions.[15] The American College of Obstetricians and Gynecologists (ACOG), which has a big influence on the way in which obstetrics is practised in North America, adopted a position in 2003, justifying caesareans conducted on non-medical grounds for *ethical* reasons.[16] This recommendation astonished Nicette Jukelevics, web editor of the website www.vbac.com, given the scientific data on risks associated with elective caesareans, and given that the risks of having a caesarean are emphasised in other ACOG publications[17], particularly when a caesarean is carried out before 39 weeks.[18] What's more, it is widely agreed that women who have a caesarean are not necessarily aware of the risks, or that they haven't understood them well.[19] It seems to me that we should be helping women who are overwhelmed by fear of birth to work through this fear, rather than immediately agreeing to their desire to have a caesarean. Studies have shown that support in the form of counselling or therapy can change women's perceptions.[20]

> Studies have shown that support in the form of counselling or therapy can change women's perceptions

The current situation 13

For some women, the caesarean operation has become a way of avoiding having to live through labour, with the painful contractions which generally accompany it. (This was confirmed by the sociologist Maria De Koninck, when I interviewed her.) With some astonishment, De Koninck confirmed that by the 1980s a caesarean had become a means for some women to have an experience of birth like that of their partners. Like him, these women claimed, they didn't have any pain (thanks to the use of anaesthesia), and like him, they 'attended' the birth. Some women are even convinced, like many men, that the caesarean section is the best way of giving birth, even when the baby is in no danger at all. In an interview published in *Mothering* magazine[21] the anthropologist, Robbie Davis-Floyd, said that *not* having technology used during labour and birth makes many women feel they've had care of a lower quality.

Clearly, society's values influence our way of seeing birth. On a personal level, we need to be aware of how we've been led to consider birth as a medical event and also why—for about 40 years—people have even considered it a surgical event. We live in a society which is full of people in a hurry, where everything has to happen quickly, where every kind of difficulty is sorted out by technology, where every health problem has either a medical or a surgical solution. We like to be masters of our lives and our bodies, and on certain levels, we're better off than ever before. But the complexity of an event as wonderful as birth won't necessarily accommodate itself to interventions carried out for the sake of convenience. In fact, some people, such as Michel Odent, are seriously concerned about the current interventionist climate. (It is particularly interesting that this man was a surgeon, who was in charge of a maternity unit at Pithiviers in France for 23 years. For the last 24 years or so, he has been helping women have home births in London.) Many medical associations are also worried about the high rates of interventions such as caesareans, which explains why groups such as the NCT (the National Childbirth Trust), the RCM (the Royal College of Midwives) and AIMS (the Association for the Improvement in Maternity Services) are all working to promote normal birth—which is often defined as being vaginal birth without induction or instrumental delivery.

Paradoxically, the 'humanisation' of the caesarean operation, which has taken place in hospitals as a result of pressure exerted by individual women or groups of women who support caesareans, have helped to make this surgery seem more commonplace. There is even a name for this humanisation: it is called having a 'natural' caesarean! Nowadays, in most hospitals it really is possible for a woman to have a caesarean 'in the heart of the family', remaining conscious with her partner at her side, and epidurals are widely available. This is infinitely more satisfying for many women than suddenly finding their womb empty (several hours after surgery) with a baby whose birth they didn't witness. (Of course, this was often the case 30 years ago.) Nevertheless, even though improvements have been made, we can't get away from the fact that a caesarean involves more risks than a vaginal birth, both short- and long-term, for the mother, the baby and her future babies too. (We shall consider these risks in detail in the next chapter.)

Reasons for promoting normality, and ways of doing so

Even though the caesarean is now an operation with infinitely fewer risks for both mother and baby than existed in the past, and even though women recover from it much more quickly now than they did 30 years ago, it is still major abdominal surgery which requires the use of an anaesthetic. For this reason alone, we should only take recourse to this operation in cases where it is medically necessary, i.e. when the safety of either the mother or baby is in question. There are other reasons why we should promote normality too... Having a caesarean deprives the baby and even the mother of the advantages of labour and significantly reduces or delays early mother-baby contact and affects its quality, as well as the potential success of breastfeeding. Lastly, we must not forget that a caesarean is a traumatic, saddening experience for many women.

> Having a caesarean deprives the baby and even the mother of the advantages of labour and significantly reduces or delays early mother-baby contact and affects its quality

If the problem is that professionals are over-extended (because of staff shortages), there must be other solutions, apart from the caesarean operation. This point was emphatically made in a Canadian daily newspaper in December 2007.[22] In this article it was suggested that the number of midwives could be increased, the role of nurses could be extended to include pregnancy and birth, and even GPs could become more involved in maternity care again. For decades, pregnant women have been told they need to be looked after by a consultant for the sake of their own health, as well as that of their baby, and for several decades in many places doctors and other specialists have been marginalising or even actively opposing midwifery services (particularly in the USA). However, most births do not require extremely specialist care.

Diane Francoeur, when she was the president of the Association of Obstetricians et Gynecologists in Quebec, noted in the article 'Pregnant women, neglected women' that a full-qualified gynaecologist is not needed for the care of a normal pregnant woman.[23] Nevertheless, we do tend to forget that a pregnant woman who is in good health does not need to be looked after by a specialist, even when she has gestational diabetes, when she's expecting twins or in any situation where she simply needs to be carefully monitored.

When the ratio of consultants (obstetricians) to ordinary people in a community is high, the caesarean rate is bound to rise.[24] This is to be expected because consultants are basically trained to intervene in cases where there are complications. When GPs are in charge, this is not the case, and it is even *less* the mindset of a midwife, who is used to attending normal births and who is therefore much more likely to have plenty of patience. The patience of midwives tends to prevent complications—because, as Klein *et al* stated in one study:[25] "There is a correlation between the rise in maternal and neonatal mortality rates in normal pregnancies and the number of interventions that are carried out during labour." Between 1990 and 2006 the maternal mortality rate in Canada rose from being the second best in the world to being the eleventh best, while the infant mortality rate went from sixth place to 21st place. In other places too, there have been rises in mortality rates. For example, in the USA while the caesarean rate has been rising, maternal mortality rates have also been increasing.[26]

Changing trends from a historical perspective

According to historical records, Jacob Nufer, a Swiss farmer, carried out a caesarean on his wife in the 16th century after she'd been in labour for several days. This legend is one of the most commonly repeated stories and it's supposed to refer to the first caesarean carried out on a live woman. Most significantly, perhaps, the legend includes the details that this woman not only survived her caesarean, but that she also went on to have four vaginal births afterwards—four VBACs, in fact.[27] Also, in the book *The VBAC Experience* (Bergin & Garvey, 1982)[28] a woman relates how she had a VBAC in 1933 in France. Her first baby had been a forceps delivery and her second a caesarean, with a classical incision. After a much easier third pregnancy (without any antenatal care, since it didn't exist in those days), and after working right up until she went into labour, this woman went into labour spontaneously, when contractions began. She went into hospital at that point and her daughter was born after a short, relatively painfree labour. The baby weighed 8lb or 9lb. It never occurred to this woman not to have a vaginal birth.

According to Dr Yolande Leduc of the Pierre-Boucher hospital in Canada, giving birth in the 1980s in Europe meant experiencing contractions and expulsion, even after a previous caesarean section (unless the medical circumstances suggested this should not happen). This was not the case in the USA, though. There, women who'd previously had a caesarean were expected to have further caesareans for any future births. This was the case until the beginning of the 1980s (after a decade in which VBACs had actually been forbidden), when people once again began to allow women who requested a vaginal birth after a previous caesarean to give birth normally. In Europe, traditionally, women had been encouraged to give birth vaginally after a caesarean—but the term 'VBAC' didn't exist for a long time, and only appeared in the 1990s. All this means that even though the caesarean rate has risen in recent years, in some countries, such as the UK, VBAC rates are much higher than in other countries. In these places women are more likely to choose a VBAC rather than an elective repeat caesarean. The current VBAC rate in the UK is almost double that of Canada, for example, but a three-month check done by the National Sentinel Caesarean Section Audit revealed that rates varied between 6% and 64% in maternity units. (See www.msss.gouv.qc.ca.) Nevertheless, rates are not as high as they perhaps should be. NICE Caesarean Guidelines (2004) mention a 2001 study that found that the VBAC rate in England and Wales was only 33% and the VBAC rate in Scotland was only 27%,[29] despite a target rate of 40% (which was subsequently lowered to 33%).

VBAC rates

Until fairly recently, no statistics on VBAC rates were available and this situation continues to this day in most countries around the world—even though some European countries have declared VBAC rates at certain points. At the present time, even though caesarean rates are fairly easy to obtain for most developed countries, the same cannot be said for VBAC rates. This data is very rarely available from official sources and even when it does exist, since rates are collected using different criteria in different places, a comparison of statistics is impossible.

Considering data which is available, it is useful to examine whether countries which have the most caesareans and the least VBACs also have lower rates of infant mortality. It seems that they don't. Here are VBAC rates for a few countries in the mid-1990s.[30]

VBAC and caesarean rates compared with mortality rates (1994-5)

VBAC rate (listed lowest to highest)	Caesarean rate	Infant mortality	Country
33.4%	17.6%	6.2 per 1,000	Canada
35.5%	20.8%	8.0 per 1,000	USA
40.4%	15.4%	4.7 per 1,000	Finland
43.2%	15%	6.2 per 1,000	UK
54.1%	12.5%	5.2 per 1,000	Norway
70%	27%	4.3 per 1,000	Singapore

As you will see from this table, the two highest VBAC rates occur in countries with fairly low infant mortality rates (Norway and Singapore). It is also notable that the Scandinavian countries (Norway and Finland), where midwives are the primary caregivers in birth, not only have some of the lowest rates of infant mortality, they also have comparatively low caesarean rates and fairly high VBAC rates.

The two highest VBAC rates occur in countries with fairly low infant mortality rates

Around the mid 1970s, when caesarean rates started growing substantially, women started requesting VBACs more often. Women's groups were founded and these emphasised the provision of information about caesareans, before moving on to provide advice about how to prevent them. A little later on, in the early 1980s, specific VBAC support groups were set up in North America.

The current situation   17

Nowadays, mysteriously, women wanting a VBAC are encountering more and more obstacles, in every country around the world. In Canada—the country where I am based—the situation is particularly worrying. Here, VBAC rates have more than halved in less than 10 years. In one single year between 2005-2006, 81.9% of the 330,000 babies born to women who'd previously had caesareans were born by caesarean—making the Canadian VBAC rate for that year 18.1%.[31] In Quebec, the province where I live, the VBAC rate went from 38.5% in 1997-1998 to 18.8% in 2005-2006.[32] In the States, meanwhile, in 2004 less than 10% of women who previously had a caesarean had a VBAC and in 2006, it had gone down to 8.5%.[33] No official statistics appear to be collected for the UK, but—as in the USA—many women are simply not offered the option of having a VBAC, or don't realise they can. This is perhaps because many hospital-based consultants (i.e. obstetricians) refuse to allow women to give birth vaginally after one or more caesareans.[34] This, of course, has the effect of negatively influencing women's own desire to have a VBAC.

As we shall see, the basic risks associated with VBAC have not changed since the 1980s, and we now know much more about the situations which are associated with risk. Nevertheless, the general obstetric climate has changed in the last 30 years all over the world and there are shortages of midwives in many places too. People are less and less attracted to the fields of midwifery and obstetrics, which means that those who are passionate about the speciality have many clients and too little time, and many are about to retire. It's not unusual today in some places for a woman to have to wait several months before she can see a caregiver for the first time, after becoming pregnant, and sometimes she might even have difficulty finding a midwife or consultant during her pregnancy.[35] What's more, fewer and fewer GPs are becoming involved in obstetrics,[36] and this might also have contributed to the constant rise in caesarean rates.[37] On the other hand, after many years of midwifery-led campaigns, many more midwives are able to practise, birth centres have opened up and others are due to open over the next few years.[38] Midwives can attend home births, as well as hospital births, when agreements to this effect are in place. Nevertheless, in the UK and elsewhere around the world, there is a real shortage of maternity staff, which also has an impact on obstetrics. Hospital-based midwives and nurses who practise as midwives have less and less time to support women in labour, a fact which has been confirmed by studies conducted over the last 10 years or so. (In one study, only 6-9% of midwives' or nurses' time was spent supporting labouring women).[39] There have also been budgetary cuts, which have affected the services on offer to all pregnant women because some hospitals have been closed down or merged with other establishments over the last few years. (According to 2010 data from the Valuation Office Agency, published in the *Reader's Digest* in May 2010, between 1997 and 2010 Britain lost 32 hospitals and clinics.) Even if women have easier access to information, thanks to the Internet, they are perhaps less well prepared before they go into labour and they have less support. Perhaps this is why there has been an increase in demand for doula services (see Glossary). The rise in the use of doulas is an invaluable development for women with no previous experience of vaginal birth.

Changing feelings about pregnancy and birth

Views of pregnancy and birth have changed quite dramatically. This explains why antenatal tests have become more common during pregnancy, why babies are even operated on while they're still in the womb and why attempts are made to save babies who are increasingly premature. (Perhaps, in fact, we should question the ethics of saving babies born prematurely, who are hardly viable, given the significantly increased risks of their experiencing health problems later on in life.) Even though certain interventions (such as episiotomy or instrumental delivery) have become less common, others have become more frequent. Examples of interventions which have become commonplace include the use of induction, epidurals, caesareans and even the use of some drugs which were not developed for use in labour or birth, but which are now being used within the field of obstetrics (e.g. Misoprostol). In addition, techniques for carrying out caesareans have been modified and, as we shall soon see, some of these changes have had an impact on VBAC rates. One element which is becoming increasingly present in our society, which affects many people's view of childbirth, is *fear*. This was emphasised by GP, Vania Jimenez, who also offers obstetric care:[40]

In obstetrics, we are constantly hearing the muzak of fear. We live in a culture of risk, even if we are only neighbours ... with the people who invented the concept of risk in obstetrics. Obstetric risk is an American invention. We're caught up in it and can't really escape its clutches without first really becoming aware of it.

In fact, a number of studies have concluded that the increase in caesarean rates could be linked to the climate of fear which now pervades the field of childbirth in the modern world and many articles have been written on this subject.[41] An atmosphere of insecurity exists not only in the field of obstetrics, but also in other areas of life, ever since September 11th in the USA and July 7th in London. This cannot fail to have an effect on younger people, whether they happen to be pregnant women, midwives, consultants or maternity assistants. In my opinion, the atmosphere is bound to also have an impact on women's feelings about whether or not to have a VBAC. The increasingly high levels of stress, which are part of our modern lifestyle, perhaps also partly explain why women resort to drugs, such as those in epidurals, while they're in labour.[42] In any case, caesareans take place so frequently that they have become a banal fact of modern life. In some places, the caesarean section is considered to be a cure for many ills and necessary attention is not given to the risks which this operation poses for both mother and baby. People insist on informing women of the risks of a VBAC, without necessarily informing them about the risks associated with a caesarean. In the 1980s it was necessary for a consultant to justify himself or herself when suggesting a caesarean, but for around 30 years, the opposite has been the case. In medical and legal respects, consultants consider themselves to be protected when they take action—their training prepared them in this way—but this is unfortunately not the case when they avoid intervention.

The current situation 19

It seems to me that nowadays women are becoming more and more afraid of labour[43] and, at the same time, they are losing confidence in their ability to bring their own babies into the world. One midwife confided to me that she had observed this change in attitudes amongst her pregnant clients, even in cases where women were preparing to give birth at a birth centre. She emphasised that a lot of 'reconstructive' work needs to take place during antenatal appointments if women are to regain confidence in their ability to give birth. For these reasons, it seems that women nowadays are more ready to accept interventions during their labours than they were around 30 years ago.[44]

Changing patterns of information transfer

In any case, in recent years the Internet has become part of our lives. It has given us increasing access to all kinds of information, including medical information about pregnancy and birth. You would have thought this easy access to information would have helped pregnant women prepare and allowed them to make better-informed choices. Unfortunately, this is not the case, as I demonstrated in a review of the relevant literature in 2004 and as I showed in my doctoral thesis, which I completed for my PhD. Until recently, it was in fact difficult to find information on the negative effects of procedures routinely used during labour or about obstetric interventions, even when various studies had been carried out on these very topics, so women using the Internet are not getting balanced information.[45]

Fortunately, two publications and recent reviews have recently signalled a turning point. In 2004, a book finally looked at the impact of labour practices on breastfeeding and it concluded by emphasising the key dyad in the whole process, i.e. it emphasised the importance of the mother-baby relationship. (This was Kroeger and Smith's book *Impact of Birthing Practices on Breastfeeding—Protecting the Mother-Baby Continuum,* published by Jones & Bartlett.)[46] Then, in 2007, a systematic review appeared,[47] which detailed the studies relating to the 10 steps of the Mother-Friendly Childbirth Initiative—an American initiative, based on the Baby-Friendly Model (World Health Organization). This review looked at the scientific foundations which allowed us to understand why labour practices need to become demedicalised. And now, over the last 30 years or so, more and more studies have been published suggesting the importance of avoiding such-and-such an intervention or obstetric procedure. These studies have exposed many interventions as unscientific and it is specifically these interventions which the movement of the humanisation of childbirth has campaigned to change. This movement began in Britain (with people such as Sheila Kitzinger) and in the USA (with people such as Suzanne Arms and Doris Haire) in the 1970s and continues today.

Despite all this, the information provided in antenatal classes is unbalanced and, in any case, not all women have equal access to classes. Often, women are not aware that they can give birth with a midwife in attendance, or even that they can give birth outside a hospital.[48] They often do not know they can have a GP follow their pregnancy and be responsible for the birth.[49] And women don't know about the side-effects of drugs administered during labour.

Several factors could explain the lack of information provided to pregnant women. Doctors and consultants usually have very little time to give women adequate information. And midwives in birth centres or maternity units are hesitant about giving information when women are in labour and in pain. Usually, they believe this information should be given to women during pregnancy. Even antenatally, midwives or nurses are afraid that information on possible side-effects will make women feel guilty if what they explain can happen actually *does* happen.[50] Secondary effects of epidurals are therefore silently forgotten. In 2009 the number of women having an epidural during labour (as reported in *The Guardian* on 12.07.09) was 36.5% and in the USA in 2006, three quarters of American women gave birth with an epidural (Centers for Disease Control).[51] In Canada, in 2005-2006, 54% of women giving birth had an epidural.[52] These women wanted to have an epidural for pain relief but they didn't necessarily know that this would involve more routine procedures, or that an epidural could have an impact on their labour (as has been shown by various studies)... They probably didn't know that it could slow down their labour, increase the likelihood of an instrumental delivery (i.e. a delivery with forceps or ventouse), and have a negative effect on the baby's position or on its ability to rotate its head, amongst other things... (There will be more on this in Chapter 6.) As for caesareans, during pregnancy women are given little or no information about the risks they involve, compared to the risks of VBACs.

The need for change

In the 1970s, 80s and 90s, it was only women's groups and a few caregivers who campaigned for change in the field of obstetrics. They campaigned about certain obstetric practices, about caregivers attending women in labour and giving birth, about birth places, and about attitudes towards labour. Since then, several organisations, sometimes even the prestigious World Health Organization (WHO), or the governments of certain countries, have taken a stand on what constitutes best practice in childbirth. For example, in the UK significant efforts have been made to respond better to women's needs during labour (following the report *Changing Childbirth* in 1993) and to make sure that changes are implemented, so as to make this possible. In 2008 a report appeared, which was unanimously endorsed by the Royal College of Midwives (RCM) and by the Royal College of Obstetricians and Gynaecologists (RCOG). It was called *Making Normal Birth a Reality*.[53] In 2007 NICE (the National Institute for Clinical Excellence, a government organisation), had published guidelines for obstetric practice. Other organisations in other countries also regularly take a stand on different subjects, including VBAC. For example, in Canada, the equivalent organisation to RCOG (the Society of Obstetricians and Gynaecologists of Canada) has set up training programmes for its members, among which the MORE[54] programme was set up in 2005 to reduce risk, using a multi-disciplinary approach. A randomised controlled trial was also set up in Canada in 2008 (QUARISMA), with the aim of testing measures to help reduce the caesarean rate in 32 hospitals.[55] In the USA, a similar initiative to the Baby-Friendly Initiative (launched by the WHO in 1992) was launched in 1996: the

Mother Friendly Childbirth Initiative. This initiative, was endorsed by more than 50 organisations, representing more than 90,000 members, as well as by numerous individuals concerned about practices affecting childbirth—and many organisations have since added their support. (See www.motherfriendly.org for more information on the Mother Friendly Childbirth Initiative.) In 2006, an international Internet survey was carried out as part of the Mother-Friendly Initiative and responses came from some 275 organisations in 160 countries (in English, French or Spanish). More than half of the organisations were in Europe, almost a quarter were in Latin America, 12% were North American, 9% were African, 9% Asian and less than 2% came from the Middle East and Australia. Results showed that:[56]

- 87% of respondents felt that induction rates should not exceed 10%
- 87% felt that the episiotomy rate should not exceed 20%
- 84% felt that VBAC rates should be 60% or more
- 83% felt that the caesarean rate should be 10 or 15% lower

Barriers to achieving better rates were thought to be, in order of importance: opposition from medical staff, the belief that interventions reduce complications in labour and the belief that women actually *want* interventions. Furthermore, in order of importance, conditions which would support an improvement were thought to involve having:

- the opportunity to choose a close companion for labour and birth
- information on the benefits and risks of procedures
- freedom of movement during labour and birth
- evidence-based practice
- early interaction with the baby
- The Baby-Friendly Initiative 10 Steps in place
- care which is sensitive to cultural differences
- non-pharmacological methods of pain relief
- openness about rates of interventions and birth outcomes
- inter-institutional collaboration

The Mother Friendly Childbirth Initiative was taken to an international level and the International MotherBaby Childbirth Initiative was launched in March 2008. The text of the Initiative had been approved by several international organisations representing different players in the field of obstetrics and perinatology. (See www.imbci.org.) Its aim is to ensure that the IMBCI becomes the model to follow when it comes to practices in labour, just as the Baby-Friendly Initiative became the guide for conditions favouring breastfeeding and mother-baby contact in the immediate postnatal period.

The significance of recent changes for VBACs

These changes and initiatives mean that we have now come much further forward in terms of the support given to practices which favour vaginal births, particularly practices which facilitate physiological births (i.e. births that involve no drugs or interventions). This can only be beneficial to women who choose to have a VBAC.

Since a VBAC has again become more difficult to arrange in recent years, women who previously gave birth by caesarean need to be particularly well prepared, especially if they choose to register with a consultant at a hospital. For some women, the idea of a VBAC immediately arises after having a caesarean, while for others the choice is less easy to make, given the 'muzak of fear' (to use the words of Dr Jimenez) which forms a backdrop to not just birth in general but VBAC in particular. In this way, it isn't always easy for a woman to make the decision for herself and her baby... a baby for whom she and her partner will, of course, need to make important decisions for 18 years or so, until he or she grows up. In any case, as far as VBACs are concerned, we do now have a great deal more information than women had only a short while ago. A few decades ago some people were only just beginning to become aware of the possibility of vaginal birth after one or more caesarean, and relatively few studies had been published, compared to those existing today.

Official policies

As a result of certain initiatives, some official bodies pronounced themselves to be in favour of VBAC in the 1980s. At the beginning of this decade for the first time in North America it was officially declared that vaginal birth after a previous caesarean was safe and that it presented few risks when the uterine incision for the caesarean had been low transverse (i.e. horizontal, along the lower part of the uterus). Even WHO came on board (at a conference held on technology appropriate for birth in Brazil in 1985), unanimously stating that there was no evidence suggesting a caesarean needed to be automatically scheduled after a first caesarean. WHO recommended that VBAC be encouraged in any place where a team was available for emergency obstetric care.[57]

> In the 1980s, for the first time in North America it was officially declared that vaginal birth after a previous caesarean was safe

In Canada in 1986, the national conference consensus on aspects of the caesarean recommended a so-called 'trial of labour'—not a very encouraging expression—for women who had had a low transverse incision, in cases where the fetus was presenting head first, provided there was no absolute contraindication for a caesarean (such as severe placenta praevia, where the placenta completely covers the cervix).

In 1988, as we've already noted, ACOG in the USA revised its policies on VBAC and declared that women should be encouraged to give birth vaginally after one or more caesareans, emphasising that no special measures were required for these births—nothing more than should exist everywhere, i.e. the facilities to proceed with a caesarean within 30 minutes, if necessary. ACOG did not oppose the use of epidurals or syntocinon for these VBACs at that time. Even later on, in 1994, ACOG did not advise against the use of prostaglandins. (These are artificial hormones which are sometimes used to soften the cervix as a first step in induction.)

The Canadian group did not consider it essential for a consultant to be available during a VBAC labour or for there to be any need for continuous electronic monitoring. This group also did not stipulate that only a consultant should attend a woman having a VBAC; a generalist was considered equally capable as long as a consultant (an obstetrician) and anaesthetist were on call and as long as a consultant had carried out an antenatal assessment. This group concluded that these recommendations were adequate for reasonable, justifiable clinical care. In other words, they suggested these parameters could serve as norms.[58]

After these policy statements , caesarean rates went down...

After these statements of policy were made, caesarean rates went down in the USA (and also in Canada) between 1989 and 1996. And ACOG continued to encourage VBACs until July 1999,[59] when it published ambiguous and controversial guidelines, with a new emphasis, *discouraging* VBACs unless an operating theatre was available in case of emergency. There was no scientific evidence to back up this requirement... only experts' advice.

Women started having fewer and fewer VBACs...

Not surprisingly, perhaps, the 1999 guidelines affected VBAC rates and transatlantic discussions may have influenced practice in the UK too. According to the Health Care Research and Quality report, published by the US Department of Health in 2003,[60] the US is now in a state of crisis which is linked to a fear of legal proceedings and staff shortages—meaning that women there probably now have fewer options, less access to care and a higher risk of having complications.

We are in a state of crisis which is linked to a fear of legal proceedings and staff shortages

In many places around the world maternity services (especially obstetrics) are in a state of crisis, particularly in rural or remote regions. In urban centres it is usually possible for a woman to find a consultant who will agree to attend a VBAC, as well as a hospital where it can take place, or a midwife might agree to attend a VBAC at home. Nevertheless, medical reactions to any one woman's situation can vary enormously. For example, medical staff may respond differently depending on whether a woman has had more than one caesarean before and on the reason for the previous caesarean (or caesareans)... Was it for dystocia? Or cephalo-pelvic disproportion? Or was it for twins? Outside big urban centres the situation isn't very encouraging at all. Many hospital protocols forbid VBACs in many cases because of guidelines developed by NICE or the Royal College of Obstetricians & Gynaecologists (RCOG) in the UK, or ACOG in the USA.

Some medical guidelines vary depending on the type of hospital women give birth in. In Canada, for example, there are three types of hospitals: Level I, II and III. A Level I hospital only deals with low risk cases. Although births take place there, there may well not be any obstetric staff so any caesareans are undertaken by a general surgeon. In a Level II hospital (which is often a regional hospital) women with certain risk factors are accepted and there are consultants, anaesthetists and paediatricians employed there, although they may be on call from home. In a Level III facility specialists are on duty on site 24 hours a day, but because there are bound to be gaps between shifts at times, the level of care provided can vary. This is relevant because a study carried out in Nova Scotia in Canada[61] (where similar categories of hospitals exist) showed that women giving birth in Level III hospitals were twice as likely to have a VBAC. Even though VBAC is mostly authorised in big cities, some hospitals in more rural areas do continue to offer VBAC. This is because it has been shown that having a VBAC in a low-volume hospital is not riskier.[62]

A first consensus development conference on VBAC is organised

More recently, in March 2010, a consensus conference on VBAC was organised by the National Institute of Health (NIH) and held in Maryland, USA. The conference included the results of a systematic review of the literature on VBAC. These results were presented to a panel along with presentations from 21 experts from pertinent fields, and input was invited from the general public (in person or by email), over the three days this event took place. The goal of the conference was to answer the following six questions and make recommendations:

1. What are the rates and patterns of utilisation of trial of labour after prior caesarean delivery, vaginal birth after caesarean delivery, and repeat caesarean delivery in the United States?

2. Among women who attempt a trial of labour after prior caesarean delivery, what is the vaginal delivery rate and the factors that influence it?

3. What are the short- and long-term benefits and harms to the mother of attempting trial of labour after prior caesarean versus elective repeat caesarean delivery, and what factors influence benefits and harms?

4. What are the short- and long-term benefits and harms to the baby of maternal attempt at trial of labour after prior caesarean versus elective repeat caesarean delivery, and what factors influence benefits and harms?

5. What are the nonmedical factors that influence the patterns and utilization of trial of labour after prior caesarean delivery?

6. What are the critical gaps in the evidence for decision making, and what are the priority investigations needed to address these gaps?

The goal of the conference was to answer six key questions

I attended this conference and it proved to be very interesting, if a little frustrating. Although all the available scientific evidence on VBAC was reviewed and not really challenged, except by some delegates who pointed out a few additional studies or ones which needed questioning, the conference's final recommendations were disappointing. While acknowledging that risks for a VBAC are not higher than for any other labour, the conference report didn't really strongly recommend the VBAC option, as such, apart from saying that "given the available evidence, trial of labour is a reasonable option for many pregnant women with one prior low transverse uterine incision."

Although all the available scientific evidence on VBAC was reviewed and not really challenged, the conference's final recommendations were disappointing

This was very different from the outcome of the NIH concensus conference on caesareans which took place in 1980, which opened the way to changes in VBAC policies, which was then more or less 'forbidden' in the USA. Most of the 2010 conference's report focused on the *risks* of VBAC, as well as on non-medical factors which influence the uptake or otherwise of VBAC opportunities, like the medico-legal climate that prevails in obstetrics, in particular regarding VBAC. Nevertheless, the final recommendation of the report to ACOG was that it should review its statement that an operating theatre and staff should be 'immediately' accessible in case an emergency caesarean is needed—a recommendation which restricts the availability of VBAC. In the box overleaf you can also see the other conclusions from the conference.

When considering these conclusions I sense a confusion as to whether the focus should be on the mother or the baby... As we will see soon, repeat caesareans carry risks and advantages which are different for mother and baby, but in my view (and in the view of some VBAC organisations) neither pregnant women nor mothers should ever have to 'choose' the safety of either the mother or the baby. Having said that, the conference discussions certainly did seem to be focused on problems that pregnant women face in trying to arrange a VBAC and caregivers are encouraged—in the recommendations—to adopt a much more evidence-based approach when assessing pregnant women for a so-called trial of labour. In addition, they are encouraged to share the decision-making process with the women themselves, after sharing relevant information which includes an evaluation of risks which the woman herself can understand. Finally, when considering the conclusions of the conference, it's worth noting that hospitals are encouraged to reveal their policy on VBAC and that all major players were told they should collaborate in the development of policies which make it easier for women to arrange a VBAC... and *even* to prioritise adequate financial measures so that the system overall is more effective in terms of offering women choices and real possibilities for success.

Caregivers are encouraged to share the decision-making process

> ### Conclusions of the NIH Consensus Development Conference on VBAC (held in Maryland in the USA on 8–10 March 2010)
>
> Given the available evidence, TOL (trial-of-labour) is a reasonable option for many pregnant women with a prior low transverse uterine incision. The data reviewed in this report show that both TOL and ERCD (Elective Repeat Caesarean Delivery) for a pregnant woman with a prior transverse uterine incision have important risks and benefits and that these risks and benefits differ for the woman and her fetus. This poses a profound ethical dilemma for the woman as well as her caregivers, because benefit for the woman may come at the price of increased risk for the fetus and vice versa. This conundrum is worsened by the general paucity of high-level evidence about both medical and nonmedical factors, which prevents the precise quantification of risks and benefits that might help to make an informed decision about TOL versus ERCD. We are mindful of these clinical and ethical uncertainties in making the following conclusions and recommendations.
>
> One of our major goals is to support pregnant women with a prior transverse uterine incision to make informed decisions about TOL versus ERCD. We urge clinicians and other maternity care providers to use the responses to the six questions, especially Questions 3 and 4, to incorporate an evidence-based approach into the decision-making process. Information, including risk assessment, should be shared with the woman at a level and pace that she can understand. When both TOL and ERCD are medically equivalent options, a shared decision-making process should be adopted and, whenever possible, the woman's preference should be honoured.
>
> We are concerned about the barriers that women face in accessing clinicians and facilities that are able and willing to offer TOL. Given the level of evidence for the requirement for "immediately available" surgical and anaesthesia personnel in current guidelines, we recommend that the American College of Obstetricians and Gynecologists and the American Society of Anesthesiologists reassess this requirement relative to other obstetrical complications of comparable risk, risk stratification, and in light of limited physician and nursing resources.
>
> Healthcare organisations, physicians, and other clinicians should consider making public their TOL policy and VBAC rates, as well as their plans for responding to obstetric emergencies. We recommend that hospitals, maternity care providers, healthcare and professional liability insurers, consumers, and policymakers collaborate on the development of integrated services that could mitigate or even eliminate current barriers to TOL.
>
> We are concerned that medico-legal considerations add to, as well as exacerbate, these barriers. Policymakers, providers, and other stakeholders must collaborate in the development and implementation of appropriate strategies to mitigate the chilling effect of the medico-legal environment on access to care.
>
> High-quality research is needed in many areas. We have identified areas that need attention in response to Question 6. Research in these areas should be prioritised and appropriately funded, especially to characterise more precisely the short-term and long-term maternal, fetal and neonatal outcomes of TOL and ERCD.

These conclusions make it clear that vaginal births after one or more previous caesareans continue to be controversial in medical circles. On the positive side, though, this conference did lead ACOG to relax its guildelines. ACOG now state that VBAC is appropriate for women who've had two caesareans, women expecting twins and women with an unknown type of incision, as well as for women with only one previous caesarean in low risk categories.[63]

The current situation 27

Reasons why so many caesareans take place and so few VBACs

One reason which is often mentioned is that women nowadays are having first babies later on in life, which means that the births are more likely to be complicated in some way. Another reason given is that women of certain ethnic groups tend to prefer caesarean births. Nevertheless, one nationwide census in North America revealed that caesarean rates are increasing amongst all groups of women, of any age, irrespective of the number of babies they are having, irrespective of their state of health, their race or ethnicity.[64] Of course, this data contradicts the reasons generally given for the rise in the caesarean rate, which were previously mentioned. In Quebec, the average age of a woman giving birth has risen by only two years—i.e. if in 1990 women typically gave birth at the age of 26 when they had their first baby, they are now only 28. Can we reasonably believe that two years could make such a big difference? Yet another report included the comment from researchers that the caesarean rate is rising faster than medical conditions or demographic factors would justify should be the case.[65] So reasons for rising rates are certainly mysterious...

We must conclude that there has been a change in obstetric approaches over the last 10 years or so... Health care providers just seem more inclined to go down the caesarean route.[66] Sometimes people say the caesarean rate has increased because fewer VBACs are occurring. If that really is a factor, it is certainly not the only one. In fact, as ACOG have confirmed, the caesarean rate for first-time caesareans has also risen. ACOG stated in 2006 that the increase in first-time caesareans took place alongside the global rise in the caesarean rate. They contend that the global increase cannot be attributed to the decline in VBAC rates.[67] If birth is surrounded by a climate of fear in every society, there must be other reasons to explain this important change. Reasons are perhaps more related to the so-called convenience of caesareans and to the medico-legal climate which infuses the field of obstetrics (i.e. the fear of litigation) than to an increased demand from women, who—according to several studies—prefer to give birth vaginally.[68] After conducting a study into maternity care, the American researcher Eugene Declercq suggested that the fact that fewer consultants now attend the births of their own clients might be a factor.[69] The increase in the number of caregivers attending any one birth could also have had an impact... Perhaps, in fact, the presence of every additional caregiver during a woman's labour increases the caesarean risk by 17%, as one American study suggested.[70]

Here are a few reasons, which might explain the dramatic changes in rates.

THE 'CONVENIENCE' FACTOR

In 1988, a Canadian consultant, Dr Usher, who was then a neonatologist at the Royal Victoria Hospital in Montreal, told me that VBAC should become the norm because that was what women were demanding. He explained that this should be the case despite the fact that it is much easier for a consultant to carry out a caesarean than it is to wait for a vaginal birth. After all, births usually take place in the middle of the night, which is as inconvenient as anything can be, and there is never any way of predicting when labour will start.

> **It's possible that consultants exert a certain amount of pressure on women so that they accept caesareans**

As a recent American study confirmed,[71] it is possible that consultants exert a certain amount of pressure on women so that they accept caesareans. In fact, a quarter of subjects in this study said they had sensed pressure of this kind from their consultants. In Brazil, it was revealed that consultants manage to persuade their clients to agree to a caesarean for false medical reasons, or they simply do not justify why they are taking recourse to this operation.[72] There is an imbalance of power between doctors and clients and research into the way in which decisions are made has not looked at how care is offered, nor has it examined conversations between women and their health providers.[73]

WHO suggests that economic reasons might be behind the variations in caesarean rates.[74] Nevertheless, in cases where medical care is provided free of charge (e.g. with the NHS), the economic factor is less likely to be more significant than the convenience factor, or the fear of legal consequences. In some other countries, financial differences between vaginal and caesarean births may not be enormous. In Quebec, for example, there is only a 25 dollar difference between the money provided for a vaginal birth and that provided for a caesarean.[75]

In other countries, though—i.e. in most places around the world—cost must certainly be an important factor, since caesareans not only involve more specialist staff, they also result in longer postnatal hospital stays, with higher costs for medical supplies.

The NIH Consensus Development Conference on VBAC (2010), in its final report, listed the following non medical factors as influencing practice and utilisation patterns of VBAC:[76]

- Professional association practice guidelines
- Professional liability concerns among physicians and hospitals
- The nature and extent of informed decision-making
- Provider and setting issues
- Health insurance status
- Patient and provider preferences.

Overall, when considering reasons for rising rates, one important factor—the last one in the list above—is the attitude of women towards their doctors. In most parts of the world doctors are some of the most respected people in society. As a result, doctors often have a great deal of influence on their patients. Their opinion is valued by the vast majority of women so any recommendation for a caesarean is likely to be accepted as a matter of course in many cultural contexts.

> One factor affecting rates is women's attitudes to doctors...

THE FEAR OF LITIGATION

One woman who contacted me in 2002 asked why we women do not allow ourselves to participate in decision-making when we give birth. She said it's our body affected, after all, and—speaking for herself alone—she said she was no featherbrain. "If it had been proved to me that a VBAC would be impossible or dangerous for me or the baby I would have understood. But I was given no valid reason for being refused a VBAC—apart from the 'fact' that it wouldn't work." Her doctor told her he'd passed her medical records to two consultants who had both refused her a VBAC. He also told her that he wanted to protect himself from possible legal consequences if the birth turned out badly. The woman in question, whose two previous children had been born by caesarean, was refused a VBAC at 39 weeks, although up to that moment her GP had told her that a VBAC would be possible. Perhaps all this is understandable when we consider the estimate that a consultant obstetrician in the USA is taken to court once every three years. Elsewhere, there are fewer court cases, but what happens in the States also influences the practice of other doctors. Insurance premiums have also increased substantially in recent years in North America. And in the UK litigation is increasingly becoming a problem, so here too fear may well be a motivating factor when it comes to the recommendations medical staff make to women about choices for their births.

He told her he wanted to protect himself from possible legal consequences, if the birth turned out badly

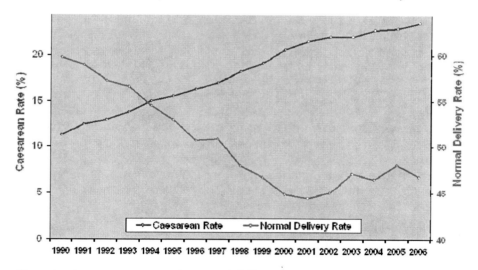

Changes in caesarean and normal delivery rates in England

Source: BirthChoiceUK.com [Note: The rising line refers to the caesarean rate, while the falling line, which rises again in later years, refers to the normal delivery rate.]

To summarise...

Recent changes in attitudes
- The caesarean is an operation which is becoming increasingly trivialised.
- The phenomenon of 'elective caesarean' without any medical reason has been fuelled into a trend by the media.
- Our modern view of childbirth is linked to our deep-seated values, particularly in relation to the emphasis on technology, the control of our lives in every respect, the avoidance of pain and our frenetic lifestyles, etc.
- In places where there is a shortage of consultants, midwives, maternity assistants and other staff, this may mean that things are hurried up during labour, that fewer normal births occur and more caesareans take place.
- The caesarean rate has risen dramatically all over the world.
- Approximately a quarter women now give birth by caesarean in many developed countries (and almost 40% in Italy). As many as 90% or 95% of women may have caesareans in private hospitals in some other urban centres in China or Brazil.
- In some places, such as Africa, a lack of resources means that caesareans cannot be performed when they're necessary.

Changing rates of VBAC
- VBACs are now a common occurrence in Europe, while in North America, they only started being encouraged at the beginning of the 1980s. However, after a sharp rise in VBAC rates in North America at that time, rates have been going down since the second half of the 1990s.
- The policies of medical associations were initially encouraging, but between 1999 and 2010 they became more restrictive. However, in July 2010, following the NIH Consensus Conference on VBAC in the USA, the influential American College of Obstetricians and Gynecologists relaxed its guidelines.

Reasons why so many caesareans take place and so few VBACs
- Increasingly, high rates of caesareans can be explained by the 'convenience factor'.
- Many caesareans are performed unnecessarily out of fear.
- The legal climate of medicine, i.e. the fear of litigation, has had a significant impact on the number of caesareans performed.

In the next chapter...

- Risks relating to VBAC for mother and baby
- Factors which increase the risk of uterine rupture
- The role of subjectivity when considering a repeat caesarean
- Risks associated with caesareans for both mother and baby
- A comparison of risks associated with caesareans and VBAC

Birthframe 3
Caregivers who were very reluctant to support a VBAC

During my first pregnancy, my consultant informed me at 32 weeks that my baby was presenting breech. After we tried turning him manually at 37 weeks I finally had a caesarean in April 2004. It wasn't a surprise and I had time to prepare myself mentally for this event.

The caesarean went well. All the same, I found it difficult having to wait two hours after my daughter was born before I could hold her. Those two hours seemed to last forever. And I can't forget how, after the operation, I wasn't in a position to take care of her. The pain was considerable and it was difficult for me to move around. Breastfeeding was painful because no position was comfortable for me. I became dependent on my husband and the midwives.

My second pregnancy was two years later. I immediately asked if I would have to have another caesarean. My consultant explained to me that it would be preferable, giving as her reason the risk of uterine rupture. I saw myself once more strapped to a bed, incapable of taking care of my newborn baby. I decided to get some more information and I became more and more convinced that I would be able to give birth vaginally. My baby was in a good position, so I saw no reason for a second caesarean. At each appointment, I talked to my consultant about this, but every time she succeeded in sewing seeds of doubt in my heart. She even told me about a baby who'd died during a VBAC.

I spoke to everyone close to me and they all knew, without exception, about my desire to have a vaginal birth and they all left me to decide on my own. I thought about this day and night, not knowing what to do. I read this book that you're reading now [the French edition] and by the time I got to the end of it I was resolved—and no one was going to change my mind. I believed in my ability to give birth, even though I knew there was a tiny risk of complications.

I informed my consultant, who succeeded one last time in sowing seeds of doubt— but only for a few seconds. I wanted to know what it felt like to give birth normally and since I felt it would be my last pregnancy, it would be my last chance.

On 8 November 2006 I went into hospital. It was 11 o'clock at night. I was accompanied by my sister, who I'd told about my intention to have a VBAC. We'd often talked about it and she knew it was my most cherished wish. On arrival at the hospital I informed the midwife on duty that I was going to try for a VBAC. First surprise... She said that whether or not I'd be able to depended on which consultant was on duty. She'd have to phone him at home. She came back saying I wouldn't be able to, not during the night. I insisted I would, so she phoned him again. She returned, listing various conditions. Second surprise... Conditions?! I just wanted to give birth and my contractions were becoming stronger and stronger and more and more painful. I was no longer able to reason with her. I said I would agree to any conditions ... I just wanted to give birth.

She said whether or not I'd be able depended on which consultant was on duty

Even after all I'd read, which had made me expect this kind of thing to some extent, I became more and more surprised

At midnight I was finally settled into my room. And that's when I found myself subjected to the first condition: the anaesthetist would come in to give me an epidural. Next, I was informed of the second condition: I would be attended by a midwife, who would stay at my bedside until I gave birth. Then I heard the third condition: I would be put on the electronic fetal monitor. Even after all I'd read, which had made me expect this kind of thing to some extent, I became more and more surprised. Finally, the consultant came to explain the procedure to me and to tell me about the fourth condition: he would not allow any fetal heart rate decelerations and, most importantly, the operating theatre was ready for use, just in case.

Then I had a new surprise, one which was rather worrying. The consultant consulted my records and couldn't find any record of how my caesarean had been performed the last time. Without that, he said he couldn't let me give birth vaginally. He explained that since I hadn't had my caesarean at that hospital, unfortunately, it wasn't possible to obtain the kind of information he needed during the night. I still insisted, all the while explaining to him that my own consultant had obtained this information, because we'd discussed it. Then, he saw in my records the note: "Protocol, OK." Good, that was all right then... He authorised my birth. It was about 1 o'clock in the morning and the consultant and midwives finally left me in peace. Of course, one midwife was there, but she was discrete.

It was about 1 o'clock in the morning and the consultant and midwives finally left me in peace

Two hours later, I was 10cm dilated and the midwife went to find the consultant. At around 3.30am I started pushing. On the second push, there were some slight decelerations in my baby's heartbeat. The consultant informed me that the baby would absolutely have to come out with the next push or else... and he said the word I didn't want to hear. He got out the ventouse and was about to give me an episiotomy, but I pushed with all my strength, feeling more determined than ever. I knew I was very soon going to see my little baby. And, in fact, the consultant didn't need to do anything. It was 4.06am and my baby had arrived. The consultant asked me to hold out my hands so I could hold my baby. I took him and put him on my stomach. He looked at me for the first time. I was living the most beautiful moments of my life. What a feeling it was to feel this little being snuggling up to me, skin-to-skin, on my chest. I felt so proud. I'd done it.

A few hours later, I got up. I had no pain. My baby boy cried and it was me who went to pick him up—I was capable of doing that. I settled in a comfortable position to breastfeed him and that went wonderfully well. I'd torn a bit and had haemorrhoids, but after only 24 hours I was already hurting much less. On the second day I left the hospital in great shape... No , it was nothing like my first birth.

A few hours later, I got up. I had no pain. My baby boy cried and it was me who went to pick him up. I was capable of doing that.

The current situation   33

Birthframe 4
Very different responses from different consultants

Towards the end of my first pregnancy (I was 41 weeks and 3 days) it was agreed that I would be induced on the following Monday. My cervix was 80% effaced and 1cm dilated. After talking with my partner, I took some castor oil. My hindwaters broke, but there were no contractions. My baby's head wasn't engaged. As soon as I got to the hospital I was asked to lie down and they put me on a syntocinon drip. The baby's head became engaged and one of the midwives broke my waters. Contractions became stronger and stronger. My partner arrived. At one point I started finding contractions very difficult to bear. The contractions had two phases, neither of which gave me any respite at all. So I made up my mind I would ask for an epidural if I wasn't at least 7cm dilated. Well, it turned out I was 4cm...

An hour after the epidural had been sited, I was fully dilated but felt no urge to push. Nevertheless, I tried to push for three and a half hours, all the while wondering if my baby was in a posterior position. He just wasn't coming down. Then I saw the consultant on duty for the first time and he told me my baby was only 1/5 engaged. My doula suggested I change position. In the end, when the doctor came round again to check on me, after pushing for more than three hours, he confirmed what I'd been suspecting all along: my baby was posterior and he was too high up for forceps to be used. I was informed I would have to have a caesarean. I felt very disappointed and very sad.

He said I could have a VBAC if I obeyed hospital protocol...

When I got pregnant the second time my consultant said I could have a VBAC on condition that I obeyed hospital protocol. This involved being on a drip and having continuous electronic fetal monitoring (EFM). When I asked if the monitoring could be intermittent, the consultant told me that EFM was essential because it would allow her to immediately detect any variation in the baby's heartbeat, which might indicate that the baby was in distress. She added that a VBAC was risky and that it would put both my own and my baby's life at risk. She seemed very shut off and said: "If you're thinking of giving birth in your bathtub, with candles all around, forget it! We're talking about a VBAC here, which is possible, but very risky for both you and your baby. We need to follow strict protocols." I found her attitude very upsetting. Since a friend had already had a VBAC at this very hospital, with no drip or continuous monitoring, I knew it was possible. When I told my consultant this she said, "That's impossible! Sometimes women give birth, then forget how it all happened." I was completely staggered by this response. When I insisted that my friend would have remembered her birth correctly, the consultant added: "I'm the professional here. Trust me. This kind of thing happens a lot." No discussion was possible. It wasn't even possible to find out why those particular hospital protocols were in place.

I talked everything over with my husband and was planning to change hospitals and consultant, because I no longer wanted to have this consultant looking after me when I gave birth

I talked everything over with my husband and was planning to change hospitals and consultant, because I no longer wanted to have this consultant looking after me when I gave birth. When I'm giving birth I certainly don't want anyone telling me I could die. As an intelligent person, I just wanted people to explain to me clearly the reasons behind any protocols. What's more, during my labour, I wanted to have a doctor present who would encourage me and understand me. My husband was enormously hesitant. He would have preferred me to stay at that same hospital, which specialised in high risk pregnancies—but he did understand that the doctor's attitude had been unacceptable to me. He tried to persuade me to stay registered there, emphasising that it was unlikely that that particular consultant would be on duty during my labour. So I agreed to see this consultant again and, once again, I was disappointed by her attitude. She treated me like someone who was both irresponsible and lacking in intelligence... I just didn't find that acceptable. She didn't object to the idea of me getting a second opinion, but she said: "Ask another consultant all the questions you want. Perhaps you *need* a second doctor to tell you the same thing." Once again, I felt I was being treated with contempt.

I met the second consultant and he confirmed I would be an excellent candidate for a VBAC

I met the second consultant at the same hospital and, after measuring the thickness of my scar, he confirmed that I would be an excellent candidate for a VBAC. This consultant took the time to answer all my questions and explained in detail the risks and also the reasons why the first consultant wanted to respect the particular protocols she'd mentioned. The second consultant even admitted that in my case such strict protocols weren't obligatory. I was very happy with this consultation. Nevertheless, I still didn't want to give birth under the original consultant or indeed at that same hospital. I'd been too deeply wounded by my first experience of giving birth and also by my consultant's attitude.

After numerous discussions with my husband, I registered with another doctor who was a GP who only dealt with obstetric cases. She attended almost all her clients' labours personally, and the births took place in a large maternity unit (with consultants who can carry out caesareans, anaesthetists, paediatricians, etc). This doctor, who was warmly recommended by my doula, reassured both me and my husband. She took as much time as we needed to answer our questions. Everything would be ready in case of the emergency which my husband was worried about, but everything would also be done to ensure that my labouring environment would favour a natural birth.

In contrast to my first labour, my contractions started naturally the day before my due date, at around 11.00pm. After I'd had a long bath, we decided to leave for the hospital at around 1.00am. When I got to the hospital I was already 7cm dilated but my waters hadn't broken. The doctor soon arrived, as well as my doula. Knowing the baby's position had been a problem in my first labour, my doctor used a Sonicaid to check how the baby was lying. It was round to my side. The doctor wanted to let my waters break naturally and suggested a position for me, which might encourage the baby to get well positioned.

The current situation   35

With gentle music playing in the background, while the sun slowly rose, I took each contraction one at a time—all the while encouraging my baby to become well positioned. My husband, the doula and the doctor (who visited frequently) encouraged me and made me feel perfectly confident in my ability to give birth . Everything was going well. At around 5.00am I was fully dilated but my waters were still refusing to break! In the end they did break partially, but even then my doctor preferred to wait patiently for them to break completely on their own. Then, at around 8.00am, my doctor, who was very much 'with' me, suggested I go and sit on the toilet seat for a few contractions. Suddenly we heard what sounded like a cannon shot as my waters exploded. Immediately, the doctor checked that the cord wasn't compressed and that my baby was fine.

That's when I started pushing—a stage which only lasted 30 minutes. I gave birth naturally to a beautiful little girl at 8.35am. She weighed 7lb 13oz (3.54kg). I just had a little superficial tearing. The fact of having birthed this baby naturally gave me an incredible surge of energy. It was one of the best moments in my life. What's more, my postnatal recovery was much faster than after my first birth and the pain was much easier to bear. Since my eldest demands my time and attention now that the baby's arrived, this improvement is much appreciated!

Birthframe 5
Preparing properly, but seeing it all from various points of view

The first time, I'd had a beautiful pregnancy. They foresaw no problems for the birth because they said I had a wonderful pelvis. At that time Gilles, my husband—who, like me, is a doctor—was already attending home births so we decided to have a home birth. But things just didn't go as planned. First, I was overdue. Gilles used a complementary therapy to induce labour. That brought on irregular contractions—some of which were strong, some weak. Then I developed a fever, so off we went to hospital. There, I was given a pelvic exam and I was told that although I had a great pelvis, the baby was too big and was a 'face' presentation. He was high up and after 12 hours of labour my cervix hadn't even opened to 1cm. The consultant on duty decided to do a caesarean because, quite apart from anything else, I had a fever. They didn't want Gilles to be present, even with him being a doctor. I thought he would be there and I waited for him right up to the moment when they put me out. Naturally, he was worried and they took their time before they told him everything was OK. When I woke up, I didn't want to know anyone and I don't even remember seeing Gilles then. I was not bothered about seeing my baby. In the end, someone came in with the baby and I told myself it must be mine. For Gilles—who had experience in obstetrics—that experience was a failure. We didn't talk about it much, although I knew his heart was heavy...

For my husband that experience was a failure. We didn't talk about it much, although I knew his heart was heavy...

One and a half years later, I found I was pregnant again. I heard a nurse where I work talking about VBAC and she invited us to a meeting run by the most senior consultant. We met him afterwards and he seemed nice. Then I signed up for some antenatal classes which focused on VBAC and we decided to have a go at having a VBAC ourselves.

I went into hospital when I first started having contractions, although I probably wasn't really in labour then. From 9 o'clock in the morning until midnight I was left to my own devices. I was making very slow progress so the consultant decided to break my waters. I then had better contractions but I didn't dilate any further than 3cm. I carried on for several more hours, without making any more progress. The baby still wasn't engaged. Eventually, it was decided I'd better have a caesarean under regional anaesthetic, with Gilles present. I thought that was marvellous. It didn't hurt and I saw my baby. (For me, the important thing is to have a healthy baby.) But as far as Gilles was concerned, it was also important for a vaginal birth to take place.

Not long after that—to our surprise—I found I was pregnant again. This time, Gilles said: "You're going to do something. It's not normal to keep having caesareans." He wanted me to go and see an osteopath. I agreed on condition that he'd come with me this time, wherever I went. It's just as well we did go and see an osteopath, actually, because I'd been told I had a pelvis which made a normal birth impossible. The osteopath advised us to take a course at a kind of personal development centre which specialised in pregnancy—because he felt that Gilles was somehow not 'with me'. Three weeks before I went into labour we spent the weekend on a personal development course. I thought it might be a load of rubbish because I was convinced it was a mechanical problem with me, but I thought: "If this is what we have to do, let's just get on with it. Let's get rid of whatever's in the way and let's do even more than that, if necessary." Over that weekend we had to talk about how births took place in our families. In mine, it hadn't always been a dramatic thing. My mother gave birth at home to babies weighing from 9lb (4kg) to 11lb (5kg). Perhaps the fact that my mother's first baby (who was born just before me) had died three hours after its birth and the fact that she'd talked to me about this a lot had something to do with my problems giving birth. Perhaps—as the course leader suggested—for me, giving birth meant the possibility of death. I must say, when I studied medicine I hated everything we did on birth. I was afraid of it.

The course leader advised us to have a doula with us during labour—so we found one to support us. Nevertheless, I felt awkward with someone I didn't know very well. I felt more comfortable with an osteopath friend, so she also came to keep me company during my labour. She helped me a great deal.

When we were thinking about having a VBAC (for our second baby), I was afraid that if we forced things it'd be bad for the baby. However, I had a lot of confidence in the consultant, who was supposed to provide care along with another consultant too.

When it came to it, during one of our last antenatal appointments my waters broke. I dilated pretty quickly to 5cm. But then I took a long time to get to 8cm. Fortunately, the atmosphere at the hospital was very good and I was encouraged to keep going. The doctor suggested I take a walk. I spent almost all my labour standing up, half squatting every now and then, because I found that helped. But when I got to 9cm I'd had enough. I just wanted to lie down on my stomach! The consultant suggested I have either synthetic oxytocin (syntocinon) or a relaxant. I accepted the latter, which made me go numb. Since I wasn't getting anywhere, the doula suggested I do a drawing to show what was wrong. Drawing two circles, I showed my fear that the baby's head wouldn't be able to get through. That did help, actually—at that moment I realised that the head really would get through, in actual fact. Meanwhile, the doula was saying too many encouraging things and I was fed up with listening to her. Gilles and my friend went out, feeling discouraged. I told the doula to stop talking to me and I locked myself in the toilet.

My contractions became stronger. I took them more gently and just let myself go. Gilles and Nicole came back and were amazed to see me carrying on. I asked them for some cold compresses and refreshed myself with the humidifier I'd brought along, which let out cold air. In the end a midwife came in to examine me and announced that I was completely dilated. I was so happy I gave her a kiss! It was just after midday and I was beginning to push. When the baby's heart rate slowed down a bit—to 90—they were a bit worried. The consultant attached a fetal scalp monitor to the baby's head. I felt confident, but I was also a bit wary. The consultant then suggested I lie down on my side and I pushed with my knees drawn up. Pushing in that way, the head came down pretty fast. But the baby's heart rate wasn't great—it was wavering between 70 and 90 beats a minute. The consultant said: "Look me in the eye! This time, this baby just *has* to get out!" I gathered up all my energy and pushed for all I was worth and I felt the head move down. (It hurt!) Then the shoulders came down—it was as if they were greased with butter. My daughter weighed 9lb 12oz (4.42kg)—she was my biggest baby! It was when she was passing under the symphysis that she had the most difficulty. I felt her moving down and it hurt all the time—to the point where I thought I was having a uterine rupture. But pushing didn't even last three quarters of an hour, after 16 hours of labour. Afterwards, I had three or four stitches and since I was exhausted, they left us alone, taking all the hardware with them, which they'd brought along for a caesarean 'just in case'.

While I was in labour I was afraid of all kinds of terrible things happening, but afterwards I felt free. I felt a bit like I'd just run a marathon. I'd done it, at least in my eyes. My husband was very touched. I went to sleep after about four hours, had an excellent night. Then, the next day I felt great—better than either Gilles or Nicole, who were both exhausted. I should also say that during my labour I had some homeopathic medicine so as to help me get better afterwards. And after I'd given birth I didn't hurt anywhere.

I don't think there's any difference in my relationship with my three children. What was important for me was to have healthy babies. But if I got pregnant again I would have a VBAC again because postnatal recovery is so much easier. However, it is hard giving birth—and it hurts! This is what I told Gilles, who thought it was more 'normal' to give birth vaginally: "Yes, it is. But you weren't the one who had to do it!"

After I'd given birth I thought about my mother and, my God, how I understood her! If she'd given birth today, she would have had a caesarean for her first baby."

CHAPTER 2:

The risk element, whatever your decision

In terms of human existence, there is nothing new about having a baby and there is also nothing new about experiencing fears around this time in life. Nevertheless, as we've already noted, women's anxiety has probably increased substantially since the 1970s and 80s, when a multitude of antenatal tests were developed. Although the objective in developing and carrying out these tests was to reassure pregnant women, the tests create anxiety when women decide whether or not to have them and when they are waiting for the results of each test, one after the other. The sociologist Anne Queniart has called our modern-day concept of pregnancy a 'constant awareness of risk.'[1]

Not only have antenatal tests increased in number, there has also been an increase in the amount of discussion about risk and now—early in the 21st century—pregnant women are strongly advised to behave in certain ways, to avoid eating or drinking various things, to take certain vitamins... the list goes on indefinitely.

In addition, the medicalisation of birth has transformed our perception of this event in a woman's life and we are therefore losing confidence in a woman's ability to give birth. Various people have commented on this and it seems that as many as three in every four women have one or more interventions when they give birth. Dr Michael Klein has argued that all this intervention is a consequence of our understandable preoccupation with the safety of both mother and baby.[2] However, he also said that the end result is no improvement in maternal or infant outcomes, an increase in the use of surgery and a loss of confidence amongst a whole generation of women...

> **Increased intervention has not necessarily resulted in an improvement in maternal or infant outcomes**

In this chapter, risks associated with VBAC will be considered, as well as risks associated with caesareans, when compared to vaginal births. Knowing the risks of the two options available to you is important, if you want to make a fully informed choice. It is particularly important because—as we saw in the last chapter—for several years the medical profession has generally been less inclined to let women who've previously had a caesarean have a vaginal birth afterwards. These days, if you choose a VBAC you need to be well-informed in order to make real choices.

I would suggest you read this chapter and discuss its contents with your consultant, your midwife or your doula and that you also follow up on what you read here by consulting websites mentioned in the Useful contacts section of this book. You will then be able to make a choice based on what feels most comfortable to you.

Risks relating to VBACs for mother and baby

In order to consider the possible risks of a VBAC, researchers have compared what happens with women who have a VBAC with those who have another caesarean. In order to do this, they usually track how many women have what is called a uterine rupture—i.e. a separation of the uterine incision, which is the basic risk of a VBAC. They also consider in numerical terms what the consequences are (with either a VBAC or a caesarean) for the health of both mother and baby.

It's long been widely accepted that having a VBAC is a safe option in the majority of cases

Since before the 1950s, it has been widely accepted that having a VBAC is basically a safe option in the majority of cases—except in North America—and that the specific risk which a VBAC presents is that of uterine rupture. The assessment of the basic risk a VBAC involves has not changed since scientific reviews of research were carried out in the 1980s. At the first consensus conference at that time,[3] VBAC was recommended in cases where the woman had previously had a single, low, transverse incision, and when she was expecting just one baby in her subsequent pregnancy, which was in a head-down position. WHO emphasises that it is not necessary for a woman to have a repeat caesarean in the majority of cases.[4] In Britain, NICE states that "Pregnant women who have had a previous caesarean and who want to have a vaginal birth should be supported in this decision."[5]

Understanding what a rupture really is...

In order to consider this risk for this book I looked mainly at the kind of scientific evidence which is considered most 'robust' and reliable in medical circles: systematic reviews of research, meta-analyses and large-scale studies—i.e. studies which look at large numbers of people—which were carried out from 1990 onwards. I also consulted key people in professional, medical or paramedical associations.

Before considering this research, let's consider what uterine rupture actually is... Here, we are talking about the situation where the uterine incision (from a previous caesarean) opens up. This is a serious—but rare—problem, when it occurs, because it can cause complications for both mother and baby. In fact, when it occurs, it's a real emergency and the mother has to be taken into surgery immediately so that her baby can be extracted and her uterus repaired.

Next—before considering the research relating to the risk of uterine rupture during a VBAC—we need to remember that, in fact, the risk of the uterus rupturing exists in any *pregnancy* where the woman has previously had a caesarean. Many people don't realise that having a repeat elective caesarean does not protect women from this risk... After all, although the risk is very low, a uterine rupture could occur even before the woman goes into labour.

Before we turn our attention to the research, we also need to recognise that most separations of uterine incisions, which were for a long time the focus of research studies, are actually cases of 'dehiscence.' This means a *defect* or opening in the uterine scar, rather than a separation of all layers. Several studies failed to differentiate between rupture and dehiscence, which makes it difficult to clearly interpret the research data.[6] The term 'fenestrated' also occurs in the research data, a term which means that a 'window-like' opening exists—which is the most benign type of opening up. This is a hole in the uterine incision which occurs when scar tissue is forming and it is not problematic. It is nevertheless detectable during an examination of the uterus during a subsequent caesarean. The separation of tissue which is called 'dehiscence' means that in one place the layers of the uterus are no longer welded together—a little like the layers of a flaky pastry! (This can be seen in cross-section, by ultrasound.) Nevertheless, in this kind of 'rupture' muscle tissue remains, even though it is thin—and there is no real separation of the uterine incision. Usually, the membranes do stay intact, there is no bleeding, no pain and the fetus remains inside the uterus. A dehiscence is therefore not dangerous in the same way as a rupture and does not necessarily need to be repaired. Like fenestration, it is again usually only detected during a repeat caesarean. Other expressions are also used to refer to other things (apart from rupture), but less frequently, such as thinning of the uterine wall because there could be an increased risk of rupture when the thickness of the uterine wall (at the uterine incision scar) measures less than 2.3mm to 2.5mm.[7] But, again, studies do not differentiate between these when they consider the prevalence of rupture.[8] But if it is a real rupture, what does it actually involve? The risk for the mother in the case of a real rupture really relates to the risk of haemorrhage and of having a hysterectomy.

You might ask at this point how it is possible to differentiate a real rupture from one of these other, less dangerous types... What are the symptoms of a real uterine rupture? According to Flamm (2001),[9] the most reliable sign that a uterine rupture is occurring is one or more prolonged deceleration of the fetal heartbeat (bradycardia)—for example, a decrease to 60-70 beats per minute or less, over a period of several minutes, with no variation when the fetal heart is stimulated by a maternal change of position. Other signs include a significant regression in the fetal station (i.e. the baby's amount of descent through the pelvis) or substantial vaginal bleeding. Flamm emphasised that other symptoms which have been the focus of attention are only weak signs of rupture—e.g. maternal tachycardia (when the mother's heart beats faster than normal), lowering of blood pressure (i.e. arterial pressure), blood in the urine and severe pain. However, he notes that we should not forget that 15 minutes after an epidural has been administered a significant lowering of the fetal heart rhythm may occur. This usually improves quickly, but may be frightening to parents-to-be and medical staff. Beyond these signs which can be observed at the moment a rupture is occurring, as yet, no way has been discovered of determining in advance whether or not a uterine rupture is likely to occur.

The level of risk: 0.2%—0.6% for spontaneous labour

Since studies failed for a long time to differentiate between these various types of rupture, some researchers, such as Beckett and Regan,[10] argue that the risk of uterine rupture should be considered to be lower than is usually stated to be the case. After all, a real uterine rupture means a rupture of the whole thickness of the uterine segment—i.e. *all* the layers, including the uterine membrane (the serosa). (This is why RCOG defines a rupture as "a disruption of the uterine muscle extending to and involving the uterine serosa".)[11] When a real rupture occurs, there are symptoms and/or a repair is needed[12]—and it is this kind of rupture which is dangerous for both mother and baby. In order to demonstrate the importance of differentiating between true uterine rupture and dehiscence, in one other study,[13] the rate of real rupture was 0.3% and that of dehiscence 0.5%. What's more, in this study, induction doubled the risk of 'real' rupture, relative to that of dehiscence.

The actual risk of a real uterine rupture occurring during a VBAC (i.e. a rupture which causes symptoms and is dangerous), rather than when a woman is having a repeat caesarean, is in any case lower than was previously thought to be the case. Studies have revealed that the risk varies between 0.2% and 0.6% when there is neither induction nor augmentation of labour.[14] The overall risk shown in the UK Landon study is 0.74 %.[15] These percentages mean that 1 to 3 women in every 500 attempting a VBAC may experience a uterine rupture. One study carried out in a birth centre showed that the risk was 0.2% for women who had only had one previous caesarean, provided they gave birth before 42 weeks. The overall risk—including other situations—was measured as being 0.4%—a rate which has been confirmed by other studies.[16] (It is worth noting here, too, that in birth centres rates of uterine rupture and perinatal death are lower than rates that have been recorded in hospitals—or at least they are no higher.[17]) Other studies have demonstrated a rate of uterine rupture of 0.6%[18] and the recent and first NIH Consensus Development Conference on VBAC talks about 0.3% for all gestational ages, and 0.77% for women who attempt a VBAC at term (compared to 0.047% and 0.022% respectively for women undergoing an elective repeat caesarean).[19]

Another way of calculating the risk in numerical terms, according to one group of researchers,[20] is to say that it would be necessary to make 370 women have a repeat caesarean in order to prevent a single uterine rupture which produced symptoms. In other words, it is perhaps useful to remind ourselves that the risk of uterine rupture is comparable to the risk associated with some antenatal tests... which some caregivers have no hesitation in offering pregnant women. After all, the risk after some tests (such as amniocentesis) can be fairly high.[21] Overall, the risk of uterine rupture is comparable to other important obstetric risks, as emphasised recently by the NIH Consensus Development Conference on VBAC in the USA (which we discussed in the last chapter). For instance, an emergency caesarean is usually required in cases of cord prolapse, serious haemorrhage during the birth, or when acute fetal distress occurs.

In the case of a real uterine rupture, there is also a risk for the baby because its body, or part of it, may escape from the uterine cavity, which means it can suffer from oxygen deprivation. There is a risk of fetal death of approximately 5%[22] when uterine rupture occurs, or 1.5 in 10,000 live VBAC births. It is therefore estimated that it would be necessary to carry out between 3846 and 7142 repeat caesareans in order to prevent a single baby's death following uterine rupture.[23] In fact, as the 2010 NIH VBAC Conference guidelines emphasise, the mortality rate for the baby (during a VBAC) is the same as the rate for the baby of any woman who is having her first child.[24]

> NIH (and RCOG) VBAC guidelines emphasise, the mortality rate for the baby (during a VBAC) is the same as the rate for the baby of any woman who is having her first child

Looking at the risks overall, the picture conveyed by the media over the last decade or so has been inconsistent because certain studies which were published created unnecessary and unjustified fear in the medical community. For example, one study published in 2001 had a great influence on VBAC practices.[25] But while it managed to trigger alarmist reports in the media, criticism came from clinicians, researchers and women's groups who all claimed the study gave a false impression of real risks. They argued that the research was based on a flawed research methodology, involving diagnostic codes which were poorly understood at that time and inconsistently applied.[26] Furthermore, although the study included details of women who'd had a uterine rupture, the researchers did not make it possible for the records to be checked, they failed to specify what kinds of prostaglandins had been used (for induction) and also what kind of synthetic oxytocin had been used. To make matters worse, the study included 105 women with a classical uterine incision, the type of incision which involves the highest risk of uterine rupture, so the results inevitably presented a distorted picture of the level of risk for the vast majority of women, who have a low transverse incision. (As we shall see later, when women have a classical uterine incision a VBAC is, in fact, contraindicated.) According to Dr Bujold,[27] three of the authors of this study wanted to exclude classical incisions from the analysis (since they involve an increased risk of uterine rupture), but they were not successful in arguing their case. So, although this study was clearly flawed in its setup and methodology, it did manage to cause a big stir in the media and it also led to changes in hospitals' and consultants' policies, which disadvantaged women wanting a VBAC. There were also problems with another study published in 2004...[28] This study revealed increased risks of complications for babies after a VBAC birth—particularly after induction or augmentation of labour. However, in this study it turned out that the VBAC women were often from disadvantaged social groups—so their pregnancies were disadvantaged right from the outset. In addition, the group again included women who had had a classical uterine incision for their previous caesarean. Unsurprisingly perhaps, this study was also criticised.[29]

We must conclude that the apparently significant risk of rupture during a VBAC is perhaps overstated, particularly when compared with the risk that the mother might die if she has a repeat caesarean. But if the risks of a real uterine rupture occurring really are small, why is it that the risks are so often presented as being high and even as increasing over time? The answer is simple... the reason is because of the interventions which became common with VBACs in the 1990s and which still continue in some places, particularly induction of labour. Other recent changes in practice have also increased the risks of a real uterine rupture occurring and—as already mentioned—the 'wrong' type of incision at the time of the original caesarean, or the 'wrong' kind of suturing, can also have an impact on the likelihood, or otherwise, of a rupture occurring in a subsequent pregnancy or labour.

Factors which increase the risk of uterine rupture

INDUCTION AND AUGMENTATION OF LABOUR

Recent research has shown that fewer and fewer births are taking place at weekends, for reasons of convenience. (This explains why more labours are now induced and why more women have elective caesareans. In England since 2005, the induction rate has been rising, after a downward trend between 1999-2000 and 2005.[30] In 2007-2008, 1 in 5 women had their labours artificially induced.) Two studies carried out in Germany and Switzerland showed a marked decrease between 1988 and 2003 in the number of babies born at weekends because of a) an increase in inductions occurring on weekdays and b) an increase in the number of elective caesareans occurring on weekdays. It is clear that the timing of a birth is increasingly being influenced by non-medical factors and this has had a negative impact on the perceived risks of VBAC.[31]

In fact, research shows[32] that the risk of rupture is greater after induction in VBAC births and it has even shown that induction increases the risk of uterine rupture for *all* women, including women who did not have a caesarean previously.[33]

Induction is, of course, one way of ensuring that births happen at certain (convenient) times but using prostaglandins so as to 'soften' the cervix and therefore prepare the way for induction (as is often the case) substantially increases the risk of uterine rupture. It has been noted[34] that prostaglandins used for induction correlated with the highest number of uterine ruptures. This is because prostaglandins cause biochemical changes which weaken the uterine scar and create favourable conditions for rupture.[35]

In Europe, since the early 1990s, the approach to VBAC has been different from in other parts of the world.[36] Rates of induction have been lower than in North America and prostaglandins have been used far less frequently. This perhaps explains why rupture rates in Europe have been lower, ranging from 0.2 to 0.4%. Nevertheless, induction has been used more often in Europe in recent years and the risk of rupture has increased along with rates of induction.[37]

Of all the prostaglandins used, Cytotec (misoprostol or E1), a drug which was not developed for obstetric use, is particularly dangerous, even when used on women who have not previously had a caesarean.[38] In case reports it has been linked to an increased incidence of uterine rupture, maternal death, fetal or neonatal death and an urgent need for a hysterectomy.[39] In its clinical directives of 2004 ACOG advised against the use of prostaglandins for VBAC and SOGC recommends limiting its use to clinical trials for all women giving birth vaginally.[40] As a result, in some parts of the world Cytotec has stopped being used for induction of labour in some hospitals.

Risk of uterine rupture (according to Lydon-Rochelle 2001)

• Without experiencing labour	0.16%
• With spontaneous labour and birth	0.52%
• With labour induced without prostaglandins	0.77%
• With labour induced using prostaglandins	2.45%

Guidelines around the world vary in the advice they give regarding the use of syntocinon for induction, but some advise against syntocinon being used in the case of a VBAC. Here is what NICE guidelines state for caesareans:[41]

Women who have had a previous caesarean can be offered induction of labour, but both women and healthcare professionals should be aware that the likelihood of uterine rupture in these circumstances is increased to:
- 80 per 10,000 when labour is induced with non-prostaglandin agents
- 240 per 10,000 when labour is induced using prostaglandins

Regarding the use of synthetic oxytocin for inducing labour—often simply called 'oxytocin' in hospitals—research has suggested the risk of rupture increases to 3.1% in this case.[42]

But what about *augmentation* of labour, i.e. speeding a woman's labour up? Does this have the same negative impact? And is the negative impact the same with induction of labour?

How does augmentation compare with induction of labour?

Several well-regarded studies (including one systematic review) have in fact demonstrated that *augmentation* of labour with syntocinon increases the risk of uterine rupture.[43] However, the 2010 NIH Consensus Development Conference on VBAC concluded that there does not appear to be an increased risk of rupture with synthetic oxytocin augmentation of spontaneous labor. In the USA in 2002, more than half of all women had their labour artificially augmented (accelerated) with artificial oxytocin, administered through a drip.[44]

(Giving women syntocinon through a drip increases the frequency, length and strength of contractions, so it is not surprising if risk of uterine rupture increases.) The American expert, doctor and researcher Bruce Flamm[45] warned against augmenting women's labours when they had previously had a caesarean, as another study also concluded (Landon et al, 2004). However, the Canadian researcher and physician Emmanuel Bujold (who wrote one of the forewords to this book) believes that augmenting labour with syntocinon is reasonable and unproblematic after 5cm dilation.[46] Nevertheless, this and other interventions perhaps need to be used with care in the case of a VBAC—which perhaps explains why RCOG VBAC guidelines say that "it should be preceded by careful obstetric assessment..."[47] After all, sometimes, simply breaking a woman's waters (i.e. performing an amniotomy), particularly after the use of syntocinon, and with the use of more syntocinon afterwards, can have a negative effect on the baby's heart rhythm. It is possible that the use of syntocinon during the latent phase of labour increases the risk too[48] but since few studies differentiate between induction and augmentation, we cannot know for sure. Some research has already suggested that the sequential use of prostaglandins and syntocinon may increase the risk of rupture three-fold.[49]

Finally, we need to consider 'alternative' approaches because a fair number of women, doulas, midwives and some consultants, prefer to try out natural methods to induce labour. Without exception, these methods—which include acupuncture and using concentrations of plant extracts (e.g. black cohosh)—have not been evaluated as to possible risks. Nevertheless, if you have never had a vigorous heel massage, (at both sides of the heel) I suggest you try giving one to a *non-pregnant* friend who is experiencing early menstrual pains. I guarantee she will feel the effect in her uterus! This is why it may be wise to avoid stimulating certain energy points in the body either when you are pregnant or in labour. I discovered the power of massage when I had a shiatsu massage every Friday for a while in my second pregnancy, during the second trimester... My uterus would then be hard all through the weekend! When I realised that the massage might have caused this, I stopped having massages and the contractions diminished. Since a scarred uterus is more susceptible to rupture than an unscarred one, you need to be even more careful about alternative methods of induction than you might otherwise be. In fact, it might be wise to avoid them altogether.

In summary, what seems to be important—if not essential—when having a VBAC, is to avoid having an induction with prostaglandins, so as to soften the cervix. It also seems to be important to avoid induction with syntocinon, even if the risks with this kind of induction are smaller—and to exercise caution with any other kind of induction too. Not only is uterine rupture a concern (particularly when the cervix is not soft, i.e. when it is long, closed and hard),[50] you also need to remember that induction increases the risk of ending up with another caesarean.[51] Induction is also associated with high numbers of non-reassuring traces in fetal heart rhythms, shoulder dystocia and forceps or ventouse deliveries—none of which are helpful for your baby.[52]

TYPES OF INCISIONS

Apart from induction and augmentation of labour, as we've already noted, having had a classical incision for a caesarean can also make a separation of the uterine incision more likely. A classical incision is a vertical incision in the 'body' of the uterus and is the type which was used at the beginning of the 20th century, when caesareans were first carried out routinely on labouring women. This type of incision is no longer common and is only used in 5%–10% of caesareans—when the baby is extremely premature (less than 28 weeks of gestation, when the lower part of the uterus has not yet formed), sometimes when the baby is presenting breech, transverse or oblique, or when there is a case of placenta praevia—when it is necessary to perform the caesarean extremely quickly (for the baby's sake)—or when there is a malformation of the uterus.

The risk of rupture in the case of a previous classical incision is generally estimated at being between 10% and 12%[53] so it is widely agreed that it is inadvisable for women with this kind of incision to have a VBAC. (Medical associations specifically consider it to be a reason not to have a VBAC.)

Other types of incision are associated with far lower rates of uterine rupture. The kind of uterine incision which involves the lowest level of risk is a low transverse incision (i.e. a horizontal incision, which is often called a bikini-line incision)—which 90%–95% of women have. It is named after the Scottish doctor, Dr Kerr, who showed in 1921 that this kind of incision resulted in fewer cases of infection, bleeding and adhesions. Another type of incision is the low vertical incision (in the lower segment of the uterus). The risk of uterine rupture could be lower because this part of the uterus has fewer veins (so there is a lower risk of bleeding[54]). Cases of T-shaped or J-shaped incisions (where the incision is low horizontal and vertical too) are rare and there are not really any studies looking at risks associated with these kinds of incision.[55]

Different types of incision

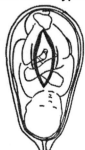 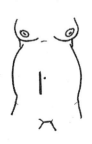 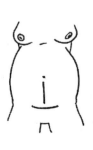

Classical uterine incision and the corresponding incision in the skin

Low transverse uterine incision and the corresponding incision in the skin (horizontal or vertical)

So that you can assess your own personal level of risk, it is helpful if you know what kind of uterine incision you had when you had your caesarean. Usually, your medical records—which you have the right to see—should indicate the type of incision, but medical records are not always clear... If you are unable to find out what kind of incision you had from your medical records, it is highly likely it was low transverse. (In fact, your consultant may be able to tell you if you explain why you had to have the caesarean last time.) In any case, ACOG latest guidelines state that there is no increase in the rate of uterine rupture in women who do not know what kind of incision they had.[56]

SINGLE SUTURING AT THE TIME OF THE CAESAREAN

The risk of uterine rupture may also increase—although research is inconclusive—in the case of women who had a suturing technique which started to be used more and more during the 1990s, i.e. a technique which involves a single layer of suturing.

A two-layer technique was the technique predominantly used up until the middle of the 1990s and after that, the single-layer technique became the technique which was most commonly used. The suture which is called 'single-layer' (or 'one-level') is a continuous suture made on the lower uterine segment, in addition to the sutures made to inhibit bleeding, which are added as necessary. The 'two-layer' suture (or 'two-level') involves a second continuous overlapping suture, which is made above the first suture. The skin suture is called the Pfannenstiel.[57]

The single-layer technique was perhaps first used in Germany or in Eastern Europe, from 1972 onwards.[58] When it was first used, various advantages would have been noted,[59] such as a slight decrease in operating time and less blood loss; in addition fewer cases of endometriosis would have been observed and the hospital stay would have been shorter. However, it was introduced without having been sufficiently evaluated and some research has suggested that more uterine ruptures may occur when women previously had this single-layer suturing... One very recent study[60] showed that there was a six times greater risk of uterine rupture after a single-layer suturing technique had been used (3.1% compared to 0.5%) and another randomised controlled trial is currently in progress (the CAESAR study).[61] On the plus side—if you are concerned about this—is the fact that there is little scientific evidence to support this concern. Results of studies are contradictory and the quality of some studies leaves something to be desired.[62] Nevertheless, it is certainly possible that the suturing technique and also the material used for suturing could affect the risk of uterine rupture, so you may want to take this into account. If you want to find out more about your own situation, again you should consult your medical records because just as the type of incision should be noted, the type of suturing technique used should also appear.

You may want to take these factors into account

The role of subjectivity when considering a repeat caesarean

Official positions on repeat caesareans and VBAC vary from time to time depending on subjectivity, not only objective research data. According to a joint statement by medical associations,[63] clinical directives mention recent breakthroughs and clinical or scientific progress when these are published but they can be modified from time to time. These associations also warn that their directives should be considered with this in mind, and that practice can sometimes not respect guidelines because "local institutions can dictate amendments to these opinions." However, if healthcare professionals should wish to do otherwise, they need to document what they do and why.

Nevertheless, health care professionals certainly are guided in their practice of medicine by the official positions adopted by their medical associations. In the UK, clinical practice is guided by NICE (the National Institute for Clinical Excellence), the recommendations from the NMC (the Nursing & Midwifery Council), the RCM (the Royal College of Midwives) and RCOG (the Royal College of Obstetricians and Gynaecologists). In the USA, it is the American College of Obstetricians and Gynecologists (ACOG) which guides the practice of a consultant and their recommendations may well also have an impact on practice in other countries, such as Canada or even the UK, given the frequency of transatlantic exchange in general, as we've noted before.

As a result of recommendations from professional associations, practices relating to VBAC have been modified over the last 20 years or so around the world. Since the end of the 1990s, policies in some places (e.g. the USA and Canada) have been that in hospitals where women are trying to have a VBAC there should be the staff necessary to carry out a caesarean 'immediately', if necessary,[64] or guidelines state that a woman who previously had a caesarean section should deliver in a hospital where a timely caesarean section is available.[65] Both these recommendations are, in fact, based on what is generally considered to be weak 'evidence' (Level III of scientific evidence, which is considered less valid than evidence provided by scientific studies)—i.e. they are based on either the results of consensus or the opinion of experts. After all, no study has demonstrated that the immediate availability of a medical team and an operating theatre improves outcomes for either mothers or babies. This perhaps explains why these recommendations have triggered reactions from women's groups, and from some consultants and doctors.[66]

The guidelines themselves are inconsistent and perhaps difficult to implement. A recent study comparing guidelines in six countries (the UK, the USA, Canada, New Zealand and Australia) concluded that not only were they citing expert opinions and consensus as evidence for some recommendations, but that they widely varied in their recommendations, which undermined their usefulness in clinical practice.[67] They have widely been interpreted in medical circles as meaning that medical teams need to be present and ready to operate, if a woman is attempting a VBAC. RCOG guidelines in Britain, and

American and Canadian ones insist on this. Nevertheless, the maximum delay generally recommended in obstetrics[68] for an emergency caesarean is not more than 30 minutes (from the time of the decision is made to perform a caesarean, until the operation starts)—although some authors have specified that the delay should not exceed 15 to 18 minutes because within this time period that the baby should not suffer any damage.[69] The Canadian association (SOGC) does, in fact, recommend a maximum delay of 30 minutes for VBAC 'for the preparation of an emergency laparotomy', but this in itself seems to contradict its position that it is necessary to do a caesarean 'at an appropriate time'. (In case you don't know, a laparotomy involves a surgical opening of the abdomen, using a large incision, so as to look inside.) Furthermore, while some people interpret these recommendations as meaning a medical team must be present and ready to operate (with an operating theatre available round the clock), other people interpret the guidelines more broadly to mean that an operating theatre only needs to be *available* within 30 minutes. In any case, the idea that these times can be respected has been challenged by some. American doctor, Pixie Williams, made the following comment: "A caesarean carried out within 15 minutes is a myth. I was trained in some of the best hospitals in Boston and New York and I never saw an emergency caesarean carried out within less than 30 minutes."[70]

Whatever people's interpretations of the guidelines, perhaps because of difficulties implementing them since they were becoming increasingly restrictive, more than 300 hospitals banned VBACs altogether in 2005 in the USA.[71] In addition, some American insurance companies refused to insure consultants whose clients had a VBAC.[72] Needless to say, perhaps, this was in stark contrast to the situation in the 1990s, when some companies were refusing to insure repeat caesareans carried out for no medical reason.

The real increase in risk... the risk of litigation?

When considering reasons for these changes in policies, we need to ask ourselves again whether a fear of litigation could possibly be influencing obstetric practice... One American consultant made the point that the risk which has increased is not actually the risk of uterine rupture, but the risk of litigation.[73] In fact, the challenge when discussing informed choice, is to manage to clearly separate risks for the client and her baby on a clinical level from the medico-legal risks which exist for caregivers. After all, there is a tendency to confuse these two types of risk in hospital documents for informed consent, in the scientific literature and in documents produced by professional and administrative associations—and the confusion is also obvious within media reports. The consequence is a distorted portrayal of risks to pregnant women and less real informed choice for the client.[74]

We need to ask whether a fear of litigation could
possibly be influencing obstetric practice

Some people do in fact believe that the change in attitude in medical associations has more to do with fear of court cases brought against consultants and hospitals than with the risks associated with VBAC.[75] The person who set up the American VBAC website www.vbac.com emphasised this possibility, quoting the Vice President of ACOG, Dr Stanley Zinberg, who said that consultants who are sued can best defend themselves if they were present when complications occurred in a particular case.[76] Since a consultant working in the USA is likely to have an average of one legal case to deal with every three years this must be a very real concern, particularly since certain cases which took place in the 1990s created fear amongst the medical community. Nevertheless, despite the possibility that fear of legal consequences may be a factor when caregivers talk about increased risks for VBAC, very little is said to a woman requesting a VBAC about any fear of litigation and very little research has been done on this subject.

It is also possible that some countries' recommendations to use electronic fetal monitoring (EFM) for VBACs—including UK RCOG VBAC guidelines—have more to do with protecting members in potential court cases than with any scientific evidence indicating that the continued use of this machine in VBAC cases is helpful... particularly since EFM has been associated with a fairly high rate of errors.[77] In fact, some people emphasise the lack of studies on this subject[78] and the use of the supine position (i.e. the woman lying on her back), which EFM usually implies, is particularly mystifying. After all, when a woman lies on her back the vena cava is compressed and this negatively affects oxygenation of the placenta, which can in turn cause decelerations in the rhythm of the fetal heartbeat—the very problem we need to avoid, which continuous monitoring is supposed to detect! Intermittent monitoring using a Sonicaid, which is far less invasive, is considered an adequate alternative to continuous monitoring, but it is often not used in VBACs... If a policy to use EFM is a particular stumbling block for you when planning a hospital VBAC, one useful option may be to request the use of telemetry to track the fetal heartbeat. This involves using a portable device to track the fetal heartbeat and it's useful because it wouldn't stop you from walking around. (It is already being used in some hospitals.)

Subjectivity on this and other issues is clear because of the wide range of variation of opinion amongst doctors, midwives and consultants. While some caregivers are very cautious, as we have already detailed, others like to help their clients have a VBAC. For example, there are even some GPs who refuse to take on women who do *not* wish to have a VBAC. They send these women to consultants in hospitals in order to optimise the use of their own resources (so that they don't have to spend time on procedures relating to women who are having repeat caesareans).[79] One general practitioner association in America is even challenging the ACOG recommendations. The American Academy of Family Physicians (AAFP) made a pronouncement on VBAC in March 2005,

The risk element, whatever your decision   51

after a systematic review of studies carried out by a US government health department (the Agency for Health Care Research and Quality) looked specifically at maternal health. The AAFP now recommends that professionals in maternity care should offer VBACs to their clients. This is not in line with the restrictions issued by ACOG, which require that access to VBAC should be restricted to institutions with medical teams present during the whole of labour. The AAFP stated that they had found no scientific evidence to suggest that these additional resources improve the results of births.[80]

The American College of Nurse Midwives (ACNM), a professional body of nurse midwives, strongly supports the practice of VBAC, emphasising that successful VBACs offer significant advantages and fewer risks for women and their babies than repeat caesareans. They also state that midwives can help women to have a VBAC, from the moment that agreements are made with the medical community as regards consultation and transfer (when needed). They specify that help from a midwife increases the chances of women 'succeeding' in having a VBAC and that it lowers the caesarean rate, results in fewer interventions and better results for women with high risk pregnancies. Two studies which evaluated the practice of midwives and another one which focused on home birth have confirmed this.[81] The ACNM study also confirms that the incidence (the frequency) of uterine rupture is similar to that of other obstetric emergencies, which can arise in any labour and birth, as long as women planning home births have not previously had two or more caesareans and as long as they are not overdue (i.e. more than 40 weeks pregnant).[82] The Quebec College of Midwives states that: "Midwives are qualified to give care to a pregnant women who've had a previous caesarean. What's more, when women who have already had a caesarean choose to have a natural birth and be looked after by a midwife, the support of the midwife increases the chances of success." A VBAC is therefore not a reason *not* to be looked after by a midwife. As the birth accounts in this book show, many midwives are perfectly happy to attend home birth VBACs, even if others aren't necessarily at ease, when faced with a request for a VBAC outside a hospital.

Even neonatologist Dr Marsden Wagner, who was previously the World Health Organization director for Maternal and Infant Health in Europe, wrote that ACOG recommendations are not based on scientific evidence. He said that they were drawn up by consultants in a conflict of interests, since it is these consultants who carry out the caesareans. He believes that the recommendations are the fruit of a desire in these consultants to protect and facilitate their work. He says that the important thing is to increase communication between the labouring woman and the caregiver in the medical establishment in such a way that it is possible to perform a caesarean when it is needed, within an optimal timeframe. In his view, it is also necessary to pay attention to the length of labour during a VBAC, in order to reduce the possibility of rupture of the incision—and it is worth noting that he also suggests banning induction of labour.[83]

The views of this former WHO employee (now retired) and the midwives I mentioned earlier are not so remarkable when we consider the research. According to one study,[84] the outcomes of VBACs which take place under the care of midwives are encouraging... 64-100% of women ended up having the VBAC they opted for, Apgar scores of their babies at one minute and five minutes were 7.99% and 8.84% respectively (which is fine) and only 5.3% of these VBAC babies were admitted into neonatal care. Another recent study into midwifery care in Holland[85] (where approximately a third of all women give birth at home), which looked at statistics for almost 300,000 women, found there was not a single maternal death after any birth (not only VBACs). (This is dramatically different from maternal mortality rates for other countries in any kind of birth, VBAC or otherwise, particularly when we consider the view of some researchers that maternal deaths are generally *under*-estimated at birth.)[86] To gain some kind of perspective on this zero rate, in the UK the maternal mortality rate was 8.2/100 000 live births in 2008 (8.4 in 1990), in the USA it was 16.6 (compared to 11.5 in 1990) and in Canada it was 6.6 (compared to 5.7 in 1990). The lowest rate was in Sweden (4.6). (Note that rates given on page 16 were for *infant* mortality, not maternal mortality.)[87]

In any case, when choosing caregivers if we are planning a VBAC we certainly need to remember this subjectivity element when it comes to risk assessment and individual caregivers' policies.

Risks associated with caesareans for both mother and baby

For several years, a great deal of emphasis has been put on the risks of VBACs, while the risks associated with caesareans have not been emphasised. Caesareans have become so common, affecting 1 in 4 women in the UK (24.6% in 2008), that it has become a mundane aspect of life—and the clear implication is that this accepted intervention must be risk-free. Yet people almost forget that a caesarean is first and foremost an operation which involves the risks associated with any surgical intervention. Clearly, when it is a question of responding to a real obstetric emergency, when it's a question of saving a mother's life, or a baby's, the advantages which the caesarean operation offers are undeniable. But when a caesarean is not performed for urgent medical reasons, what is the level of risk—and what *kind* of risks are we talking about?

Contrary to the impression we generally have, caesareans are far from being risk-free. Risks relate to the period immediately around the surgery or in the following years, and they include risks for subsequent births and subsequent babies. Risks for the woman include death at the time of the caesarean, short-term problems (which will necessitate treatment and further hospital care), long-term problems (which may cause long-term pain), including problems with bonding and breastfeeding, psychological problems and problems with later pregnancies and births. Risks for the baby include death or injury, respiratory problems, and infections which are likely to necessitate intensive care after the birth. There is also the risk that the baby will have asthma and allergies later on in life.

THE RISK OF THE PREGNANT WOMAN DYING

Caesareans are associated with an increased risk of maternal death when there are blood clots, infections or problems with anaesthesia. One study which compared 300,000 women[88] who gave birth between 1988 and 2000 (women who'd previously had a caesarean and who later had a trial of labour and women with a previous caesarean who later had another caesarean, on demand) concluded that repeat caesareans on demand involved almost four times the risk of death for the mother than an attempt at a VBAC (1.6 per 100,000 women against 5.6 out of 100,000 women). The link between caesareans and higher mortality rates is even officially recognised in some places. For example, a document published in 2004 by a Canadian government department on maternal mortality and morbidity[89] mentioned that a rise in the number of maternal deaths due to complications of surgery or anaesthesia was anticipated, given the regular increases over the previous few years in the rates of caesarean births. In the USA in 2007, after several years of rises in the caesarean rate, it was also officially confirmed that rates of maternal death were higher than they had been for several decades.[90] A recent WHO study[91] also showed a strong association between maternal mortality, complications affecting the mother and an increase in caesarean rates. (The study also confirmed more deaths amongst babies and more admissions into intensive care (with stays of seven days or more), even when premature births weren't included in the sample considered.)

Another study concluded that caesareans on demand involve almost three times the amount of risk of maternal death than vaginal birth, and almost eight times the risk when an emergency caesarean is performed.[92] This risk can increase to eleven times greater, and is principally associated with complications of infection and accidents linked to the use of anaesthesia.[93] Even doctors and researchers do not consider the risks to be merely theoretical... One doctor confided to me that he had a client who didn't want a VBAC, but an elective caesarean instead, and she died on the operating table. He estimated the risk of dying during a caesarean on demand like this at 1 in 2000. Researchers writing a recent report on mortality connected with birth also confirmed that all the maternal deaths studied were linked directly with birth and each case was the product of a caesarean.[94]

THE RISK OF SHORT-TERM SERIOUS COMPLICATIONS

Women who choose to have a repeat caesarean experience more complications than women who choose a VBAC, particularly when they complete the VBAC.[95] One recent WHO study which looked at caesarean rates in several countries in Latin America confirmed that a high caesarean rate leads to a rise in serious complications for the mother.[96] WHO also suggest that when the caesarean rate rises above 15% of all births, the risks to health far outweigh the advantages. They also point out that the high caesarean rates in developed countries may lead to an excess of maternal deaths. Another study which looked at *all* low risk women who gave birth in one country in a 14-year period (1991-2005) showed that women who'd had a caesarean had five times more heart attacks, three times more hysterectomies, twice the number of thromboembolisms (i.e. blood clots in the lungs or legs, which can cause death), twice the number of complications linked to anaesthesia and three times more serious infections than women who gave birth vaginally.[97]

Yet another recent report[98] showed a more than 50% rise in serious maternal complications when births in 1991/1992 were compared with births in 2000/2001. Even if we do not differentiate between caesareans and vaginal births with regard to serious maternal complications, it would be easy to believe that the rise in the caesarean rate, as well as the increase in interventions of all kinds during labour and birth (epidurals, induction with prostaglandins or syntocinon, augmentation with syntocinon, etc) could have contributed to this rise in complications, since it has recently been discovered that induction of labour doubles the risk of amniotic fluid embolism, a rare complication, for sure, but one which can be fatal.[99] This is when a quantity of amniotic fluid goes into the maternal blood system during labour (and the birth) and becomes stuck in a vein. Usually, a pulmonary embolism is fatal for the mother. Other studies emphasise the negative effects of interventions. [100]

Perhaps the rise in the caesarean rate as well as the rise in interventions have contributed to the rise in complications

Short-term risks of complications include significant surgical risks and the risks are 4.5 times higher when a repeat caesarean is performed. These complications include serious haemorrhage (which necessitates further surgery), pelvic infection, pneumonia and septicaemia (i.e. a serious infection in the whole body). Just like minor complications, which affect a third of all women who have a caesarean, these complications affect significant numbers of women and may involve fever, haematomas (i.e. blood clots, usually after a haemorrhage), urinary infections, infections of the uterus or the incision, and paralysis of the intestines or bladder. Caesareans also double the risk for the mother of (re-)hospitalisation (after the birth) and are more often followed by bad pain or weakness during the postnatal period, all of which would not be without repercussions for the newborn baby.

THE RISK OF PSYCHOLOGICAL REPERCUSSIONS

A review carried out by the organisation Childbirth Connection concluded that various psychological effects were associated with caesareans. These included a less satisfactory experience of birth (when compared with women's reports after vaginal births) and the development of depression, which can lead to trauma or mental health problems and low self-esteem. (I will not elaborate on this further here, because we will return to this subject in later chapters.)

THE RISK THAT BREASTFEEDING MAY BE AFFECTED

It is possible that having a caesarean can affect breastfeeding, although researchers' conclusions on this topic vary.[101] There is a danger of confusing issues here, because lower breastfeeding rates amongst caesarean mothers could be linked to the drugs used in epidurals,[102] early mother-baby separation after the operation or to the practice of hospitals offering formula supplements in certain cases. It is also possible that the difficulties some caesarean babies experience are linked to the fact of having fewer catecholamines in their blood and fewer natural hormones, which contribute to alertness levels (all of which will be explained later in this chapter). Other hormones might play a role since the amounts of oxytocin or prolactin (this latter hormone being associated with milk production) are lower in caesarean mothers than in mothers who've given birth vaginally. Finally, after a caesarean the new mother's milk certainly comes in later, so this could also negatively affect the success of breastfeeding.[103]

THE RISK OF LONG-TERM COMPLICATIONS

Too often, it is forgotten that having a caesarean increases the risks (for both mothers and babies) during subsequent pregnancies and births. In recent years, various researchers[104] have drawn attention to the long-term consequences of caesareans, which can include abnormal attachment of organs or fibrous tissue and the formation of adhesions. Adhesions cause problems because they delay a subsequent baby's exit from the uterus (and the problem increases if a woman has more than one caesarean). More than half of all women have adhesions after a first caesarean[105] and some women feel pain at the site of the adhesions or at the incision for a long time afterwards.[106] Adhesions may also cause pain during sexual intercourse or they can cause intestinal problems. When a woman has a caesarean, there is also the risk of organs being damaged during the surgery, which obviously may also have long-term consequences.

RISKS FOR FUTURE PREGNANCIES

Studies have shown an increase in fertility problems after a caesarean and a higher rate of ectopic pregnancies (where the embryo remains outside the uterus).[107] Problems linked to the placenta are particularly important and increase with the number of caesareans performed. They include an increased risk of placenta praevia in a subsequent pregnancy (where the placenta is too low and sometimes covers the cervix).[108] Another significant risk for a future pregnancy is the risk of placenta accreta, which means the placenta does not separate from the uterus after a subsequent birth. This risk has been noted to be 44% in the case of women who've had one caesarean and 60% in the case of women who've had two caesareans. In several cases placenta accreta has led to maternal death (the risk with this condition being 7%)[109] and in almost all cases the women affected needed to have a hysterectomy.

Overall, the risks associated with caesareans rise as women have more caesareans. This is why it is never a mundane, ordinary thing to have another caesarean and why it's important not to carry out caesareans on first-time mothers unless it's absolutely necessary.

THE RISK THE BABY MIGHT DIE OR BE BORN BRAIN-DAMAGED

In everyday life and even within the field of obstetrics, it's easy to assume that caesareans are risk-free for the baby. Nevertheless, most recent studies do not show that the baby is less at risk when a caesarean is performed, whether it's a first caesarean or a repeat one. In the case of a first caesarean, the risk of death for the baby when there are no complications is high, even 69% higher than in vaginal births.[110] (It was a very recent study which concluded this, which looked at 98% of newborn deaths in the USA between 1999 and 2002. These were all normal pregnancies—i.e. they were full-term pregnancies, with singleton babies, which were presenting head-down, with no medical risks or placental problems.) If indeed VBACs do present more risks for the baby—the main risk being the risk of death after uterine rupture—we could assume that with fewer VBACs the neonatal mortality rate would be lower... but this is not the case. A US study[111] which looked at 400,000 women who'd previously had a caesarean revealed that the mortality rate for babies had not decreased between 1996 and 2002, a period in which the VBAC rate fell to almost half what it had been before.

THE RISK OF THE BABY HAVING BREATHING PROBLEMS AND NEEDING TO BE ADMITTED INTO INTENSIVE CARE

If we compare the risks for the baby during a vaginal birth and a repeat caesarean or any type of caesarean—excluding situations which could influence results, such as prematurity—we find a much higher risk that the baby may suffer from pulmonary hypertension (which increases the risk of death). In fact, the risk is almost five times higher after an elective caesarean than after a vaginal birth. Elective caesareans are associated with a four times higher rate of general respiratory problems in the baby. Of course, this is problematic not only in itself but also because respiratory problems necessitate admission of the baby to intensive care. The risk of this happening is almost three times greater in women who have a planned caesarean.[112] The WHO study on caesarean rates in Latin America demonstrated that high caesarean rates were associated with an increase in the admission of babies into intensive care.[113]

A repeat caesarean is also associated with problems for the baby, even when the caesarean is carried out after 39 weeks of gestation. Higher numbers of babies born by repeat caesarean need to go into intensive care and these babies need to stay longer in the hospital.[114] (I mention this because although it is well-known that risks increase as we move away from the due date—as we shall see later—babies born before 39 weeks are more likely to have breathing difficulties because their lungs are less likely to be developed.)

Caesareans are often performed at 37 or 38 weeks (for medical reasons)— and 'sweeping' is often done from 38 weeks on—and when the due date is miscalculated (as often happens) it is only noticed afterwards that the caesarean was carried out too soon and that the baby hadn't been ready to be born. (It is generally accepted that a caesarean should not be carried out on a woman who is less than 39 weeks' pregnant, unless there is a medical reason to do so.) Babies born at 37 or 38 weeks are 120 times more at risk of needing ventilation since they have insufficient surfactant in their lungs, compared with babies who are between 39 and 41 weeks.[115] (Surfactant prepares the baby's lungs to breathe outside the womb.)[116] In addition, a caesarean carried out at 37 or 38 weeks presents at least three times the risk of respiratory complications. Even at 39 weeks, the risk for the baby is double. Some of these babies can be very ill and others may die, according to researchers, and the risk is principally linked to the absence of labour before the caesarean is carried out. Elective caesareans (whose timing may be based on a miscalculated due date) are particularly problematic since carrying out a caesarean before 39 weeks increases the risk for the baby of being born prematurely and of suffering from low birth weight.[117] This is why it is in Brazil, where the caesarean rate is high in private clinics (up to 90% in some clinics), that it is well-off middle-class women who run the highest risk of having low birth weight babies, more than women who are socially disadvantaged, which is the case in other countries, such as the UK and Canada.[118]

The baby is at increased risk of respiratory complications, after an elective caesarean section, compared to after a vaginal birth

As mentioned in the RCOG VBAC guidelines, three studies have shown that the baby is at increased risk of respiratory complications even at term, after an elective caesarean section, compared to after a vaginal birth. (A caesarean is from two to three times riskier to seven times riskier.) Childbirth Connection concluded that the risks in this respect were 'moderately high'. Even later, children born by caesarean are at higher risk of suffering from asthma,[119] a problem which is increasing in our society at an alarming rate, and these caesarean babies may also be more likely to suffer from allergies later on too.[120]

THE RISK OF FUTURE BABIES AND CHILDREN BEING DISADVANTAGED

It has recently been discovered, without our being able to explain why, that babies gestating in women who have had one or more caesareans are more at risk than other babies. (Some people hypothesise that there may be problems with the placenta.) These babies have a higher risk of suffering from congenital malformation, lesions of the central nervous system and even uterine death,[121] a risk which is 1 in 1000,[122] which should prompt us to reduce the frequency of first-time caesareans, as well as subsequent caesareans. Strangely, perhaps, women who have had a caesarean are also likely to have fewer babies afterwards.[123]

A comparison of risks associated with caesareans and VBAC

In order to evaluate risks effectively, it is useful to first of all remind ourselves what is meant by risk and how we usually assess risk in our daily life. According to the Cambridge Online Dictionary, a risk is 'the possibility of something bad happening' and being 'at risk' means 'being in a dangerous situation'. The Wikipedia definition is particularly interesting:

Risk concerns the expected value of one or more results of one or more future events. Technically, the value of those results may be positive or negative. However, general usage tends to focus only on potential harm that may arise from a future event, which may accrue either from incurring a cost ('downside risk') or by failing to attain some benefit ('upside risk').

Both definitions imply that in certain situations there might be the increased likelihood—or *decreased* likelihood—of something happening and the second definition also reminds us that we sometimes face a risk because of the benefit we hope to obtain from a particular choice. The definitions also remind us that the notion of probability is a statistical one. This is very different from our usual understanding of the word 'probability' (when we usually think it means something is highly likely to happen). It is simply an assessment of odds for something happening, which mostly does not happen.

When you weigh up the specific risks of having a VBAC or another caesarean, you would do well to remember positive and negative aspects of the probabilities. After all, we face all kinds of risks in other areas of life, but they do not usually prevent us from continuing with our day-to-day activities.

Given this, it is interesting that people insist on emphasising the risk which a VBAC presents... The risk could be the same level of risk as a risk we would accept in our everyday life at home, without thinking, such as the risk of falling on the stairs. The risk of a VBAC could be even lower than some everyday risks, such as the risk of crossing a road, for example. Do we think about the risk of having an accident every time we use some stairs or whenever we go about our daily business? Do we think twice about crossing a road because we're afraid of being in a road accident? As far as obstetric risks are concerned, do we hesitate before deciding to have children because we're afraid of having an ectopic pregnancy?

Do consultants hesitate before suggesting interventions?

Do consultants hesitate before advising pregnant women to have an amniocentesis, for fear they will have a miscarriage? They usually don't, even though the risk of miscarriage following amniocentesis is considered in some studies to be similar to the risk of uterine rupture during a VBAC.[124] And do consultants hesitate before performing caesareans because they're afraid of the risks they present? They usually don't, even in cases where there are no specific medical reasons for performing the caesarean.

In order to help you make a decision, here is a table which will allow you to see the risk associated with a VBAC in comparison with other typical risks in life or childbirth.

Comparison of risks, according to the Paling scale[125]

	Very low risk 1 in 10,000	Low risk 1 in 1,000	Moderate risk 1 in 100	High risk 1 in 10
Risks in daily life		Risk of dying from an accident in the home	Risk of being injured on stairs	Pedestrian accident (involving death or serious injury)
Obstetric risks	Maternal death due to a caesarean	Ectopic pregnancy Perinatal mortality	Risk of miscarriage after amniocentesis	
		Uterine rupture (true ruptures and scar defects)		

Emphasis is often put on the risk of having a VBAC and people want women attempting a VBAC to give birth in conditions which are different from other women in labour. As I emphasised before, the risk of a serious, unpredictable complication occurring, which necessitates an emergency caesarean, is 2.7% in all labours (i.e. VBACs *and* other vaginal births.)[126] and the risk of uterine rupture is comparable to other important risks. It's worth remembering, though, in this respect, that many urgent situations can, paradoxically, be anticipated. The French midwife Francine Dauphin[127] said that cord prolapse can be avoided if the woman's waters are not broken when the baby is very high up; extreme fetal distress can be avoided by allowing labouring women to eat as they wish; and she said that there is no need for labour to be augmented with syntocinon (or pitocin) if waters are not systematically broken. She added that it is also possible to prevent haemorrhage by avoiding inducing or augmenting labour or even by avoiding extended labours with epidurals and syntocinon. And if it's not possible to completely eliminate the risk of uterine rupture during a VBAC, it is at least possible to reduce it by avoiding induction and perhaps also augmentation.

Given this and the other data I have detailed earlier on in this chapter, it is clear that a vaginal birth which does not involve unnecessary interventions (such as those mentioned by Francine Dauphin) involves fewer risks than a repeat caesarean... so having a repeat caesarean does involve many more risks than a non-interventionist VBAC. Obstetric experts, Murray Enkin and his colleagues (who wrote *A Guide to Effective Care in Pregnancy and Childbirth*, Oxford University Press 2000), which examines the research evidence underpinning common practices, confirmed that VBAC is a practice which is beneficial overall. In the third edition of their book they classified VBACs after one or more caesareans as being one of the 'Forms of Care Likely to be Beneficial'. After devoting a whole chapter to VBAC, the authors confirm that evidence for classifying VBAC as 'likely to be beneficial' is solid. (This chapter is available online.)[128] A detailed comparison of risks relating to caesareans (compared to vaginal births), carried out by Childbirth Connection also showed that caesareans involve a much higher number of risks, that vaginal births involving forceps or ventouse carry intermediate risks, while spontaneous vaginal births which do not involve instrumental delivery involve few risks.[129]

The advantage for your baby of letting birth start spontaneously

If, despite the low level of risk a VBAC seems to imply, you would still prefer to opt for a repeat caesarean, it is a good idea to remember that—from the baby's point of view—even when a caesarean is planned, it is preferable if your labour does begin first, before the caesarean is performed. Contractions effectively stimulate the production of hormones, which help prepare the baby physically for life outside the womb. Letting your labour begin first also increases the chances that your baby will be at term so it will increase its chances of being able to adapt well to life outside the womb. After all, research has shown that waiting until labour begins before carrying out a caesarean decreases the risk of respiratory distress for the baby. [130]

Another good reason to wait until you go into labour, whatever your choice about VBAC, is that towards the end of pregnancy, the level of endorphins rises in the baby, in preparation for the contractions of labour[131] and these endorphins decrease the perception of pain, while also increasing the sensation of well-being. There are also studies which emphasise the importance of waiting for labour to begin.[132] As Dr Julie Choquet explained, (and as early as 1986 it was discussed in the Scientific American[133]), the circulation of catecholamines in the baby, caused by labour, helps the baby to empty its lungs of secretions, in preparation for breathing after birth. The article in the Scientific American explained why contractions are beneficial for the baby and it was preceded and followed by the appearance of several studies on the lung problems affecting babies born by caesarean in the 1980s.[134] Since the 1980s, several articles have been published on the subject. The role catecholamines play during labour has been confirmed: they protect the baby from a lack of oxygen during labour and prepare its lungs for life outside the womb. These hormones facilitate the baby's respiratory functions by helping the lungs absorb liquids, and by facilitating the production of surfactant, a substance which helps to prepare the lungs to function at birth. Even in 1980, a study conducted in Sweden[135] had shown that the capacity of the baby's lungs to be used and to fill with air is linked to the level of catecholamines present in the baby's circulation at birth. This study also showed that two hours after the birth, babies born vaginally have lungs which function better than those of babies born by caesarean—and this has since been confirmed by other studies.[136] In the 1980s, it was also proposed[137] that a low level of natural prostaglandins during an elective caesarean could be responsible for breathing difficulties in babies born by caesarean.

The risk element, whatever your decision 61

Another effect of catecholamines is to increase the baby's metabolic rate in such a way that the baby conserves energy reserves in its liver and fat cells, so that it has reserves ready for when it begins to feed. These reserves also help babies maintain their body temperature. In babies born by caesarean, this mechanism functions less efficiently and there is the risk of low glucose levels in the blood. Yet another effect of catecholamines is that more blood goes to the vital organs. This means that babies born vaginally have better circulation of blood to the lungs than those born by caesarean. In short, the hormones which are called catecholamines produce a state of alertness in the baby, which can facilitate the bonding process between mother and baby from the moment of birth onwards.

Other hormones, which are produced more during labour, also have beneficial effects on the baby, according to the authors of an important Danish study, which was published in 2007.[138] The circulation of hormones favourises the mobilisation of brown fat, which is important for helping the baby maintain its temperature, and it also favourises the circulation of blood to the brain and the heart.[139]

Apart from all this, the authors of a study published in 1995[140] hypothesise that the reabsorption by the lungs of liquid is likely to be linked with argipressin, a hormone which plays a role in water retention. (Also known as antidiuretic hormone (ADH), argipressin is a human hormone that is mainly released when the body is low on water. It causes the kidneys to conserve water by concentrating the urine and reducing urine volume.)

Studies published since that time, which have compared records of babies born by caesarean with or without an experience of labour, as well as babies born vaginally, have continued to confirm the beneficial effects of labour, as we've already seen. We must conclude that contractions are beneficial for the baby even if labour ends up with a caesarean. We must also conclude that the nearer a baby is to term when it is born, the better off it is. Every week counts and the more time passes, the more we can confirm a lowering of the risk of complications relating to breathing difficulties for each week of completed pregnancy.[141] For example, between 37 and 39 weeks of gestation, the risk goes from being 14.3 times higher (than at 40 weeks) to 3.5 times higher. We also shouldn't forget that these complications are serious and mean that newborn babies have to be admitted to intensive care.

The absence of labour constitutes the biggest risk for babies born by caesarean.[142] No matter how long gestation is, the risk of respiratory complications increases when the baby does not experience labour.

We also should not forget that these complications are serious. Therefore, if you do decide to have another caesarean, try to make sure that the caesarean takes place after you have spontaneously gone into labour, since even some hours of labour have been shown to be beneficial for the baby, and if this is impossible, make sure it takes place as near as possible to your due date.

Unfortunately, it is rare that a woman for whom a caesarean is planned is allowed to go into labour spontaneously first. Why is this? Because it is less practical for caregivers and for the hospital. It is unfortunately the case that the baby's well-being can be superseded by practical considerations. Of course, it is easier to organise childcare for one's first child or other children if you plan for the presence of your partner or helper for convalescence when you know in advance the date of the operation. But is it better for the baby who is coming? No, unless there is a clear medical reason to have the caesarean early. A caesarean on demand deprives the baby of benefitting from the advantage of labour and birth at the time which would be its time to be born, and not at the time which is convenient for the hospital.

For French child psychiatrist and psychoanalyst Myriam Szejer, author of the book whose title translates as 'Women and Babies First',[143] it is important not to force birth, either through induction or arranging a caesarean. She says:

"If you monitor statistics, you will find that numerous newborns immediate display difficulties recovering from a violent birth. They experience pain, they seem distressed, upset, tearful, even anorexic or insomniac, and they are sometimes ill. Unfortunately, these symptoms, which occur alongside medical interventions, are rarely considered in a symbolic dimension and they are rarely put into words at the heart of their history and their meaning. Most often, they are only seen as manifestations of pediatric records, which people must put a stop to."

In conclusion, perhaps we need to re-evaluate the over-cautious attitude which has led to so much intervention in obstetrics. Are we becoming too cautious in this area of life, as well as in others? Only 30 years ago we used to drive around happily wearing no seatbelt or poodle along on a bicycle with no helmet... but now it seems imperative for us to protect ourselves from all possible risk, in the misguided belief that if we do everything necessary, we will remain healthy and safe. However, even though behaviour which is encouraged in the name of health and safety can make sense at times, the omnipresent obsession with risk can have the effect of increasing our levels of anxiety. Your own decision needs to take this into account, as well as your own view of the research you've read about in this chapter and your feelings about your upcoming birth...

To summarise...

Risks relating to VBAC for mother and baby
- The risks associated with VBAC are smaller than is generally believed.
- The 'basic' risk that the uterine incision will rupture at the time of a VBAC has not changed. It may occur in 2 to 6 women in 1,000, when a woman goes into labour spontaneously, and the risk increases when a woman's labour is induced.
- This risk has been exaggerated by the media.

The risk element, whatever your decision

- Nowadays, we have far greater knowledge about what can increase the risk of rupture.
- The most dangerous eventuality is when a uterine incision separates along its whole thickness, including the membrane. Note, though, that the most clear indication of imminent uterine rupture is ongoing anomalies in the rhythm of the baby's heartbeat.
- Potential risks for the mother are either haemorrhage or hysterectomy (but note that these risks also exist for women who have a caesarean).
- Potential risks for the baby (which occur in 5% of ruptures, i.e. 5% of the 2-6 women out of 1,000) involve not getting enough oxygen and death. This risk is the same as the risk of death for any baby at the end of a first pregnancy
- The risk of having an emergency caesarean (during *any* kind of vaginal labour), is 2.7%, i.e. 2 or 3 women in 100.

Factors which increase the risk of uterine rupture

- The risk increases when a woman has her labour induced, especially when induction is achieved through the use of prostaglandins (either as a gel applied vaginally, or as tablets taken orally, which soften the cervix). Misoprostol, a type of prostaglandin, increases the risk substantially and—even though the risk is lower—the risk of uterine rupture may also increase when syntocinon (synthetic oxytocin) is given (in a drip) to induce labour.
- If a woman had a classical (i.e. a high vertical) uterine incision for her caesarean, there is a higher risk of rupture. Although this type of incision is uncommon, having this kind of vertical scar is a reason not to attempt a VBAC.
- The one-layer suturing technique, which started being used in the 1990s, may increase the risk of uterine rupture in a later VBAC.
- There could be an increased risk of rupture when the thickness of the uterine wall (at the uterine incision scar) measures less than 2.3 to 2.5mm.

The relativity of the medical associations' VBAC guidelines

- American and Canadian medical associations recommend that facilities be ready for an immediate caesarean when a woman is attempting a VBAC, in case she has a uterine rupture. Nevertheless, professional associations in both these countries emphasise that information provided through hospital hierarchies should not be interpreted in absolute terms to indicate the protocols professionals should follow. They say that ways of proceeding can be adapted by caregivers, although caregivers need to document any deviation from the guidelines.
- In the conclusion of its preliminary report, the 2010 NIH Consensus Development Conference on VBAC urged the American College of Obstetricians and Gynecologists to reassess their requirement for 'immediately available' surgical and anaesthesia personnel during a VBAC, taking into account the fact that other complications have a comparable level of risk and also that there are widespread staffing shortages.

Risks associated with caesareans for both mother and baby

Significant risks are associated with caesareans, which are far from being risk-free. However, some risks do increase as a woman has repeat caesareans.

RISKS FOR THE MOTHER

- The risk of maternal mortality becomes at least four times greater.
- There is four or five times the risk of serious, short-term complications. These can include serious infection, cardiac arrest, hysterectomy, thrombo-embolism, and complications linked to the use of anaesthesia.
- There is also the risk of long-term complications. These can include problems with fertility, adhesions (resulting in pelvic pain and intestinal problems), and serious problems associated with the placenta.
- Having a caesarean can also result in having a less fulfilling experience of birth. There may be a higher risk of depression and trauma and breastfeeding may be more difficult.

RISKS FOR THE BABY

- The risk of neonatal mortality (fetal or newborn death) increases, even if the woman was considered low risk when she had her original caesarean and even when there are no complications when the caesarean is performed.
- There is a four times increased risk of respiratory problems of various degrees of severity. This means that more caesarean babies are admitted to intensive care and that more of them have interventions at birth, etc.
- The earlier the caesarean takes place before 39 weeks, the more the baby is at risk.
- There is an increased risk that the baby will suffer from asthma and maybe also allergies.
- For the baby who is born *after* the original caesarean is performed (after a subsequent pregnancy) there appears to be a higher risk of malformations, lesions of the systemic nervous system and death.

A comparison of risks associated with caesareans and VBAC

- Having a repeat caesarean involves more risks than having a VBAC.
- A fairly high number of risks are associated with instrumental deliveries, i.e. births involving the use of forceps or ventouse, so these interventions should be avoided, if possible, in a vaginal birth.
- From the baby's point of view, even when a caesarean is planned, it is preferable if the woman's labour begins first. Contractions effectively stimulate the production of hormones, which help prepare the baby physically for life outside the womb.
- There are fewer risks when a VBAC is a spontaneous birth, i.e. when the woman's labour begins spontaneously.

The risk element, whatever your decision   65

In the next chapter...

- Your decision: Are you going to have a VBAC or another caesarean?
- Reasons in favour of having a VBAC, reasons to have another caesarean...
- What are your chances of having a successful VBAC?

Are you going to have a VBAC or another caesarean?
Consider risks for and against, as well as your own situation.

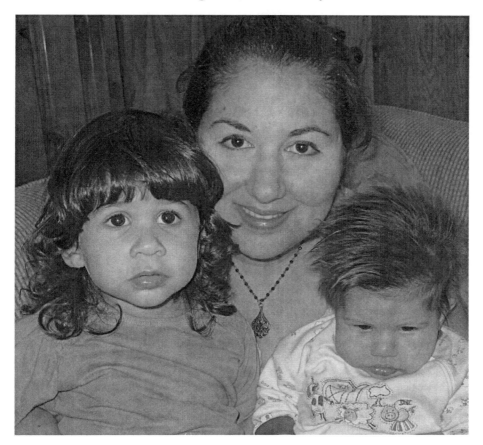

Antoinette, with her two children. You can read about her in Birthframe 6, overleaf

Having a repeat caesarean involves more risks
than having a VBAC

Birthframe 6

A scan which wrongly 'revealed' the baby was too big for a VBAC

My first pregnancy went well. I was under the care of a consultant. At 34 weeks I was told I needed a scan and this revealed that I was carrying a big baby, with a predicted term weight of 8lb 13oz (4kg). The consultant was concerned it might be a case of gestational diabetes and she practically wanted me to stop eating and restrict myself to just fruit and vegetables!

At 37 weeks and a half, my waters broke and I went into hospital in a bit of a panic. As soon as I arrived I was examined and found to be only 1cm dilated and the baby's head wasn't engaged. They decided to put me on a drip and give me antibiotics. The only nourishment they let me have was ice chips and I had to remain lying down—no movement was allowed. The next morning, I was examined again and I was still only 1cm dilated. My labour was deemed 'ineffective' and I was put on a syntocinon drip.

I then had very painful contractions all through the afternoon and the only encouragement I had was from a midwife who kept coming in and going out, spending only enough time with me to check the printouts from the fetal monitoring machine. Later in the afternoon, when I was 3cm dilated I could no longer stand the pain and I asked for an epidural. Soon, I could no longer walk because my legs were completely paralysed by the anaesthetic. After 16 hours of labour, the doctor on duty gave me his evaluation of the situation: "The baby's big and his head doesn't seem to want to come down. We're going to have to do a caesarean." I was exhausted and heard this pronouncement with a sense of relief, consoling myself with the thought that at least I wouldn't have to push out a big baby. My daughter Sabrina came into the world at 9.00pm weighing 8lb 6oz (3.8kg) and I was only able to see her for a few minutes in the operating theatre. I couldn't breastfeed her at that point because she was taken off 'for observation' since she had inhaled some amniotic fluid. Being separated from my daughter was more difficult to endure than the caesarean.

At around 3 o'clock in the morning, the midwife finally brought my baby back into my room, after almost six hours of separation. In the hospital where I gave birth I was not able to keep my baby with me after the caesarean. The midwife told me she was going to show me how to feed my baby. She took her face in one hand and my breast in the other and wanted my baby to open her mouth. My little girl cried a lot because it was obvious that the midwife was not treating her gently, just impatiently. I told the midwife that I wanted to try on my own. She told me she wasn't available all night long to show me how to do it and that the baby had to feed straight away—at that hour! That really shocked me. What's more, I was experiencing pains all over my body and they were preventing me from moving—so I just felt I wouldn't be able to manage it on my own. So I told the midwife that, just for that night, she could give the baby some supplementary feeds and that I definitely wanted her to bring the baby back to me in the morning, so I could breastfeed her. The midwife left with my baby in her arms. I had been dreaming of breastfeeding successfully for a long time but the circumstances got us off to rather a bad start. Nevertheless, I still wanted to persevere.

The next morning the midwife returned with my baby. This time I told her I wanted her to leave me alone, so I could breastfeed on my own. I then gently told my baby to open her mouth. She listened to me and was able to drink a few drops of colostrum. I felt so proud of myself! I knew I had to do it gently and calmly, following my maternal instinct. I carried on breastfeeding at the hospital day and night, using a lying down position. My milk came in about four days after the birth. When she was feeding at my breast, the first smell of milk as it came down really made an impression on me, which has always stayed with me. What a good feeling, knowing that my baby was drinking and growing thanks to milk from a mother who loved her so much!

After my caesarean I read a lot. There was Hélène's French edition of this book and a couple of other books about having positive birthing experiences. These books gave me the courage to try for a VBAC for my next birth.

I found I was pregnant a year later. I phoned a local birth centre but they had no space. At another nearby birth centre I got put on the waiting list. I then called my consultant and at my first appointment I explained to her my plan to have a VBAC. She told me I had a more than 50% chance of needing another caesarean because I'd had dystocia, which she said had been caused by cephalo-pelvic disproportion. Then she added: "Your pelvis won't let babies through and there's also the risk of uterine rupture. If you want to try for a VBAC you can always try on your own, but I think you'll end up having another caesarean." In my head I thought: "What? Am I deformed? I can't believe that. I know I can give birth normally, like the majority of women." I felt like an alien from another planet, coming to her with my request for a VBAC. I cried a lot, faced with the prospect of having another caesarean and was very sad about not having a place at a birth centre.

Then my luck changed. A place became available and I met my midwife at the birth centre. Immediately, I felt confidence rising up within me. The midwife believed in me. She encouraged me and told me that I was capable of giving birth. Suddenly, I felt more self-sufficient.

During my pregnancy, at a certain point my haemoglobin level was a bit low and wasn't coming up again, so I was in danger of having to give birth in the hospital. Luckily, my readings improved and this cloud passed. When I contemplated my upcoming labour and birth I told myself that since I was still breastfeeding Sabrina (my daughter), that would stimulate contractions and would mean I could avoid being induced with syntocinon. I had a scan at 20 weeks and then refused to have any more because I didn't want to hear any predictions of my baby's weight.

Time passed and my due date arrived. At 40 weeks, the mucous plug came out. My midwife came to visit and on examination she found I was already 1cm dilated. The baby's head wasn't engaged. I felt a bit anxious because it seemed like the same scenario as before and I was afraid I'd end up having another caesarean. But she kept my hopes up and dismissed all my negative thinking. The night passed with me having contractions and not really sleeping at all. In the early hours of the morning I was still only 1cm. So as to avoid having the whole scenario play out again, exactly as before, I tried breathing deeply and concentrating on my plan to have a VBAC. This time, I wasn't restricted to the bed. I decided to take a bath and to carry on through the day as normal, with Sabrina and my mother.

My contractions completely stopped me getting any sleep

The day passed and my labour continued. In the evening, I decided to stay at home for the second night. This time, my contractions completely stopped me getting any sleep. The next day I went into the birth centre. Then I took another bath, which I found calming. My husband was still at my side and I couldn't have survived without him there. I was given 5-star treatment, the midwife ensuring a quiet atmosphere, with dimmed lighting, candlelight, massage... All of this helped me to relax while continuing on with my labour. The midwife focused on me, and not only on the baby, unlike in my first labour. She also prepared delicious food for me, which helped me to keep up my energy and strength. What's more, I was able to rest with my husband in an intimate atmosphere without anyone disturbing us. This 'sacred magic' was also very useful, as was the room's décor, which encouraged relaxation and visualisation.

> I was able to rest with my husband in an intimate atmosphere without anyone disturbing us. This 'sacred magic' was also very useful, as was the room's décor, which encouraged relaxation and visualisation.

A third wakeful night loomed ahead. I was getting more and more exhausted. The next morning, I had the feeling I was losing all my strength. I really needed to rest and get some sleep—otherwise I just didn't see how I'd be able to push the baby out. I asked to be transferred to the hospital to have an epidural so as to get a few hours' sleep before the second stage. At that point I was 8cm dilated and the only way in which my labour had been stimulated was through breastfeeding Sabrina—and this had occurred after I'd lost the mucous plug. Breastfeeding allowed me to relax, to let go and forget about the pain of contractions a bit. My daughter Sabrina didn't hesitate to give me a few kisses and cuddles when she saw I was suffering—and that gave me a lot of comfort. My husband drove me to the hospital at around 5 o'clock in the morning. When we got there the consultant was astonished by the obvious effect breastfeeding was having on my contractions.

The consultant was astonished by the obvious effect breastfeeding was having on my contractions

After a few hours of sleep, evening came and I was 10cm dilated. My waters broke while I was being examined by the consultant. I asked the doctor why the consultant had broken my waters. (I didn't want to have a single intervention that might lead to a caesarean, especially knowing as I did that the baby's head was not yet engaged.) The consultant then told him: "Don't worry. The waters broke on their own while I was examining her. I felt the baby's head engage in the pelvis, its nose pointing down!" I was so happy I just couldn't believe it! I had achieved my objective—getting to 10cm with my baby well-engaged in my pelvis. (Me, who was supposed to have a small pelvis...) I was now ready to push and bring this baby into the world!

I followed instructions: "Breathe, stop, push..." I pushed with all the energy I could muster from deep inside me. I was supported by my husband, who kept making comments to encourage me and counting each time I pushed. My two guardian angels (my midwife and the student midwife) gave me drinks between contractions, massaged my legs and encouraged every effort I made. I told them it was very useful having them around! Towards the end of the second stage, I heard the consultant telling me I had to push harder, or she'd have to use the ventouse or forceps... I pushed harder, not letting up. Then I pushed some more, for hours and hours and I was still pushing. After five hours of pushing, my efforts were finally rewarded. You see? I managed all on my own. I gave birth to my baby and they put her on my chest. That was the most beautiful moment in my life. My daughter looked at me. It was magnificent. I heard people sobbing around me, saying, "Wow! You did it!" We were all crying tears of joy.

When she was born my 'little' Sandra weighed 10lb 9oz (4.8kg) and her fontanelles weren't even overlapping. In the end, I thought to myself, "My pelvis turned out to be much better than I thought!" I continued breastfeeding (tandem-feeding) and had no experience of the 'baby blues', which I'd had after my caesarean. After a caesarean women try to console themselves by saying that at least the baby's healthy. That's

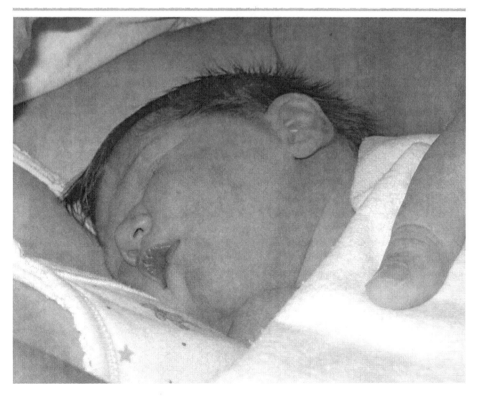

Sandra, 10lb 9oz at birth, Antoinette's VBAC baby (who you've just read about)

Birthframe 7
Being encouraged to have a VBAC, with various conditions

To my surprise, my consultant was suggesting I have a VBAC. As a nurse married to a doctor, I'd worked in obstetrics and had already seen women giving birth vaginally after previously having a caesarean.... but me? I'd had a caesarean two and a half years before, at the age of 30, because of a poorly placed placenta (placenta praevia) so my first child had been born with a regional anaesthetic. Until that point I hadn't prepared particularly well in my second pregnancy—I trusted my doctor more than the experience of seeing a few VBACs, as a nurse. But here was my consultant, suggesting I have a VBAC... After a while, I felt it was indeed important for me to prepare for a vaginal birth. Having a caesarean is often so painful and sad... I felt I had to put everything I had into preparing for a VBAC so that the birth could take place as positively as possible.

My consultant said I could have the VBAC as long as the baby didn't look like it was going to be too big, as long as my labour didn't progress too quickly... and as long as my pregnancy was normal. Everyone around me was worried, including the paediatrician. They all said I was thinking too much about myself and taking too big a risk. But I persevered and finally gave birth vaginally when I had my second baby.

My labour progressed very quickly

My labour progressed very quickly. Following my consultant's advice, I went into the hospital as soon as I went into labour and it turned out I was only 1cm dilated at that point. Fortunately, my own consultant was on duty—he was the only one to allow VBACs in the whole hospital! He broke my waters, and two hours later, with two pushes, I gave birth to my baby, who weighed 5lb 12oz (2.60kg). It was my husband, who's a doctor (as I said), who caught the baby since my consultant was actually in the operating theatre next door at that point! The staff were a bit stressed out because I was the 'VBAC case' and there seemed to be some decelerations in the baby's heart rate too. (I think that was because I was lying down.) There were a lot of people in the room—they were constantly coming and going—and none of them introduced themselves. That did nothing to help my concentration when I was in labour and giving birth!

I was very proud of myself, very happy, and at the same time a bit shocked by the speed with which everything had taken place. I hadn't had time to adjust to each stage of labour. I would have liked to have given birth like they do in the books—some hopes!—to see my baby's little head appearing, then going back in, and so on. I also had problems with the atmosphere of the birth. My partner also felt overwhelmed and he was just stuck in a corner of the room while I don't know how many people got all het up looking at the electronic fetal monitor. At one point I signalled for him to come over to me—to come and breathe with me.

Would I do it again? Definitely. I'd do exactly the same thing all over again.

I'd do exactly the same thing all over again

CHAPTER 3:

Persuasive reasons to have a VBAC

This chapter should help you make a decision about your next baby's birth. Before you even start thinking about this decision, you need to understand that the picture currently portrayed in our society favours a repeat caesarean, rather than a VBAC. This was explained and emphasised by the authors of a systematic review of scientific research, published in 2007 in *The Journal of Perinatal Education*.[1] My own personal aim in writing this book is to redress the imbalance and present a much more balanced view, which—if anything—favours VBAC, rather than a repeat caesarean.

The need for a decision, whatever people around you think

One thing you can certainly do is decide whether or not to have a VBAC. Whether your partner is for or against the idea, it is mainly the woman who'll be affected by the decision—so you are the one who needs to take control. Having your partner's support is very important, but it isn't necessarily essential for you to be successful. If you don't have his support you will obviously need to be very determined and you will need to go and find support elsewhere. Some men start worrying the moment their partners decide to have a VBAC, but as they become better informed their attitude usually changes. Sometimes the opposite happens, though, and it's the man who insists that his partner should have a VBAC. Whatever your partner's reaction, though, at whatever point, it really is your decision and your experience in the end.

Sometimes, other people around you—particularly caregivers—will try to impose their own opinions, irrespective of your legal rights. This is why in some countries which are considered free countries, although in theory it is the woman who decides whether or not to have a VBAC, in reality she is often denied this choice.[2] This is certainly often the case in the USA—and sometimes it happens in the UK too. During labour and particularly when a woman is almost completely dilated, a woman sometimes expresses the desire to have a caesarean, even when she previously chose to have a VBAC. A progressive consultant might remind her of her earlier decision and some consultants even refuse to perform a caesarean without a valid medical reason. And there are even places which are supportive of VBAC, where a woman is left to continue labouring—before having a repeat caesarean—if she has gone into labour spontaneously before the date she was booked in for the caesarean. But again, whatever people around you think, if you really want a VBAC you have a right to have one, and if you really want a repeat caesarean, you should be able to find appropriate support.

Pros and cons for the baby of either a VBAC or a caesarean

In this era—when people are constantly talking about caesareans on demand as if they were a woman's prerogative, and when people are constantly worrying about the 'dangers' of birth—they often forget that childbirth not only functions to get the baby born, it also prepares him or her for life outside the womb. This is what we were talking about at the end of the last chapter. Now we will discuss other ways in which a vaginal birth is beneficial for the baby, from the moment he or she is born.

When people are constantly worrying about the 'dangers' of birth they often forget that childbirth not only functions to get the baby born, it also prepares him or her for life outside the womb

Just as the humanisation of birth movement has long emphasised immediate postnatal mother-baby contact,[3] research into neurobiology and psychology has also increasingly revealed the importance of the first contact between a mother and her baby. Research has shown this contact to be important in terms of the baby's development, as well as in terms of optimising the bonding process. In fact, skin-to-skin contact stabilises the baby's temperature and regulates the baby's pulse, as well as his or her respiratory rhythm and temperature.

Babies who have immediate skin-to-skin contact after birth cry less and sleep better[4]—which parents tend to appreciate a great deal! Normally, there should be no separation between mother and baby straight after the birth. Early mother-baby contact also helps breastfeeding get off to a good start. What's more, it helps the baby's metabolic adaptation, it helps the baby preserve his or her energy, it stops him or her from getting cold and it minimises crying. Early mother-baby contact also improves neuro-behavioural development[5] and facilitates bonding because it causes a rise in oxytocin levels in the mother—oxytocin being a hormone which is strongly associated with loving behaviour.[6] Early contact also helps protect the baby from getting infected by hospital bacteria... Being close to the mother's skin, where the bacteria are familiar, the baby is more able to protect itself from the resistant and damaging bacteria of a hospital.[7] What's more, research shows that the intestinal flora of the baby is altered when he or she is born by caesarean and this significantly decreases the number and diversity of good bifidobacteria. This may have something to do with the later more frequent development of asthma and allergies through inflammatory mechanisms in children born by caesarean.[8]

The increased likely of immediate postnatal contact with your baby after a VBAC involves all kinds of benefits for the baby

Another reason supporting a vaginal birth, with the increased early mother-baby contact it usually involves, is that women usually enjoy it! Women who've had early contact with their babies after giving birth tend to talk about powerful emotions... They report having felt an immediate bond with their new baby, having touched and caressed him or her, having looked into their baby's eyes, and not having wanted to let the baby go. They love recalling this moment, which had a profound influence on their experience of giving birth overall.[9] No doubt it is for this and all the other reasons that I've mentioned already that more and more public health organisations—notably WHO—recommend early mother-baby contact.[10]

Interventions carried out soon after the baby's birth, such as weighing the baby, measuring his or her length and head circumference and administering antibiotics in the eyes, can all be delayed for at least an hour or two so as to make conditions for mother-baby contact as good and as undisturbed as possible. One article published in 2007[11] does in fact question any early interventions involving the baby from the time of his or her birth onwards. The author of this research project concludes that practices such as routine aspiration of the respiratory tubes and of the baby's stomach can cause complications, quite apart from being painful for the baby and being the possible cause of an increase in arterial pressure. (Routine aspiration is also not recommended by WHO.) Other routine procedures that the author of the article talked about (e.g. taking measurements, weighing and bathing the baby) also reduce the baby's reflexes and affect the baby's neurological behaviour, his or her olfactory reference points (i.e. they affect how well the baby can become oriented by smells) and they affect the baby's temperature.[12] Circumcision also disturbs early bonding processes for very obvious reasons and means that newborns drink less often and seem more demoralised.[13]

> I realised it's not always necessary to trust doctors and midwifery staff... That it's not necessary for us to literally put ourselves in their hands. That it's important to become well-informed. That we need to think calmly about decisions they make and not feel bad about making other decisions which seem best for us.
>
> *Caroline, a woman who had a VBAC after two previous caesareans*

Taking everything into account, if you choose to have another caesarean, or if you have to have one, make sure you arrange to have skin-to-skin contact with your baby straight after the birth—i.e. in the minutes following it, and in the recovery room. Even after a caesarean it is possible to arrange to spend several minutes with your baby, held up against you, even if this isn't yet a routine practice in the hospital where you are delivered. If it does prove to be impossible for you to have this kind of contact with your baby, nothing will stop someone like your partner from spending these few precious moments with your baby, pressed skin-to-skin. This will be as beneficial for your partner as it will be for your baby, if he is able to do this.[14] And if your partner is not present at the birth, perhaps a doula or other birth attendant could perform this task.

How women make a decision

As we saw in the last chapter, there certainly are objective risks involved in having a VBAC, which we know about, thanks to obstetric research. On a more subjective level, the pros and cons of the two choices (VBAC or a repeat caesarean) often depend on our circumstances or past experiences, so we need to take these into account when making a decision. Some women, for example, believe that having a VBAC will allow them to recuperate more quickly and easily postnatally. Others appreciate being able to plan support at home or childcare around the date planned for their caesarean. For some, being able to have early contact with their baby is more important than anything else and they realise that this is easier if they have a vaginal birth. Others want their partners to be with them when they give birth and they feel that having a fixed date (as is the case with a caesarean) makes this easier. Depending on where they live, some women also need to take into account that a caesarean with an epidural isn't available round the clock, so they may prefer to plan another caesarean, not wanting to risk having an emergency caesarean during a VBAC. Also, it's often the case that hospitals want to keep caesarean-born babies in a nursery, so they can keep them under observation—a practice which isn't necessarily justified—and this may make some women opt for a vaginal birth instead.

> *Women think a great deal about the effect a decision one way or the other could have on postnatal recovery*

The feelings a woman has about having a caesarean or a vaginal birth are also affected by other choices she might make. Unfortunately, studies on motivations behind choices to have a repeat caesarean or a VBAC have rarely been carried out, until very recently.[15] According to McLain,[16] women think a great deal about the effect that a decision one way or the other could have on postnatal recovery and they wonder when they will be able to return to work or they wonder when they will be able to resume a normal social life. In addition, even if the medical risks influence some women's decisions, other women are often not influenced by objective factors when they make their decision. These women also consider other advantages or disadvantages of possible solutions and are often influenced by their partner in the decision-making process. One interesting aspect of the decision-making process is that a fast return to 'normal life' after the birth is given as being as reason to justify both a VBAC and a caesarean. However, a common reason given for choosing a VBAC is easier postnatal recovery and the wish to be able to take care of other children more quickly. Women who've previously given birth by caesarean don't necessarily immediately know how they would like to give birth the next time. They get information from medical staff and some women prefer not having to make the decision themselves. Some women change their mind often during their pregnancy. What's more, women's levels of confidence in decisions made vary too.[17]

Psychosocial factors can also influence women's concerns about their health, when they've previously had a caesarean.[18] For example, a woman may choose to have a repeat caesarean because her first labour was long and painful and because she felt 'saved' by the caesarean. Another woman, having experienced similar difficulties, may make entirely the opposite decision and opt for a VBAC because she wants to give herself the chance to experience an 'ordinary' birth to put things 'right', in a certain manner of speaking.

According to the authors of the book *Pregnancy as Healing* (Mindbody Press, 1984)—doctor Lewis Mehl and therapist Gayle Peterson—your decision should be based not only on facts, but also on your feelings, after having weighed up all the evidence. According to Mehl and Peterson, making a decision is an irrational process. Recently, decision aids that have been developed to help women choose include as an important element the consideration of personal values. Studies have shown they can reduce anxiety and be helpful. You may want to use one yourself...[19] However, as I've already noted, in reality, we often decide with our heart as much as with our head and we choose the solution with which we feel safest. Elizabeth Shearer, an American antenatal teacher, suggests that if we were to make VBAC illegal in hospitals where there is no consultant or anaesthetist on duty 24 hours a day, and if women affected were directed to large maternity hospitals where these staff were available, we would also have to do the same for any women who smoke, for example. In fact, research has clearly established a link between smoking during pregnancy and additional risks for the baby. So if you want to think about risks, you need to take other risks into account too!

When conducting interviews for her research on women's reactions to birthing experiences (whether vaginal or abdominal), the sociologist Maria De Koninck confirmed that many women are afraid of vaginal birth and can even be comforted by the fact that they've had a caesarean, even when they didn't necessarily find the experience easy. Deciding to have a VBAC does not mean that you will not occasionally have periods of doubt, or that you will not come back to the question, or that you will not face anxiety about the decision you've made or that you won't worry about how you will experience the VBAC.[20] You may be worried by doubts and fears which people around you talk about.

When someone has had a difficult experience the first time, when a woman has never finished labour or even begun it, it is normal for that woman to feel as if she's facing the unknown and to experience doubts and fears. Women typically wonder if they will succeed with a VBAC. They wonder if all the energy they've invested in preparing for a VBAC will be worth the effort and they wonder if it wouldn't be simpler to just make a date for another caesarean. What's more, women are often afraid of giving birth because it hurts... A caesarean does too, but afterwards, and labours can be long. In one sense, women relive the fears that every pregnant woman experiences about her future birthing experience, but of course we have to remember that in the case of a woman who's already had an emergency caesarean, her fears proved to be well-founded during her previous labour.[21]

In order to get a clearer idea of what you personally want to do for your next birth, it's a good idea to talk through your thoughts and feelings, raise your concerns at antenatal appointments, discuss things with other women who've given birth vaginally, or who've had a VBAC, or talk through your thoughts and feelings with a consultant or midwife, or even get in touch with an organisation which can offer you support. (See the Useful contacts at the back of this book.) Getting information and expressing your fears, without being judged because of them, will help you to see things in perspective. Thinking about what your feelings might be when giving birth yourself to your own baby might also be a good way of motivating you in one direction or another.

Some women are worried about the fact that so many others choose to have a repeat caesarean and they are concerned that the caesarean operation has been trivialised in our society. On this topic, one antenatal teacher I spoke to said: "I feel devastated whenever I see someone who wants to have another caesarean at all costs. It's like someone who drinks deciding to drive nevertheless." An American doctor went so far to say, "Consenting to that kind of surgery on demand—a repeat caesarean—makes no sense at all. This kind of decision wouldn't be made for any other kind of surgery."[22] But it is almost unthinkable in our society to force a woman to give birth vaginally after a caesarean. Besides, some doctors agree to do a first caesarean simply because it suits the client or because the woman is fearful about giving birth and is afraid of pain. One study on responses from doctors to requests for caesareans found that consultants generally don't hesitate to agree when there are clear medical reasons to carry out the operation. When there are no clear-cut medical reasons for carrying out a caesarean, consultants' responses vary considerably. It is when there is no absolute medical reason for a caesarean that women can take a greater part in the decision-making process. Unless yours is an extreme case, it is best to assume that being pregnant in itself does not affect your decision-making abilities![23]

Why did you have a caesarean before anyway?

Any woman who's had a caesarean wants to know why it was carried out. Even women who don't emerge from the experience psychologically damaged, who accept what's happened, like to know what happened and why or—if the caesarean was planned in advance—they want to know the precise reasons why this was the case. It isn't always easy to find answers to these questions. Medicine doesn't have answers to everything and information on caesareans isn't necessarily easy to obtain, medical records aren't always very clear, and consultants are usually extremely busy. In antenatal classes teachers often forget to encourage participants to explore the reasons for previous caesareans. And when women who've had a caesarean before do try to find out what happened and why, the information they get may be rather overly brief or they may find that other class participants turn a deaf ear to their reporting back in class because other participants may find it difficult to imagine that it could happen to them too. Many people are very superstitious and believe that simply talking about something makes it more likely to happen. Unfortunately, though, women or couples who are ill-informed or who haven't paid attention to the information they've been given are completely taken aback when that precise thing occurs. What's more, these people have difficulty participating in any decision-making relating to that process and they are unable to indicate when they would find a caesarean acceptable. According to a survey carried out in 2005, 88% of women thought it was very important to be informed about what is happening and about choices available to them. They also wanted to participate in any decisions being made.[24] Since nowadays approximately 1 in 4 women are having a caesarean when they give birth, it's very important that information is available and well understood. If you don't have this information retrospectively, do try to find it out.

Was your caesarean necessary or not?

After getting hold of the appropriate information some women and some couples feel that the caesarean which took place perhaps wasn't necessary. This may be very difficult to deal with. Even though many consultants are worried about the current high rate of caesareans, few of them are prepared to say that a certain proportion of caesareans aren't justified. But if we examine current caesarean rates in the light of WHO recommendations (which say that the caesarean rate should not be more than 10%–15% in both centres for low risk and high risk women), we unfortunately have to concede that a large number of caesareans carried out in the UK (and elsewhere) are not necessary, since the UK rate is around 24%. In Latin America the number of unnecessary caesareans carried out annually has been estimated at almost 1 million.[25] Elsewhere in the world, more than 90% of caesareans are performed for one or other of the following justifications, listed in decreasing order of importance (the most common one first):

- Previous caesarean. This may be the reason cited for most caesareans in some places.
- Failure to progress (i.e. labour slowed down or stopped). This may have happened because the baby was poorly positioned or was not descending well. It sometimes happens as a result of disturbance, the use of analgesia or anaesthesia, or because the woman is not moving around freely.
- Breech presentation. This is a reason which is increasingly given, since fewer caregivers now than ever before have the necessary experience to attend vaginal breech births
- Fetal distress, which is monitored with an electronic fetal monitor. Unfortunately, electronic fetal monitoring is associated with many misreadings and it can also often be the *cause* of fetal distress. This is because it usually means women lie on their backs, which depresses the vena cava, thereby depriving the baby of oxygen.

None of these motives for performing a caesarean constitute a reason which is valid in 'absolute' terms. As we will see later, the policy to always arrange a caesarean in cases of breech presentation is one which is being questioned, and the other reasons can also all be avoided or challenged in one way or another.

Clear medical indications for a caesarean ('absolute indications')

Of course, there are times when a caesarean is absolutely necessary. In these cases, there should be no hesitation about the need to go ahead with the caesarean immediately. They are as follows:

- Serious deformity in the pelvis caused by polio, rickets or an accident
- Prolapse of the umbilical cord—i.e. when the umbilical cord comes down into the vagina before the baby's head; pressure of the baby's head can compress the cord and thereby deprive the baby of oxygen; this condition may occur in 1% of cases after a woman's waters break
- Bad cases of placenta praevia (malpositioning of the placenta) or placental abruption (where the placenta becomes detached)—both of which put either the baby's or the mother's life in danger (or both), because serious haemorrhage may result
- Transverse presentation of the baby (by the shoulder, with the baby lying horizontally across the womb); this may occur after a failed attempt at external cephalic version (after the baby has been detected lying breech)
- Acute fetal distress, which doesn't disappear after a change of position or stimulation of the baby's head, etc. (More on this soon.)
- Poor maternal health, such as a serious heart condition

Possible but controversial indications ('relative indications')

There are situations when a caesarean may be advisable in certain cases, depending on the precise details of the situation. Many of these 'reasons' are controversial but they cause 90% of caesareans and are the reasons listed before (previous caesarean, failure to progress, breech presentation and fetal distress). Other less frequently occurring reasons include caesareans following an unsuccessful induction by amniotomy (breaking a woman's waters), an overdue pregnancy (i.e. one which—according to the WHO definition—is over 42 weeks), pre-eclampsia, genital herpes, diabetes, a twin pregnancy... but, again, none of these can be considered clear, incontavertible reasons. (Note that all three signs of pre-eclampsia—i.e. hypertension, oedema and protein in the urine—need to be present for pre-eclampsia to be confirmed.)

It is important to consider how clear indications for a caesarean are because of our general assumption nowadays that caesareans are already carried out for a clear medical reason, i.e. to save either the mother or her baby. Although this used to be the case, it isn't always the case now. In fact, in industrialised countries a woman rarely dies in childbirth, although it must be said that the risk of this happening is higher if she has a caesarean. Also, it is not as common as people think for a baby to really be in distress. (According to the American National Institutes of Health (NIH), this is a condition resulting from a lack of oxygen to the baby in the womb (or in the vaginal passage, if that's where the baby is) and an excess of carbon monoxide. According to the NIH, fetal distress occurs when the pH level of the blood is acidic, when there is meconium (the first of the baby's poos, which is usually only released after the birth) in the amniotic fluid, and when there are irregularities in the rhythm of the baby's heart. When only one of these signs is present there is not sufficient evidence to conclude that the baby is in distress, except—obviously—when there is a serious and prolonged decrease in the baby's heartbeat.

The doctor who invented the fetal monitor said the caesarean rate as a result of fetal distress should never exceed 1% or 2%

In 1987 the doctor who invented the electronic fetal monitor said that the caesarean rate as a result of fetal distress should never exceed 1% or 2%. Above this rate, he said, caesareans are being carried out unnecessarily—so we must conclude that a certain proportion of diagnoses of fetal distress are incorrect and the result of machine-induced errors. In any case, it is not necessary to hook up low-risk women in active labour to a fetal monitor. According to NICE, intermittent auscultation (i.e. checking of the fetal heart) is preferable.[26] Auscultation can be carried out with a Sonicaid (a portable ultrasound device) and it allows women in labour not to have to lie down to be checked. There is even a Sonicaid which can be used underwater. If a Pinard is used—a portable device which uses no ultrasound—the woman needs to lie down or lean forward in order to be checked. Some caregivers also monitor by noting the sounds women are making as they labour, and by noting their general behaviour, and they find these to be reliable methods.

Breech presentation, which has usually meant a caesarean in recent years, is also not a clear reason to resort to this form if surgery, as we saw before. Thanks to some research published in 2000[27] there has been a policy in North America for caesareans to be automatically decided upon in the case of breech births. However, this study has since been heavily criticised[28] and later research (for example, a study carried out in 2006) has concluded that we should go back to allowing women with a breech baby to have a vaginal birth.[29] However, since a vaginal breech birth requires the presence of a consultant or midwife who is experienced in breech births, there is sometimes no caregiver available, since few doctors have been trained (since 2000) to assist with a vaginal breech birth and there are fewer and fewer caregivers left who still have these skills. Of course, this complicates things for a woman who does not want a caesarean for her breech baby.

A recent study concluded that we should go back to allowing women with a breech baby to have a vaginal birth

The baby's position at the end of the seventh month

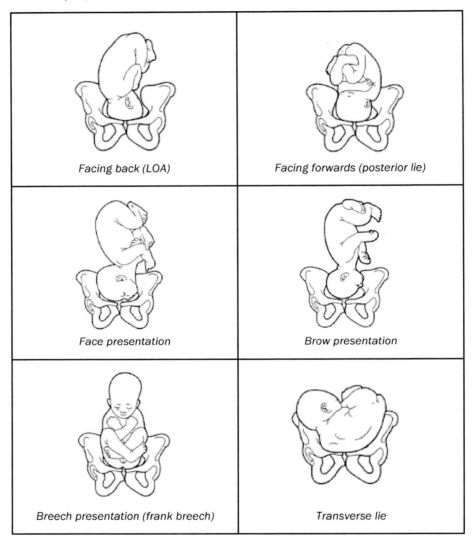

The way in which the baby is presenting is often settled by the end of the seventh month of pregnancy. The first position shown (head down, facing backwards) is the most common position and is the most favourable. LOA—left occiput anterior—simply means the baby is facing towards the mother's left side, his or head is down and his back is round the mother's front. (ROA means the baby is lying to the right side.) The other positions involve various difficulties and increase the probability of having to have a caesarean, with the exception of breech presentation, since around 2005.

Cephalo-pelvic disproportion is another reason frequently given for caesareans, but there are actually far fewer true cases of this (which means the baby's head is too small to pass through the mother's pelvis) than some people would have you believe. Most often, it is a case of poor presentation of the baby's head, which may be a very slight case of malpresentation. (This may be corrected when the mother moves around.) Also, people often forget that when the labouring woman is in an upright position, a small bone—her tailbone—moves back, actually increasing the diameter of the opening for the baby by 1cm—which may be the difference between a 9cm diameter and a 10cm one. (Of course, this is particularly relevant given that so many women who are on electronic fetal monitors are forced to lie down, or encouraged to do so by their caregivers—since the bone cannot move back when the woman is lying down.)

A considerable number of caesareans are decided upon when labour is prolonged, or when it stops altogether. There was a great deal of imprecision in the 1980s when diagnosing 'failure to progress' (which is also sometimes called 'dystocia') and this imprecision persists even to this day. The reasons for this imprecision are poorly understood, though. It is possible to try and prevent or remedy certain situations... Things which usually help include moving around during labour, walking regularly, getting down on all fours, squatting, drinking or eating. (See Chapter 6 for more details on what facilitates labour and birth).

Perhaps the problem arises because the rhythm of labour is not the same for all women. The first stage of labour, the 'latent' phase, may be very noticeable to some women, but not to others. It may last several hours or even several days, and women who are aware of this stage of labour may even wrongly believe they are near to giving birth, when really their body is only preparing itself for the second stage of labour. (In the first stage of labour, the cervix softens and elongates, drawing itself up so that it can also dilate, i.e. stretch.) In the second stage of labour, which is called 'active labour', contractions intensify and the woman's cervix dilates from 3-4cm to 10cm. Perhaps women's experience varies because different women experience different types of pain. Some women have painful contractions during the latent phase of labour, while others don't, and the length of this phase varies from woman to woman. Unfortunately, a latent phase can last a long time—sometimes several days—while other women go into active labour quickly.

Many caregivers feel that no limits should be imposed on the length of labour as long as both mother and baby are well. One exploratory study, which re-examined the tool which is very widely used in maternity units (the Friedman curve), concluded that first-time mothers may have a first stage of labour (dilation) lasting 26 hours, and a second stage (from the time of complete dilation until the birth of the baby) lasting up to 8 hours, without any negative effects for either mother or baby. This study also found that in cases where women were not experiencing their first labour, the length of the first stage could be 23 hours and the length of the second stage could be 4.5 hours.[30] These timings are much longer than those allowed for in the Friedman curve.

Myths about problems people believe a caesarean can prevent

There are several myths about caesareans which keep on circulating. One of these myths relates to incontinence, either urinary or fecal, i.e. the involuntary evacuation of urine or faeces (wee or poo). While some researchers conclude that caesareans prevent this problem, there is also evidence to show that incontinence is associated with pregnancy, having several children, and forceps births—opinions and results of research vary. The same applies to prolapse of pelvic organs (e.g. uterine prolapse). Yet another myth relates to a woman's sex life after having either a caesarean or a vaginal birth... In 20 years of looking at scientific studies on childbirth, I have found no serious evidence to suggest that a vaginal birth has a negative effect on a woman's sex life.

What are your chances of having a VBAC?

If a woman who had an elective caesarean because her baby was breech has more chance of having a successful VBAC at the end of her next pregnancy, this is perhaps because this woman's confidence wasn't eroded by the thought that her labour would go wrong. However, other women have every right to feel confident that they can have a straightforward vaginal birth.

You have every right to feel confident that you can have a straightforward vaginal birth

In 2005, while I was running a VBAC workshop I met a Jewish woman who was a member of an orthodox branch of this religion called Hasidic Judaism—a branch which promotes spirituality and joy through mysticism. She told me about her own experience... Several years before, she said she had succeeded in having a VBAC after having *six* caesareans. Her VBAC took place in a big hospital in Montreal, in Canada. She told me about her joy in having succeeded in putting an end to her caesareans. She particularly appreciated her VBAC because afterwards she later gave birth to several other babies vaginally.

To me, this story is a reminder that VBACs can happen in the most unlikely circumstances. It also reminds me of the joy women usually feel when they do have a VBAC after everything they've experienced before. Many women hesitate when they consider the idea of having a VBAC because they're afraid they won't succeed. One of the questions women often ask is precisely the question which is the title of this section: "What really are my own personal chances?" The first thing I'm going to say is that the number of women who try to have a VBAC, who succeed, is very encouraging: three quarters of women who've previously had a caesarean have a successful VBAC.[31] Also note that success rates as high as 87% have been reported and in women with an optimal profile for VBAC (e.g. low risk women attended by midwives) the rate is as high as 95%.[32]

The rate of vaginal births amongst women who plan a VBAC depends a great deal on the philosophy of the caregiver and on hospital policies relating to VBAC

Actually, according to the Coalition for Improving Maternity Services (CIMS),[33] the rate of vaginal births amongst women who plan a VBAC depends a great deal on the philosophy of the caregiver and on hospital policies relating to VBAC (in the case of a hospital VBAC). The policies and protocols recommended by CIMS' Mother-Friendly Childbirth Initiative and by the International MotherBaby Childbirth Initiative help to promote safer VBACs and higher rates of VBAC so it's a good idea, if you decide to have a VBAC, to check if the hospital of your choice accepts these policies and protocols. For more information, see www.motherfriendly.org and www.imbci.org.

If you decide to have a VBAC it's a good idea to check if the hospital of your choice accepts the policies and protocols of the Mother-Friendly and MotherBaby Childbirth Initiatives

Since I first started writing about VBAC, numerous women have written to me asking if a VBAC is possible in one situation or another. More often than not, in the first few years no particular study had focused on the situations these women were asking me about. Nevertheless, over the last 20 years or so our knowledge of VBAC has increased substantially. Studies have been published and these conclude either the probability of having a straightforward VBAC in this or that situation, or the risks that would be associated with attempting a VBAC. For example, one important study, which looked at 13,532 women, confirmed that the risk of uterine rupture decreases after a woman's successful first vaginal birth (after a previous caesarean) as well as the risk of dehiscence and other complications—whether the woman had one or more caesareans previously.[34]

Over the last 20 years or so our knowledge of VBAC has increased substantially

On the following few pages you will see everything that research has revealed so far about the risks in various circumstances linked to pregnancy or VBAC after one or more caesareans. This data includes recommendations from NICE and RCOG and the 2010 NIH Consensus Development Conference on VBAC. On the following pages you won't necessarily find answers to all your questions (because still not enough research has been done on certain aspects of VBAC)—but many situations are certainly covered. As I said, what we know now is a great deal more than only a few decades ago.

Situations linked with your previous caesarean

Notes for this and the other lists which follow:
- Classifications of risk range from 'none known' to 'increased risk'.
- When considering the factors affecting the completion of a VBAC, consider the information in the light of the fact that—according to NIH 2010—74% of VBACs are successfully completed, so 'increased likelihood' means there's even more chance of success than 74%.
- Guidelines or recommendations are from RCOG (UK, 2007),[35] NICE (UK, 2004),[36] SOGC (Canada, 2005),[37] ACOG (USA, 2010)[38] and NIH (USA, 2010).[39]

1. **PRIOR SURGERY TO THE UTERUS**

   Risk of the uterine incision separating: No known impact on the risk

   Factors affecting VBAC success: No information available

   Guidelines / recommendations:
   - RCOG: There is insufficient and conflicting information on whether the risk of uterine rupture is increased in women with previous myomectomy or prior complex uterine surgery.
   - ACOG: Vaginal birth after a previous cesarean delivery is contraindicated in women with extensive transfundal uterine surgery

2. **REASON FOR PAST CAESAREAN: BREECH PRESENTATION**

   Risk of the uterine incision separating: No known impact on the risk

   Factors affecting VBAC success: Increases the likelihood of having a VBAC[40]

   Guidelines / recommendations:
   - None specific to this situation

3. **REASON FOR PAST CAESAREAN: FETAL DISTRESS**

   Risk of the uterine incision separating: No known impact on the risk

   Factors affecting VBAC success: Increases the likelihood of having a VBAC[41]

   Guidelines / recommendations:
   - None specific to this situation

4. **REASON FOR PAST CAESAREAN: FAILURE TO PROGRESS**

   Risk of the uterine incision separating: No known impact on the risk

   Factors affecting VBAC success: Decreases the likelihood or no negative effect; this is not a reason to avoid a VBAC; dysfunction will not necessarily repeat itself in a future labour[42]

   Guidelines / recommendations:
   - RCOG: Previous dystocia decreases the chances of completing a VBAC
   - NICE: Previous dystocia decreases the chances of completing a VBAC

Persuasive reasons to have a VBAC

5. **REASON FOR PAST CAESAREAN: CEPHALO-PELVIC DISPROPORTION**

   Risk of the uterine incision separating: No known impact on the risk

   Factors affecting VBAC success: Decreases the likelihood or no negative effect; this is not a reason to avoid a VBAC; dysfunction will not necessarily repeat itself in a future labour[43]

   Guidelines / recommendations:
   - RCOG: Previous dystocia decreases the chances of completing a VBAC
   - NICE: Previous dystocia decreases the chances of completing a VBAC

6. **INCOMPLETE CERVICAL DILATION PREVIOUSLY ACHIEVED**

   Risk of the uterine incision separating: No known impact on the risk

   Factors affecting VBAC success: Conflicting evidence[44]

   Guidelines / recommendations:
   - RCOG: Limited and conflicting evidence on whether the cervical dilatation achieved at the primary caesarean for dystocia impacts on the subsequent VBAC success rate.

7. **PREVIOUS VAGINAL BIRTH (BEFORE CAESAREAN, OR A PAST VBAC)**

   Risk of the uterine incision separating: This reduces the risk; every VBAC further decreases the risks or the risk remains the same, according to other studies[45]

   Factors affecting VBAC success: This increases the likelihood of having a VBAC; every vaginal birth increases the chances of having another successful VBAC[46]

   Guidelines / recommendations:
   - RCOG: The single best predictor for successful VBAC, and is associated with an approximately 87-90% planned VBAC rate.

8. **LOW VERTICAL UTERINE INCISION OR UNKNOWN TYPE OF INCISION**

   Risk of the uterine incision separating: No increased risk[47]

   Factors affecting VBAC success: No negative effect[48]

   Guidelines / recommendations:
   - RCOG: Low vertical is associated with an increased risk of uterine rupture.
   - ACOG: VBAC is not contraindicated unless there is a high clinical suspicion of a previous classical uterine incision (in a case where the type of incision is unknown).
   - SOGC: Most unknown scars will be lower transverse incisions (92%) and therefore at low risk for uterine rupture.
   - NIH: No increased risk .

/continued overleaf...

9. **MORE THAN ONE PREVIOUS CAESAREAN**

Risk of the uterine incision separating: Conflicting evidence[49] but one very recent study concluded there was no increased risk after three or more caesareans[50]

Factors affecting VBAC success: Slightly decreases the likelihood of having a VBAC if a woman's had more than one previous caesarean (success rate is 83% instead of 87%)[51]

Guidelines / recommendations:
- RCOG: No significant difference in the rates of uterine rupture in VBAC with two or more previous caesarean births compared with (one); women with a prior history of two uncomplicated low transverse caesarean sections, in an otherwise uncomplicated pregnancy at term, with no contraindication for vaginal birth, who have been fully informed by a consultant obstetrician, may be considered suitable for planned VBAC... RCOG advises against having a VBAC after three or more caesareans
- SOGC: Not a contraindication but women should be informed about the increased risk.
- ACOG: Women with two previous low transverse caesarean deliveries may be considered candidates.

10. **SINGLE LAYER TECHNIQUE/SINGLE LEVEL SUTURE FOR UTERINE INCISION**

Risk of the uterine incision separating: Research is inconclusive on this[52] although Bujold (2010) found that it doubled the risk of uterine rupture.[53]

Factors affecting VBAC success: No information available

Guidelines / recommendations:
- RCOG: There is conflicting evidence on whether single-layer compared with double-layer uterine closure may increase the risk of uterine rupture in subsequent planned VBAC.
- NIH: Risk impossible to quantify (lack of data), with low level of scientific evidence.

11. **PAST CAESAREAN WITH PREMATURE BABY**

Risk of the uterine incision separating: Research is inconclusive; two studies concluded that a caesarean carried out when the baby was very premature increases the risk of uterine rupture (because the lower segment of the uterus was less developed)—and these studies concluded that the risk was 1% instead of 0.68%;[54] a different study showed no increased risk[55]

Factors affecting VBAC success: No information available

Guidelines / recommendations:
- RCOG: This reduces the chances of a VBAC being successful.

12. **CLASSICAL INCISION (i.e. VERTICAL IN THE UPPER PART OF UTERUS)**

Risk of the uterine incision separating: Increases the risk significantly

Factors affecting VBAC success: No information available

Guidelines / recommendations:
- This is a contraindication for a VBAC for RCOG, ACOG and SOGC

13. **PREVIOUS UTERINE RUPTURE**

Risk of the uterine incision separating: Between 6% (when the incision is in the uterine lower segment) and 32% (when it is in the upper segment)

Factors affecting VBAC success: No information available

Guidelines / recommendations:
- This is a contraindication for a VBAC for RCOG, ACOG and SOGC

Situations linked with your personal characteristics or situation

1. **BEING SINGLE**

Risk of the uterine incision separating: No known impact on the risk

Factors affecting VBAC success: Decreases the likelihood[56]

Guidelines / recommendations:
- None

2. **BEING WHITE**

Risk of the uterine incision separating: No known impact on the risk

Factors affecting VBAC success: Increases the likelihood[57]

Guidelines / recommendations:
- RCOG: Being non-white decreases the odds of completing a VBAC.
- NIH: Speaking Spanish and being Black-American decreases the odds.

3. **EXPECTING A BOY**

Risk of the uterine incision separating: No known impact on the risk

Factors affecting VBAC success: No information available

Guidelines / recommendations:
- NIH: Decreases the odds of completing a VBAC.

4. **BEING HEALTHY BEFORE THE PREGNANCY**

Risk of the uterine incision separating: No known impact on the risk

Factors affecting VBAC success: Increases the likelihood[58]

Guidelines / recommendations:
- None specific to this situation.

5. **BEING DIABETIC (TYPE I DIABETES)**
Risk of the uterine incision separating: No known impact on the risk
Factors affecting VBAC success: Decreases the likelihood[59]
Guidelines / recommendations:
   - SOGC: This is not a reason not to have a VBAC.

6. **BEING ASTHMATIC**
Risk of the uterine incision separating: No known impact on the risk
Factors affecting VBAC success: Decreases the likelihood[60]
Guidelines / recommendations:
   - SOGC: This is not a reason not to have a VBAC.

7. **HAVING HIGH BLOOD PRESSURE**
Risk of the uterine incision separating: No known impact on the risk
Factors affecting VBAC success: Decreases the likelihood[61]
Guidelines / recommendations:
   - SOGC: This is not a reason not to have a VBAC.

8. **HAVING LESS THAN 12 YEARS OF SCHOOLING**
Risk of the uterine incision separating: No known impact on the risk
Factors affecting VBAC success: Decreases the likelihood[62]
Guidelines / recommendations:
   - NIH: This lowers the success rate.

9. **BEING OBESE OR HAVING A HIGH BMI**
Risk of the uterine incision separating: May increase the risk;[63] in absolute terms the risk is low
Factors affecting VBAC success: Decreases the likelihood[64]
Guidelines / recommendations:
   - RCOG: When a woman's BMI is higher than 30 this is unfavourable for completing a VBAC.
   - SOGC: Definitive conclusions cannot yet be drawn regarding the risk.
   - ACOG: This has a negative effect on completing a VBAC.
   - NIH: Being thin increases the odds of completing a VBAC but there is a low level of evidence regarding obesity.

Being thin increases the odds of completing a VBAC but there is a low level of evidence regarding obesity

10. **BEING OVER 30 YEARS OLD**

Risk of the uterine incision separating: Increases the risk; over 30 (or in other studies 35) the risk is higher[65]

Factors affecting VBAC success: Decreases the likelihood[66]

Guidelines / recommendations:
- RCOG: 'Advanced maternal age' lessens the odds of completing a VBAC.
- SOGC: Definitive conclusions cannot yet be drawn regarding the risk.

11. **HAVING AN UNUSUALLY SHAPED UTERUS (BICORNATE, ETC)**

Risk of the uterine incision separating: Increases the risk; one small study shows the risk is higher[67]

Factors affecting VBAC success: No information available

Guidelines / recommendations:
- None specific to this situation.

12. **BEING SHORT (5 ft 4.6 inches OR LESS FOR SWEDISH WOMEN!)**

Risk of the uterine incision separating: Increases the risk; according to one study, the risk is higher.[68]

Factors affecting VBAC success: No information available

Guidelines / recommendations:
- RCOG: Short stature lessens the odds of completing a VBAC.
- NIH: Being tall increases the odds.

Situations linked with your present pregnancy

1. **HAVING A BABY WHO IS PRESENTING BREECH**

Risk of the uterine incision separating: No known impact on the risk

Factors affecting VBAC success: No information available.

Guidelines / recommendations:
- In the UK and France, this is not a reason not to have a VBAC.[69]
- ACOG: Available data are insufficient to determine the risks and benefits of a VBAC.

2. **HAVING AN EXTERNAL CEPHALIC VERSION (TO TURN A BREECH BABY)**

Risk of the uterine incision separating: No known impact on the risk[70]

Factors affecting VBAC success: No information available

Guidelines / recommendations:
- SOGC: There is no reason why external cephalic version shouldn't be attempted before a VBAC
- ACOG: Not contraindicated

3. **HAVING A PREMATURE BABY**

Risk of the uterine incision separating: Decreases the risk of uterine rupture[71]

Factors affecting VBAC success: Increases the likelihood of having a VBAC[72]

Guidelines / recommendations:
- RCOG: Women who are preterm and considering the options for birth after a previous caesarean should be informed that planned preterm VBAC has similar success rates to planned term VBAC but with a lower risk of uterine rupture.

4. **EXPECTING TWINS**

Risk of the uterine incision separating: No increased risk of either rupture or complications for the babies.[73]

Factors affecting VBAC success: Similar chance as for a singleton pregnancy[74]

Guidelines / recommendations:
- RCOG: A cautious approach is advised when considering planned VBAC in women with twin gestation.
- SOGC: This is not a reason not to have a VBAC.
- ACOG: May be considered suitable candidate for VBAC.

5. **HAVING HYPERTENSION OR PRE-ECLAMPSIA**

Risk of the uterine incision separating: No increased risk according to a 2006 study[75]

Factors affecting VBAC success: Decreases the likelihood[76]

Guidelines / recommendations:
- None specific to this situation.

6. **EXPECTING A 'BIG' BABY (EXPECTED TO BE OVER 4KG AT BIRTH)**

Risk of the uterine incision separating: Maybe a slight additional risk.[77]

Factors affecting VBAC success: Decreases the likelihood but scans or pelvimetry are not very good at helping caregivers to estimate the baby's weight, or at predicting the outcome of a birth.[78]

Guidelines / recommendations:
- RCOG: Decreases the chances of completing a VBAC; a 'cautious' approach is advised.
- SOGC: This is not a reason not to have a VBAC.
- ACOG: Suspicion of macrosomia by itself in a nondiabetic patient should not disqualify a patient from a trial of labour.
- NIH: Reduces the chances of completing a VBAC; the risk is impossible to quantify with actual data (because there's not much evidence).

7. **GIVING BIRTH AT OR BEYOND 40 WEEKS**

Risk of the uterine incision separating: Contradictory evidence;[79] one study concluded there was no increased risk (not even after 41 weeks), while another concluded that the risk is higher after 41 weeks; a third study concluded that the risk is higher after 42 weeks.

Factors affecting VBAC success: Equals of decreases the likelihood. Attempts at VBACs when babies are at or before term generally enjoy more success than babies born after 40 weeks;[80] however, it depends on the state of the cervix before the woman gives birth (i.e. on whether it's soft or not)

Guidelines / recommendations:
- RCOG: VBAC at or beyond 41 weeks of gestation decreases the chances of completing a VBAC.
- NIH: They drew the same conclusion as RCOG.
- ACOG: Gestational age of greater than 40 weeks alone should not preclude VBAC
- SOGC: Success rates and risks are comparable; postdatism is not a contraindication to a trial of labour after a previous caesarean.

8. **HAVING A THIN UTERINE SCAR**

Risk of the uterine incision separating: Some studies have concluded that having a 'thin' uterine scar can increase the risk of uterine rupture. Some say less than 2.3 to 2.5mm is risky and others state higher or lower values.

Guidelines / recommendations:
- None specific to this situation, except those in one systematic review.[81]

Situations linked with the circumstances of your VBAC

1. **HAVING A VBAC IN A RURAL HOSPITAL, OR IN A PRIVATE HOSPITAL**

Risk of the uterine incision separating: No known impact on the risk

Factors affecting VBAC success: Conflicting evidence; more recent studies conclude this increases the chances of completing a VBAC, while older studies concluded this decreases the chances.[82]

Guidelines / recommendations:
- NICE: Women having a VBAC should labour in a unit where there is immediate access to caesareans and on-site blood transfusion.
- NIH: This increases the chances of completing a VBAC.
- ACOG: VBAC should be attempted in institutions equipped to respond to emergencies with physicians immediately available to provide emergency care.
- SCOG: For a safe labour after a caesarean section, a woman should deliver in a hospital where a timely caesarean section is available.

2. **HAVING A VBAC IN A LOW VOLUME HOSPITAL**

Risk of the uterine incision separating: There is a low level of maternal mortality in high-volume hospitals (more than 500 births a year) and there are lower rates of neonatal mortality in premature infants.[83]

Factors affecting VBAC success: No information available

Guidelines / recommendations:
- NIH: It is impossible to quantify the risk with actual data.

3. **HAVING A VBAC IN A COUNTRY WHERE MIDWIVES ARE THE MAIN CAREGIVERS IN THE CASE OF A NORMAL BIRTH**

Risk of the uterine incision separating: No known impact on the risk

Factors affecting VBAC success: Increases the likelihood.[84]

Guidelines / recommendations:
- None specific to this situation.

4. **HAVING A VBAC IN A BIRTH CENTRE**

Risk of the uterine incision separating: No increased risk compared to hospital; the risk is from 0.2% to 0.4% (i.e. two or four per thousand births) after one caesarean; the rate is not lower in a hospital[85]

Factors affecting VBAC success: Giving birth in a birth centre with a midwife in attendance increases the likelihood of completing a VBAC.[86]

Guidelines / recommendations:
- None specific to this situation.

5. **BEING LESS THAN 4cm DILATED AT ADMISSION**

Risk of the uterine incision separating: No known impact on the risk.

Factors affecting VBAC success: Decreases the likelihood[87]

Guidelines / recommendations:
- RCOG: This reduces the odds of completing a VBAC.
- NIH: If the cervix is more dilated on admission or when membranes are already ruptured (the woman's waters have broken), this increases the odds of completing the VBAC.

Research shows a woman is more likely to have a successful VBAC if she goes into hospital when she's more than 4cm dilated

6. **BEING INDUCED WHEN THE CERVIX IS FAVOURABLE (i.e. SOFT)**

Risk of the uterine incision separating: Decreases the risk[88]

Factors affecting VBAC success: Increases the likelihood[89]

Guidelines / recommendations:
- None relating to this situation.

7. **HAVING A SOFT CERVIX AT THE BEGINNING OF LABOUR**

Risk of the uterine incision separating: May reduce the risk[90]

Factors affecting VBAC success: Increases the likelihood[91]

Guidelines / recommendations:
- NIH: A cervix effaced at 75%—90% inceases the odds, but when the cervix is unfavourable on admission it is impossible to quantify the risk—because scientific evidence is weak.
- ACOG: Spontaneous labour has an increased probability of success.

8. **HAVING A VBAC AT HOME**

Risk of the uterine incision separating: There may be no increased risk; in the only (small) study conducted so far, there were no cases of either rupture or dehiscence[92]

Factors affecting VBAC success: This increases the likelihood of success; between 88% and 93% of women are successful when labour begins spontaneously (i.e. without any induction)[93]

Guidelines / recommendations:
- None available for this situation.

9. **HAVING SYNTHETIC OXYTOCIN IN A DRIP TO INDUCE LABOUR**

Risk of the uterine incision separating: The evidence is contradictory; this may increase the risk (0.9% vs 0.4%),[94] or it may not.[95] See the previous chapter for a discussion of this.

Factors affecting VBAC success: Decreases the likelihood.[96]

Guidelines / recommendations:
- RCOG: Although augmentation is not contraindicated it should be preceded by careful obstetric assessment, maternal counselling and by a consultant-led decision; syntocinon augmentation should be titrated such that it should not exceed the maximum rate of contractions of four in 10 minutes; the ideal contraction frequency would be three to four in 10 minutes.
- NIH and NICE: This decreases the odds of completing a VBAC.

10. **EXPERIENCING FAILURE TO PROGRESS DURING THE ACTIVE PHASE OF LABOUR (i.e. NO PROGRESS IN LABOUR DESPITE CONTRACTIONS COMING THICK AND FAST)**

Risk of the uterine incision separating: May increase the risk of uterine rupture

Factors affecting VBAC success: One study found that three quarters of women (75%) have a successful VBAC in this case.[97]

Guidelines / recommendations:
- ACOG: Synthetic oxytocin (syntocinon) may be used for augmentation

11. BEING INDUCED IN ANY WAY

Risk of the uterine incision separating: Increases the risk[98]—can more than double it (1% instead of 0.4%), or can increase it between three to five times (2.45% vs 0.52% or 0.77%),[99] but some studies do not conclude this; nevertheless a combination of methods (methods) seems more harmful.[100] See the previous chapter for a discussion of this issue.

Factors affecting VBAC success: Decreases the likelihood of completing the VBAC (to 63%)

Guidelines / recommendations:
- RCOG: Reduces the chances of completing a VBAC. "Women should be informed of the two– to three-fold increased risk of uterine rupture and around 1.5-fold increased risk of caesarean section in induced and/or augmented labours, compared with spontaneous labours. Women should be informed that there is a higher risk of uterine rupture with induction of labour with prostaglandins.
- NIH: Reduces the odds of completing the VBAC.
- NICE: Women who've had a previous caesarean can be offered induction of labour, but they should be aware that the likelihood of uterine rupture in these circumstances is increased to 80 per 10,000 when labour is induced with nonprostaglandin agents, and 240 per 10,000 when labour is induced using prostaglandins.
- ACOG: Misoprostol should not be used and it is better to avoid the sequential use of prostaglandins and oxytocin. Mechanical induction (with a balloon) may be an option. Synthetic oxytocin use for induction or augmentation of labour is not contraindicated.

12. HAVING A BABY WITH ITS HEAD ENGAGED AND DESCENDED LOWER

Risk of the uterine incision separating: No known impact on the risk

Factors affecting VBAC success: Increases the likelihood of having a VBAC[101]

Guidelines / recommendations:
- NIH: Increases the odds of having a VBAC.

13. HAVING THE LENGTH OF LABOUR LIMITED IN ADVANCE

Risk of the uterine incision separating: No known impact on the risk

Factors affecting VBAC success: Decreases the likelihood[102]

Guidelines / recommendations:
- None specific to this situation.

14. HAVING MOVEMENTS RESTRICTED DURING LABOUR

Risk of the uterine incision separating: No known impact on the risk

Factors affecting VBAC success: Decreases the likelihood[103]

Guidelines / recommendations:
- None specific to this situation.

15. HAVING NON-REASSURING FETAL HEART TRACES

Risk of the uterine incision separating: No information available

Factors affecting VBAC success: Decreases the likelihood[104]

Guidelines / recommendations:
- None specific to this situation.

16. HAVING AN EPIDURAL

Risk of the uterine incision separating: No known impact on the risk

Factors affecting VBAC success: Decreases the likelihood[105]

Guidelines / recommendations:
- RCOG: Reduces the chances of having a successful VBAC.
- NIH: Impossible to draw conclusions about the effects of epidurals.
- ACOG: May be used.

17. EXPERIENCING LABOUR PROGRESSING WELL

Risk of the uterine incision separating: No known impact on the risk

Factors affecting VBAC success: Increases the likelihood[106]

Guidelines / recommendations:
- None specific to this situation.

The information in these lists should not make you give up on the idea of having a VBAC if you find yourself in a category where the risk of uterine rupture is higher than normal. The amount of additional risk will vary, depending on the situation. It may mean that in these situations it would be wise to take precautions, i.e. to ensure that there is no induction when the cervix is not soft, and no induction at all with prostaglandins, and also to ensure that the requisite staff and facilities are available, in case an emergency caesarean should be needed. VBAC and a repeat caesarean are two options which both carry benefits and risks, as I explained in the last chapter. Nevertheless, there are very few reasons why a woman should not have a VBAC, and professional organisations are increasingly supporting VBAC.

According to one doctor I spoke to admission criteria for a VBAC should have little to do with the reasons why any previous caesareans were performed or even with the type of scar. This doctor feels that people pay too much attention to statistics and not enough attention to the woman herself, to her lifestyle and her state of mind. In his view, what is important is that women are determined and motivated and that they have good lifestyle habits (because this will mean there is a smaller likelihood of complications arising). This particular doctor spends a lot of time getting to know his clients. He has helped women have VBACs after one, two or even more caesareans, with different types of scars. For him, the conditions in which the VBAC takes place are the most important thing. In his view, a supportive environment and the absence or minimal existence of restrictions are the key to a successful outcome.

What if a woman refuses to have a VBAC?

When I interviewed people for this book, and on other occasions since then, several doctors told me that often women refuse to try for a VBAC. One even told me that this is the case with half the women he sees and another said that 1 in 3 women refuse to go for a VBAC. Some women just don't want to experience labour again. Others prefer to have a repeat caesarean with the same consultant, rather than change consultants in order to have a vaginal birth. Since VBACs are often (unnecessarily) the preserve of consultants, some women prefer to stay with their usual GP, who is more available to them, even if it means living through another caesarean.

On the one hand, as another doctor pointed out,[107] decisions that either a woman or a couple make are strongly influenced by the way in which their caregiver tackles the subject of VBAC. (This factor was also emphasised at the recent NIH Conference on VBAC.) On the other hand, I wonder if women are really offered the support they need during pregnancy and labour, so as to make a decision which is right for them and so as to go through with it. Are women being encouraged to have normal births? Is their confidence in their ability to succeed being undermined? Are they given full information about the risks that another caesarean will involve, and are they being told about the advantages for their baby if they have a vaginal birth? Are they given the support they need to have a successful VBAC, including permission to have a doula during their whole labour?

It's strange how caregivers working in institutions where VBAC rates are high have no trouble persuading women to have a VBAC. On this note, another doctor stressed that in the hospital which he's in charge of, most women to whom he suggests a VBAC and who receive information on this agree to have one. Yet another doctor, Barry Schiffin (who is quoted in *The VBAC Experience*) said that if a woman chooses to have a repeat caesarean, she should be informed (for both medical and legal reasons) that she is choosing the most dangerous of the two options. This doctor offered women meetings to help them and their partners make a decision.[108] It is actually the restrictions that so many hospitals put on women that really limit the choice to have a VBAC. (Sometimes, these are simply routine protocols applied to all women: drip, EFM, limiting the length of labour, etc. Sometimes, it's a question of an atmosphere of fear reigning in the maternity unit, when it comes to VBAC.) Caregivers say to women when they come to hospital in labour, "Oh, so you're the VBAC case?" And it gets worse... In reality, even in some places where VBACs often take place, a woman might occasionally find herself with a midwife who panics, or with a nervous consultant or midwife, and that does nothing to facilitate the whole process. This is what one doula told me... When she was attending a woman in labour in a hospital where VBACs had been going on for at least two years she was horrified to see—and angry too—that a registrar was approaching her client, saying: "Don't be frightened, but your womb might explode." All the woman's desire to have a VBAC instantly vanished and the birth ended up being another caesarean. There is a lot of work to do to ensure that all health professionals are appropriately informed about VBAC. Unfortunately, more than 25-30 years after the first official recommendations in North America on VBAC in 1980 and 1985 (which stipulated that women can have a VBAC if they want one) it's still possible to hear this kind of comment made by either consultants or midwives. I've had other women tell me about similar experiences by email.

On a more positive note, some consultants, known for having helped numerous women have a VBAC, never meet clients who refuse to go ahead with a VBAC. This was the case with James King, who told me he'd never had a client refuse a VBAC. If ever it happened, he said, he would explain to the woman that the safest course of action (if she would only give up the idea of having a caesarean) would be to wait for labour to begin on its own. He said he would add that if she needed help during her labour and if it all proved to be too difficult for her, she'd be able to have a repeat caesarean after all. As for Dr Bujold (who we've mentioned before), 80% of his clients decide to have a VBAC.

Personally, I have never met a consultant who would refuse a woman a caesarean if that's what she wanted, and if that's what she'd had before. But some of the consultants I've spoken to would certainly inform the woman of the risks involved and would encourage her to go into labour first.

What if you're refused a VBAC?

Since a VBAC isn't possible in all hospitals or with all consultants or midwives, you might be wondering what your options are if you encounter refusals. For your part, you also have the right to refuse a caesarean if you don't want to have one, even if this refusal meets with disapproval and even if your caregivers put you under great pressure to change your mind. In fact, in the UK, you have the right to refuse any treatment and although it is the duty of caregivers to make you aware of risks relevant to any decisions you make, it is also the duty of caregivers to act as your advocate.

In the USA one group started to protest about the unavailability of VBACs, and they started offering advice to women who faced refusals—for example, they helped them take legal action, if necessary.[109] Even though some of their recommendations are only applicable in the States (because the American healthcare system is different from ours), some of their recommendations can be adapted to the UK. Before you give birth (in almost all cases) or afterwards, if necessary, you are advised to do the following...

- Complain to the hospital administration or the hospital where you're registered for care.
- Consider your options for alternative birthplaces—checking how caregivers at each place feel about you having a VBAC. You can do this by logging on to www.birthchoiceuk.com. (No phone number is available. If you don't personally have access to the Internet at home or at work, you can always access it at your local library, with help from a member of the library staff, if necessary.)

- If you've requested midwifery care, tell your midwife you would like to see her Supervisor of Midwives—or contact your local Primary Care Trust to arrange this yourself, if necessary.
- If you can afford to pay for private care, contact the Independent Midwives Association (www.independentmidwives.org.uk, Tel: 0845 4600 105).
- Get more information and support from the VBAC Information & Support Group (www.vbac.org.uk, Tel: 01243 868440), ICAN (the International Cesarean Awareness Network (www.ican-online.org, no phone number available), or the homebirth website (www.homebirth.org.uk—no telephone number available) if you're thinking of having a VBAC at home. Alternatively, contact the NCT (National Childbirth Trust) for information and support (www.nct.org.uk, Tel: 0844 243 6000).

Get more information from VBAC support groups

- Check out your personal situation (in terms of relevant research and rights) by contacting AIMS (the Association for Improvements in Maternity Services at www.aims.org.uk, Tel: 0300 365 0663.
- If you're thinking about this after the birth, contact the Patients' Association (www.patients-association.org.uk, Tel: 0845 608 4455) or the Nursing & Midwifery Council (the NMC) (www.nmc-uk.org, Tel: 020 7333 9333) if you feel dissatisfied with nursing or midwifery care you've received.
- If you just want to talk through what has happened to you, contact Birth Crisis (www.sheilakitzinger.com/BirthCrisis.htm, Tel: 01865 300266).

If after contacting any relevant organisations antenatally and exploring all options, you are still having problems getting someone to attend a VBAC (which, it must be said, is unlikely given the current climate of promoting evidence-based care, which supports VBAC over unnecessary repeat caesareans), you are advised to get legal advice. In the USA, by taking appropriate action, some women who've been forced to have a caesarean have succeeded in getting compensation for post-traumatic stress after the birth—which makes the likelihood of repeat cases lower.[110] In Latin America, in Brazil—a country where the caesarean rate is very high, as we've already noted—one VBAC organisation has demanded public meetings on the abuse of the caesarean operation, and members of this organisation have enlisted support from the Attorney General after a report (which included full scientific references) was produced describing what was happening in the country.[111]

If after contacting any relevant organisations antenatally and exploring all options, you are still having problems getting someone to attend a VBAC, get legal advice

Hospitals which are focused on increasing the VBAC rate

Fortunately, there are institutions which are trying to improve access to VBACs. For example, in the USA, some health centres have done important work to increase accessibility to VBAC. Two examples are the Dartmouth-Hitchcock Medical Center and Fletcher Ellen Health Care. In collaboration with the University of Vermont, they have included ACOG guidelines in the *Vermont/New Hampshire VBAC Project* on ways of avoiding the situation where all women who want a VBAC end up in the 'high risk' category (even though ACOG didn't speak about 'high risk' in its guidelines). This group has also developed a clear consent form and a leaflet which is designed to help women obtain all the information they need to have, not only on the advantages and risks of VBAC but also on those associated with repeat caesareans.[112]

There are places which are trying to improve access to VBACs

This initiative resulted from the observation that access to VBAC had decreased considerably in the region because of the confusion about national standards, because of negative articles in the media, and because of court cases which resulted in compensation amounting to enormous sums of money. Half of hospitals in New Hampshire and several hospitals in Vermont had stopped offering VBACs. A group of almost 200 people met up in 2002 to establish this project. The project specified three levels of risks associated with VBAC and specified appropriate guidelines for each of these levels for women wanting to have a VBAC. Incorporating later research, they would be as follows:

- **Level 1:** This is the lowest level of risk, when a woman has previously had one caesarean, when her labour starts spontaneously and is not augmented with syntocinon or pitocin (synthetic oxytocin), when her baby's heart rhythm is satisfactory or when this woman has already had a VBAC. This level of risk would be the same for any pregnant woman who is considered low risk. In this case, a hospital without specialist care is adequate.
- **Level 2:** This is a moderate level of risk, associated with induction or augmentation of labour, two or more previous caesareans, a previous single layer uterine suture, or an interval since the last caesarean and the due date of less than 18 months. This level of risk requires, in this project's recommendation, the presence during the active phase of labour of a consultant who is capable of carrying out a caesarean, as well as an anaesthetist, and the availability of an operating theatre (with the necessary staff and equipment).
- **Level 3:** This indicates high risk and applies a) when there are repeated non-reassuring traces of the baby's heart rhythm (when the baby does not respond to clinical intervention, such as the mother changing position), b) when bleeding indicates problems with the placenta, and c) when there is failure to progress during labour (i.e. no change in dilation) over a two-hour period in the active phase of labour, despite the woman experiencing adequate contractions.

Protocols were established for antenatal appointments, for labour, and agreements were also made between hospitals. This initiative received a prize awarded by ACOG. The authors of the project emphasise that it would cost enormous sums of money (7.5 million US dollars) to prevent every case of damage to babies, connected with uterine rupture, without taking account of the fact that many more babies—if most women were forbidden to have a VBAC—would need intensive care due to breathing difficulties, which caesarean babies often have.

One birth centre attached to a community hospital in Oregon, the Family Birth Center of the Three Rivers Community Hospital, decided that they would not officially offer women the option of having a VBAC, but they would help women who refuse a repeat caesarean. The consultants responsible for these clients have agreed to remain at the hospital during VBACs and an anaesthetist is on duty 24 hours a day. This hospital was the first large American hospital to be awarded the label 'Mother-Friendly Hospital.'[113]

The Cowansville Hospital in Quebec, the first Canadian hospital to obtain certification as a Baby-Friendly Hospital, found a way of honouring the SOGC's recommendation about EFM during VBACs... The administration bought a portable appliance, which works with the use of telemetry, and this allows the labouring woman to continue to move around and walk, and does not confine her to a bed, as is the case with conventional machines. Since their initiative, other hospitals have bought these types of appliances.

When hospitals are really concerned about a woman's right to bring her baby into the world herself, there is a way of finding solutions which respect guidelines from medical associations

These examples show that when hospitals are really concerned about a woman's right to bring her baby into the world through her own efforts, there is a way of finding solutions which respect guidelines from medical associations. SOGC does in fact specify that health professionals need to take into account individual needs, patient resources, the limits of institutions and types of practice. This professional association also adds that it is permissible to adapt practical guidelines to local conditions, and that if this is done, it should be noted in writing. NICE guidelines make the general recommendation that "Pregnant women who have had a previous caesarean and who want to have a vaginal birth should be supported in this decision." As far as monitoring is concerned, NICE states that women should be offered electronic fetal monitoring during labour, but they don't specify whether EFM should be used throughout labour, or whether it should only be used at certain points.

Given these initiatives and the balance of research, which generally indicates that VBAC is a safe choice for most women who've previously had a caesarean, I would encourage you to keep on checking out your own personal options if you decide to go ahead with a VBAC. If you receive a refusal initially, it's quite possible that another caregiver or institution will be supportive.

Persuasive reasons to have a VBAC

Photo © Rachel Yellin

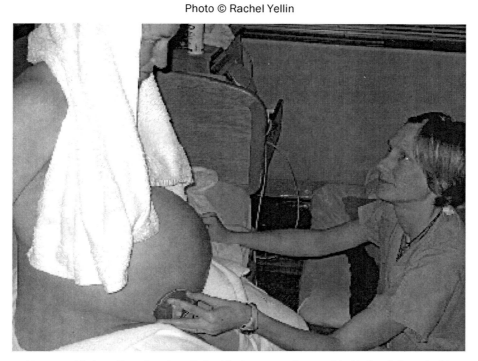

Above and below: *Even in a hospital setting care can be provided intimately and with low technology. Increasingly, this type of very humane care is available.*

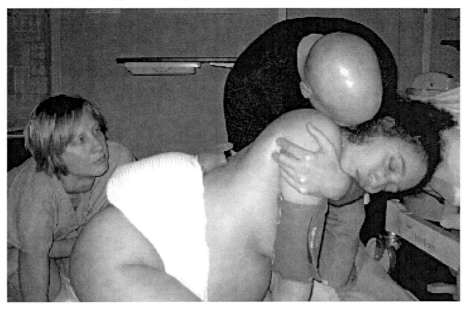

Photo © Michelle Welborne

To summarise...

Your decision: a VBAC or another caesarean?

- In order to decide, women identify what's important for them. Sometimes they change their mind during their pregnancy. Often, they make a gut decision, after reading through all the facts.
- It's normal to have doubts or anxieties.
- Women's decisions are influenced by the opinions of their caregivers (GPs, midwives or consultants).
- The decision women make should also be informed by the reasons why the original caesarean was performed. It is important for women to have the questions they have about their caesarean(s) answered.

Sometimes women change their mind during their pregnancy. Often, they make a gut decision, after reading through all the facts... It's normal to have doubts and anxieties.

Reasons in favour of having a VBAC...

- Almost all women are capable of having a VBAC.
- A vaginal birth is beneficial for your baby because it prepares him or her for life outside your womb. It prepares both the lungs and the metabolism.
- The closer your baby is to being 'term', the better it is for him or her.
- The first contact mother and baby have, just after the birth, is important for the development of the baby and for bonding.

What are your chances of having a successful VBAC?

- On average 75% of women have a successful VBAC and In good conditions, the percentage of women completing a VBAC successfully rises to 95%.
- We now know much more about factors influencing the risk and 'success' of a VBAC. They relate to the circumstances in which the woman had her original caesarean, the circumstances of her previous labours, the personal characteristics of the woman concerned, her pregnancy and the circumstances in which the VBAC takes place.
- If you think about your personal level of risk, this should help you identify the best conditions for having a VBAC. While you do this, you also need to bear in mind that you can change your mind at any time, remembering too that some institutions create more favourable conditions for VBACs, than others.

On average 75% of women complete a VBAC and up to 95% do so in a favourable environment

Birthframe 8
Persuaded of the reasons, but still unsure... her body decided!

My wife Coleen was seven months' pregnant with our second child when an article on VBAC appeared in a magazine. We read and re-read the article and discussed it with our GP. Our first son had been born by caesarean because his head hadn't engaged properly. Scans had revealed that our second child would be a big baby. We'd therefore been booked in for a caesarean. Coleen, who dreaded having contractions, had no trouble with the idea that the caesarean would mean she could avoid them altogether. As for me, I only had one regret: I was sorry I hadn't experienced a normal, vaginal birth with her, like everybody else. But it was up to her to decide.

> Coleen, who dreaded having contractions, had no trouble with the idea that the caesarean would mean she could avoid them

Between reading the article and her booking-in date, Coleen felt there was not enough time to prepare for such a radical change of course. Once a caesarean, always a caesarean, after all...

> Coleen felt there was not enough time to prepare for such a radical change of course

Three days after a beautiful weekend touring round a local area, Coleen woke up at 5 o'clock one morning, astonished to find she was having contractions. They soon became much stronger so by 7 o'clock we were at the hospital. She was already 2cm dilated. Coleen's consultant wasn't there, but he nevertheless talked to the consultant on duty over the phone, who then came to see us. He told Coleen in a reassuring, but firm tone of voice: "Since you've gone into labour on your own, you can get through to the end of it on your own too." There was a flash of panic in my wife's eyes in a break between two contractions but the midwife, the consultant and I all managed to reassure her a bit. The baby, who was premature, would be small so it should be able to get through without too much difficulty...

> Coleen's face went red each time she pushed—she was obviously keen to get it all over and done with

At around 10.30am Coleen was taken to the delivery suite and I followed her, feeling a bit worried but also totally thrilled. Coleen's face went red each time she pushed—she was obviously keen to get it all over and done with. Apart from that, everything went well. At 11.02am after a routine episiotomy, Coleen pushed one last time and Patrick was born, weighing 6lb 5oz (2.85kg). Today we're both happy we experienced this unexpected VBAC. And if you were to ask Coleen what she liked least, she would reply: "Getting stitched up again!"

> Today we're both happy we experienced this unexpected VBAC

Birthframe 9

A successful VBAC, despite a family history of caesarean birth

Where should I begin? My story really began more than 33 years ago, when I was born by elective caesarean because my big brother had been born in the same way three years before. From then on, my mother—having had two children without experiencing a single contraction—never stopped going on about her regrets on the matter. 29 years later, without ever having asked myself if I'd like to have children some day, I found myself looking at a pregnancy test which had registered positive. I was in a complete panic—speechless, incredulous and overjoyed. For as long as I could remember I'd been worried about the idea of having children. Oh, it wasn't the mysteries of pregnancy or the responsibilities of motherhood that frightened me, just the unbearable pain of labour. From a very early age I had decided I'd have an epidural when I got to 39 weeks of pregnancy, so I could be sure of feeling nothing at all during this terrible event. Nevertheless, on 20 October 2003, faced with the reality of a 'fait accompli'— especially in the light of what I still had to accomplish!—a little voice in my head told me that not even an epidural would be able to mask the enormity of what I was about to experience...

My change of heart started when I went looking for a book. I needed to know what was happening to me and what was awaiting me. I remember going to a bookshop and having terrible trouble finding a book which didn't adopt a tone which seemed, to me, to be patronising, as if it was for children. Eventually, I found a book which suited me and as soon as I got home I read Chapter 10 all in one go—it was called 'Labour and birth'. When I'd finished reading, I thought: "Well, there you go. That almost seems doable!"

I remember going to a bookshop and having terrible trouble finding a book which didn't adopt a patronising tone

A week later I announced the news of my pregnancy to my parents. I did this first because I wanted to share my happiness, but also because I wanted to find out what I had to do! Since I hadn't yet even decided whether or not I wanted to have any children (it had been decided for me) I was light years behind, when it came having developing a 'birthing philosophy'. I'd always thought these questions would resolve themselves during pregnancy, but I realised the matter had now become complicated...

She gave me a list of consultants... I picked one at random

My mother gave me a list of consultants at the local hospital. I picked one at random and telephoned so as to make an appointment for six weeks later. That seemed an eternity away! Meanwhile, I found a rich network of midwives and somehow found myself on two long waiting lists for two birth centres. I began to realise that an enormous number of pregnancies ended up on the operating table and that the vast majority of women seemed to need drugs to start labour off, to augment it, to stop it, to bring pain relief, or to stop bleeding... and that all seemed absurd. I began to have a vague idea of what I was hoping for in my own labour, but I discovered one very important thing: I should have thought about that famous 'birthing philosophy' much sooner... What was going to happen to me? What kind of labour would I have? I realised that we were living in a culture of terror as far as childbirth is concerned, but what exactly are we supposed to be afraid of? More to the point, I thought, what choices are available to me?

It took me just one five-minute visit with my doctor to determine that the word 'choice' was meaningless in my particular situation. At the end of my second doctor's appointment (which lasted at most four minutes) I asked for my records to be transferred to a nearby hospital, which I'd heard a lot of good things about. It was there that a birth plan was suggested to me. And it was there that I was asked to share my thoughts during my appointments—to express my fears... my philosophy, in fact. But in any case, after that appointment with my doctor I had the impression that things were changing. Mostly, I began to feel confident. Nevertheless, a phone call to a local birth centre let a new cat among the pigeons and I spent a good week feeling doubtful again. Did I have enough courage to (try to) give birth a long way away from the availability of an epidural? Was my body capable of giving birth? Not having been 'birthed' myself, how could I know if I'd be able to do it? I even liked my consultant! By some miracle, it was just at that time that I had the honour of attending a cow in labour, which belonged to my parents' neighbours. The cow went into a calm, peaceful state of mind. It was so simple. Plop! The calf fell onto the straw, all slimy. Its mother licked it, it got up and then started to suckle. I had a revelation: that was exactly how I wanted to give birth...

I had a revelation: that was exactly how I wanted to give birth...

I met my midwife one month later, when I was 25 weeks' pregnant. I adored her and I was happy to finally find myself at the 'nerve centre' of my feelings. I could talk to her about my hopes and fears. At last I was exactly where I wanted to be and I couldn't believe my good fortune! But at 34 weeks my midwife announced that my baby was breech, just as my mother and brother had been.

Suddenly it seemed entirely logical to me that my baby would present himself 'badly'. A black cloud had appeared above my head. My midwife told me in vain that there was still time, that there were things we could do—in short, that there was still plenty of hope—but I just heard thunder rumbling overhead. I was devastated. In one moment, all the confidence which I'd had such trouble finding dissolved into thin air. I tried everything possible to bring back my hope: acupuncture, visualisation, putting an ironing board up against the sofa (women who've been there know why)—but my cards were on the table. In my head it was impossible for this baby to turn. And, just as you might expect, my baby kept her head high, her ear pressed up against her mother's beating heart—which was pumping away crazily! I was transferred to a consultant at another hospital at 37 weeks after the original consultant, who was famous for 'turning' babies successfully, refused to try and turn mine. (It seemed there wasn't enough amniotic fluid, space, time, inclination to do so... I don't know.)

On 3 June the consultant and I (yes, it was me) chose 9 June 2004 at 9 o'clock in the morning as the date my baby should be born. At this stage I was floating in a kind of cloud of resignation: I was going to have my stomach opened up in order to become a mother and there was nothing I could do about it. I was terrified, but caught in a trap.

On 9 June I got up very early in the morning and had a shower, using a little disinfected sponge which I'd been given the day before, for the occasion. Then I looked at my intact body in the mirror for the last time. I have neither the space nor the courage to tell you about that horrible morning—the moments of anxiety and panic, the cold sweats and trembling which I experienced before an enormous needle was inserted into my spinal cord and they started cutting into my flesh. In reality, those are the moments I prefer to forget—and I'm not talking about sadness here, but about the most animal kind of terror. On the other hand, the moment they put my daughter on me all the fear, sadness and bitterness disappeared. OK, so I was still on the operating table, with my arms attached (strapped down?) as if on a crucifix, with a large bleeding slit, gaping open across my abdomen. But my baby was lying on me and I laughed with happiness. When the baby-doctor-turned-stomach-opener shook my hand I thanked him, feeling genuinely happy!

From then on, my only aim was to take care of my daughter

From that moment on, my only aim in life was to take care of my daughter Greta as well as I possibly could—and in order to do this I had to heal up physically. As for the psychological wound, I quite simply had neither the time nor the energy to focus on it. Breastfeeding was easy (I'd been breastfed myself) and in physical terms, I got back to normal fairly quickly, considering the substantial mutilation I'd been subjected to. The 'shock of motherhood'—that sudden and violent realisation that comes after the birth of a first child, when we realise the enormity of the task ahead of us—that shock temporarily wiped out the emotional pain of what I'd experienced. Life was beautiful and I was in love again.

But slowly, after a few months, sadness started to haunt me again. It crept up on me. I took to reading again, encouraged by my midwife... and I learnt that not only was I not alone in having had a caesarean, I was also not alone in having suffered so much as a result. After a year I had a whole library of books on caesareans, VBAC and natural birth. My daughter had learnt how to walk. My periods had come back. And I suddenly noticed that my body seemed to belong to me again, that I recognised it—like an old friend. But I wanted to have another baby.

I had no trouble whatsoever persuading my partner, and for three months my periods didn't arrive as expected. I was assured a place in every birth centre and I carried on with my life as I waited. Finally, I realised I was attending appointments without ever having done a pregnancy test... I just KNEW I was pregnant.

My first appointment was at my local birth centre, with my old midwife. But as soon as I went into her consulting room I felt uncomfortable—as if I'd been pushed into a place which I knew too well, where I had too many sad and recent memories of confusion and loss of control...

When I went to see another midwife, I told her my history and she briefly told me her own—and we had a good old laugh. She didn't listen to my baby's heartbeat using a Sonicaid, but we still knew I was pregnant. The beginning of this pregnancy was so much more instinctual than the first one. And I had a ferocious desire to find answers to questions on my own and to build some confidence in myself. In order to do that the most important thing was for me to *listen* to myself.

The most important thing was for me to *listen* to myself

I started trawling through studies on VBAC—rates of uterine rupture, symptoms and risk factors, the effects of various interventions on risks of uterine rupture, mortality rates for both mother and baby after uterine rupture... and so it went on. I always arrived at the same figure of 0.5%—or 1 in 200. And at that point I would turn the numbers on their head and tell myself that I had a 1 in 199 chance of NOT having a uterine rupture. In the end, I put these numbers into perspective: my daughter had a 4% risk of being breech at the end of my pregnancy, or a chance of 1 in 25. I was therefore 'only' eight times more likely to have a uterine rupture in a trial of labour! In short, I filled my head with useless numbers and mathematical logic and did all this with the aim of defending myself when faced with critics.

I had a less 'magical' pregnancy than the first time round. I had quite a lot on my plate, with a little girl of 18 months, who was curious and stubborn. And, unlike the first time, I'd already had a taste of motherhood—in fact, I was experiencing it morning, noon and night. Although I was anxious to get on with things, the idea of having another child, who I'd have to devote myself to, filled me with anxiety. When I was around six months' pregnant, I started desperately feeling my abdomen: I wanted to be certain how my baby was positioned as early as possible. When I was about 30 weeks' pregnant my desperate attempts to find out were becoming manic. I was absolutely convinced the baby was once again head up! Neurotically, I went to see an acupuncturist, who gave me moxa treatments. Then one day, when I was lying on the floor with two telephone directories under my hips, my baby suddenly gave me a solid kick in the ribs—something I'd never experienced before. I took out the books, which had been lifting up my pelvis and remained lying down, with my arms held out in a cross-shape. I forced myself to stay attentively calm for a few minutes, in order to establish my baby's position once and for all, without touching my abdomen. After analysing what was going on, I concluded that this little imp was well and truly head down—and I really believed that. I waited for my next midwife's appointment. She took a long time palpating me—an eternity, in fact!—before declaring what I already knew: "Your baby's perfectly positioned!" I was up in the clouds! So I continued along on my way...

But another anxiety soon appeared in my heart... My God, I was going to have to birth this baby for real! At that point I carried on from exactly where I'd left off in my first pregnancy... I stopped reading about studies and statistics, because that hadn't helped at all. I had no choice but to follow my idea through to its conclusion, come what may. I was really in for it not. It wasn't that I preferred to give birth in hospital or to have another caesarean—not on your life! I simply had stage fright. I knew that whatever came of this whole thing was going to be my life's main event.

I remember that while I was working on a contract all through the winter I would come home on the Metro every evening. The walk from the station to my house lasted about eight minutes, and every evening as I emerged from the underground Metro station, I re-enacted my labour in my head. It was very difficult: I was in pain and sweating, but also calm and confident. And then, with one final push, my baby was born, all hot and slimy—pop! Out she came, onto the straw! I'd done it! It was inevitably on the railway lines, just after the supermarket, that this would happen and I'd then burst into tears every evening, day after day, birth after birth. It was like a secret crime and I was convinced that I would never be allowed to experience such happiness. And during the three minutes it took me to get home, I would formulate a prayer to God to allow me this one wish—to know what just one contraction felt like. That's all I asked.

I don't remember very well what the end of my pregnancy was like but I do remember that at my appointment on 17 May 2006, the date when it had been decided I would have the baby, my midwife, my partner and I had a good old laugh. The atmosphere was relaxed and sparkling with excitement. Then on the evening of 22 May, my partner put our little girl to bed and it happened. Me, Céline Bianchi, with a scarred uterus and the daughter of a woman who had two scars on her uterus... I felt the first contraction to be experienced in two generations! I wasn't sure at first, but after five minutes a second pain lasting about 45 seconds took hold of me at the base of my stomach, so I knew. My wish had been granted. Thank God!

> Then on the evening of 22 May, my partner put our little girl to bed and it happened. Me, Céline Bianchi, with a scarred uterus and the daughter of a woman who had two scars on her uterus!

I slept very well that night and woke up at about 6 o'clock the next morning, on 23 May, having a delicious contraction which lasted a minute. And it came back again five minutes later. I was in another dimension, feeling both extremely excited and also completely lucid. My mother arrived at about 11 o'clock so as to look after our daughter and my partner and I went off to have a coffee. (OK, it was a peppermint tea!) When we got back home I decided to lie down for a while, to have a rest. A big contraction appeared. Then another. And another. Up until that point the little contractions had taken up my attention, and had (almost) stopped me from talking, but they'd been perfectly bearable. But this time it was something else. My mother left with our little one and I spent a long time sitting on the toilet seat, which I found relatively comfortable. My mucous plug came out and then my waters broke. I vomited. Then I called my midwife. It was 5.00pm and I was beginning to want to be at the birth centre, not knowing too well how much longer I'd be able to manage the journey. However, it was bang in the middle of the rush hour and the radio traffic news was advising us every five minutes not to venture onto the motorway, particularly if we were going in a westerly direction...

> I was feeling both extremely excited and also completely lucid

At around 7.00pm we were finally on the road. It was good weather for the first time in ages. I was on the backseat and groaning gently while I was experiencing contractions—with my husband scrutinising me in the rear view mirror, counting in his head. When we arrived at the birth centre a room was prepared for me and the midwife asked me if I needed anything. I said I'd really love some lasagne... A quarter of an hour later a plate of steaming lasagne was on my bedside table. We spent the whole evening and a good part of the night alone, my partner and I, working through contractions. My midwife came in to see us about every 45 minutes to listen to the baby's heart and she would sit down and keep us company through a few contractions. Then she'd be off again. It was all very calm.

Then... I heard the woman in the room next door give birth

At around midnight, I heard the woman in the room next door give birth. That made a big impression on me and I was anxious for it to be my turn... A little later on, I finally got into the bath. That did me a world of good. An hour and a half later, I got out of the bath and my midwife checked me and declared that I was 5cm dilated. I was discouraged because the whole process seemed to be going on for ever... At around 5 o'clock in the morning, my contractions became more spaced out, then faded away altogether. I thought, "That's it! They're definitely going to take me away now and transfer me, because of failure to progress." And I finally took the opportunity to get a bit of sleep. Really, I didn't give a damn... or at least, I almost didn't... and I cursed myself for having let myself believe that I'd be able to give birth all on my own, like a grown-up. My midwife reassured me that by the time the sun rose, my contractions would have started again. I didn't believe her. I was convinced that babies are always born during the night and it was slowly becoming daylight.

A little later, I woke up and my partner said: "Come on, Céline. Your labour must move forward. Hey, let's go to the kitchen!" This expedition proved to be difficult but also my saving grace. When I opened the door to leave the room, I saw my midwife dozing on a couch in the corridor. She opened one eye and followed me into the kitchen, where she made herself a cup of coffee. One image will remain etched in my mind till the day I die... I was leaning on the sofa in the kitchen, while the midwife was sitting at the table, drinking a steaming mug of hot coffee and eating a bowl of cereal, looking at her watch, while I had a contraction. I felt incredibly lucky to be able to lie down in an atmosphere which was so peaceful and 'normal'.

I then ended up returning to my room, where I continued to labour, with contractions becoming more and more powerful as each ray of sunshine streamed into the room. And after having bobbed about on the waves for ages, like a furious buoy in the sea, I was completely dilated. I was in the bath for the second time when I started slowly pushing. For a long time, we'd been waiting for me to spontaneously start pushing, but after a while my midwife suggested I get out of the bath and push intentionally. It took me a few contractions to get the hang of it, but in just a short while my body knew what to do. But, my goodness, how it hurt! Between each contraction I cried as if it were the day I'd been born myself.

110 birthing normally after a caesarean or two

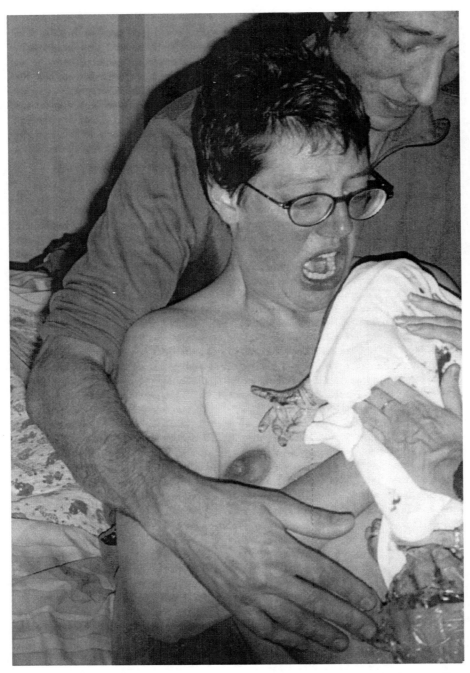

Céline, the mother, shouts out a moment after she's given birth, completely normally

After several contractions, my midwife encouraged me to touch my baby's head. It was 1cm away from being born, shrivelled up like a Morel mushroom. I remember thinking at that precise moment: "It's not possible. I won't be able to do it. I want to go back home. We'll forget all about this, OK?"

A little later—apparently it was at about 12.11pm—the midwife suddenly put the baby in my arms, as if it was a hot potato she didn't want to hold! I didn't even know the head had come out! And that was when I let out a cry I'll never forget. It was a bit like a hen when it lays an egg. And this cry lasted an eternity and came from the deepest part of my being. I can't describe the emotion which produced this cry: it wasn't simply joy or relief, but what I'd now call a kind of 'super-emotion'—something more powerful than victory, more profound than happiness... Something I just can't explain. And in a flash, I was returning from my journey, feeling completely lucid and present.

I took a shower while all the guardian angels at the birth centre busied themselves clearing up my room. I telephoned my mother and we kissed and cuddled our little boy before going to have dinner in the kitchen—which was heated up lasagne. Then we had a little siesta.

We went home again at around 7pm, where we presented our baby boy to his big sister, granddad and grandma, as well as my aunt and uncle. We all had supper together. Then, finally, we went to bed, exhausted. I slept straight through until early the next morning, dead to the world, without dreaming, without feeling any pain and without even wanting to go to the loo.

Then we got up and life went on as usual...

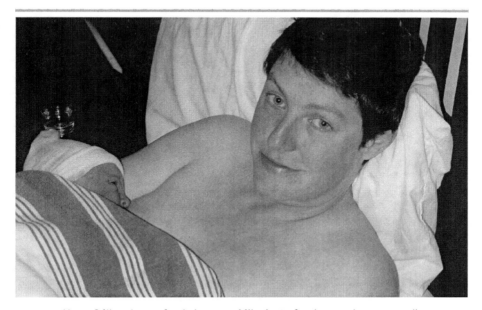

Here, Céline, breastfeeds her son, Milo, just after he was born normally

Part 2:

How to prepare for a safe, successful VBAC

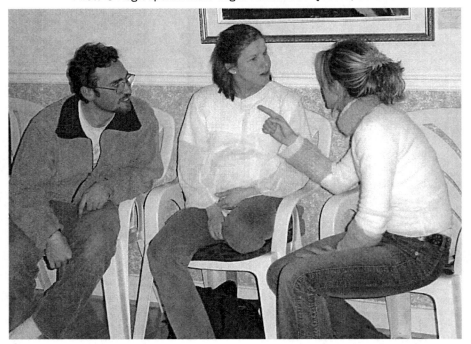

Photo © Regroupement Les Sages-Femmes du Québec, Canada

A couple discuss an issue which is important to them during an antenatal class

How do you and your partner usually reach decisions?

In the next chapter...

- The emotional impact of a caesarean
- Surviving a previous caesarean and creating a positive mindset

CHAPTER 4:

Consider the emotional aftermath

Consider your own feelings

It's easy to underestimate what childbirth means for a woman. Even though we give birth less and less often in the modern world, this event is so intense for a woman that she usually remembers it for the rest of her life, even down to the tiniest detail. In recent years some first-time mothers have been expressing the desire to have a caesarean because they're afraid of giving birth, but others feel differently. For some women, a difficult labour which ends up being an emergency caesarean is a shattered dream—their dream of having a normal birth. The labour the woman was working through as a team with her partner is interrupted... They are no longer in control of events... Sometimes, as a result of the unexpected interruption which the caesarean represents, the couple are also deprived of some precious moments of contact with their new baby in the hours after the birth. And that's saying nothing about the more difficult and longer postnatal recovery which are an inevitable part of the caesarean experience.

There has not been much research on the psychological impact of having a caesarean. However, in 2008, a book was published in Germany, after the authors had interviewed and taken pictures of 162 women aged between 22 and 77, who had had between one and four caesareans each.[1] Most of the women felt that the media under-represented the impact of caesareans and they experienced their caesarean(s) as disappointing, unnatural birth experiences, and as a failure of motherhood, which they needed to grieve over. The authors stressed that almost half the women experienced difficulties bonding with their babies when they'd been born by caesarean.

According to Rahima Baldwin, author of *Pregnant Feelings* (Celestial Arts, 1986), childbirth is a major event in a woman's life. A positive experience will raise a woman's self-esteem, while a negative experience can leave her with a bitter taste in her mouth. Unresolved emotions may stay with her for her whole life and these may colour her relationships with her partner and children.[2]

Some people might object that not all parents react in this way. That's true, and it's particularly the case when a caesarean has been planned and explained thoroughly in advance, when it's been carried out with a regional anaesthetic (usually an epidural) with the woman's partner present, and when contact with the baby has been established immediately after the birth. Nevertheless, even a necessary caesarean, which was performed in good circumstances, can be difficult to come to terms with. One woman reminded me of this. (She'd had three caesareans because her pelvis had been damaged in a car accident.) She said: "I was asleep for my first caesarean—

I had a general anaesthetic because the epidural hadn't worked—and I was conscious for the other two. It wasn't easy because the epidurals never completely took effect. But I preferred the epidurals to the general anaesthetic. At least my partner and I were able to consciously welcome our last two babies when they were born. But the medical staff chatted about food and their favourite restaurants, perhaps because it was a mealtime when they were performing the caesareans. What an atmosphere for giving birth!"[3]

In fact, it's likely that surgeons and other medical staff are unaware the effect their behaviour or speech may have, because women rarely tell them about their feelings. One woman called Josée[4] said that when she read a book about 'happy birth', she cried her eyes out. "I was crying because I realised that the terrible, intimate suffering I'd been carrying inside me since I'd had my first baby two years before had a name: robbery. I'd been robbed of my ability to give birth normally, as well as of my right to a happy birth, and I was stripped naked... And this was all because of my inexperience, my good faith in my caregivers, and my naïvety."

Many consultants simply don't know if their clients are satisfied with their birthing experience. What's more, in the few cases when surveys are carried out (on vaginal or caesarean birth) because of the constraints of the surveys themselves women are rarely able to express their real feelings about their births. In fact, when a new mother is still in hospital she is still in shock about what's happened. She is relieved to have 'survived' and happy that her baby is healthy. She probably doesn't feel entirely free to say what she's thinking while she is still in the care of medical staff. And it's rare for a woman to realise what's happened and to understand how she experienced everything straight after giving birth. This is why the inconvenience a new mother experiences as a result of an episiotomy (i.e. a cut made to the perineum), a forceps delivery (which will probably have caused considerable bruising) or even a caesarean don't weigh heavily on the woman's heart. Even when it was a case of an emergency caesarean, the woman will still be in a state of shock and it will be difficult for her to think back and be critical about what's happened. It is often only several months and even several *years* later, particularly in a subsequent pregnancy, that questions, emotions and feelings bubble up to the surface of a woman's consciousness... and this process is often unexpected. Personally, it was only when I got pregnant again and watched a film about birth that I became aware of my feelings. I was so overcome with emotion that I almost got up and left the cinema—my first birth had affected me that much. Up to that point, I thought I'd accepted my caesarean without any problems.

In one email I received, a mother of a baby who was almost seven months old told me about her feelings... "I am a mother who had a caesarean for a breech baby. My baby is now six months old. I want to have other children and I hope they'll be born in a birth centre or at home. I don't feel comfortable in a hospital environment. I am therefore beginning to prepare myself mentally for my future births, while I do the housework... Feeling afraid and sad, I keep having the feeling I've missed out on something in having a caesarean. Physically, I'm beginning to recover. Emotionally, I'm beginning to forgive myself... I'm getting there."

Isabelle Brabant, who's been a midwife for 30 years, told me she'd found that many women who've had a difficult birth find it hard to talk about it in the first year afterwards. In general, if a woman talks about her birth, it's with her friends, her mother, her antenatal teacher... but it's rarely with her consultant or GP. After a caesarean, women often spend years wondering if their caesarean was really necessary or if it could have been avoided. Hundreds of women have written to me or phoned to tell me about the difficulties they've had accepting their situation and about the questions which have continued to haunt them on this subject. Some women, even if they had a vaginal birth before their caesarean, may have found the experience of the caesarean painful and they may have only one wish: to give birth normally again afterwards.

In 1986 Fay Ryder, women's representative at a national consensus conference on caesareans,[5] told me about something that happened... At the conference, one of the biggest surprises the doctors on the panel experienced was when women (who'd had caesareans) came to talk to them about their feelings: the consultants were completely taken aback. They asked Fay if these women's reactions were representative of all women who'd had caesareans, or if they were just a minority of women who were capable of expressing their feelings. She told them she didn't know—at that time there was no research on the topic—but she said that if 50,000—60,000 emotionally-affected women had written to Nancy Cohen, antenatal teacher and author of *Silent Knife* (Bergin & Garvey, 1983), if hundreds of women had revealed their difficulties to the Maternal Health Society in Vancouver, where she herself worked, if hundreds of thousands of others had written to American organisations such as Cesarean Support, Education & Concern or the Cesarean Prevention Movement, wasn't all that sufficient for them to take notice of what these women were saying? Did these women who were complaining absolutely *have* to represent the majority of women and did they have to produce scientific proof about the numbers they represented? The consultants concluded that even if these women who'd been profoundly affected by their caesareans did constitute a minority, it was a substantial problem.

Consultants or doctors who attend women giving birth vaginally *after* a caesarean are more aware of the impact the surgical birth had. GP Philippe Shea told me that more than half the women who go to see him to arrange a VBAC are in tears in his office during their first antenatal appointment. Dr James King, who was previously in charge of maternity services at a large hospital, told me he'd heard countless women tell him about painful experiences which had occurred at the time of their caesarean.

Caregivers who attend women having VBACs are more aware of the impact the surgical birth had

A small study of women who had a caesarean (2005)[6]

- 52% of women say they didn't participate in the decision-making process
- 45% had post-operative pain
- 39% were not given sufficient information postnatally
- 35% took a long time to recover (experiencing tiredness and having difficulty functioning)
- 35% were not informed about risks
- 26% were not satisfied with their caesarean experience
- 19% regretted having a caesarean
- 16% felt unprepared for the caesarean
- 13% experienced physical and psychological after-effects
- 13% declared themselves incapable of looking after their children

Sometimes women also rationalise the experience of having a caesarean because they are unable to face the emotions they experienced or because the birth was just too painful. Caroline Sufrin, who set up a VBAC group in Ontario, told me how much time she spent trying to convince her doula that she'd had 'fantastic caesareans' and that she didn't want a VBAC so as to be able to have a satisfying experience of birth. However, after this, an enormous amount of anger bubbled up inside her and resulted in shouts of rage. This made her realise how much she'd suppressed her anger. She hadn't even been aware of it until she went into labour. She said: "My god! I decided my caesareans had been fantastic. How blind I was! They made me fall to pieces. I didn't even realise that my heart had been sobbing in silence for five years. Now I feel whole again. Joyful."

I decided my caesareans had been fantastic. How blind I was!

Women don't have much time to adapt to motherhood and reflect on their birth experience, particularly after they've had their first baby. In addition, some women don't have the support they need if they're to face up to painful feelings. And also we mustn't forget that some women—or couples—may well be filled with joy about the arrival of their new baby, without necessarily feeling the same thing about the birth itself.

Giving birth either affirms or invalidates a woman's ability to bring a child into the world. It's an act which has a profound subconscious impact—an issue I'll come back to later. And giving birth the very first time is a rite of passage towards a new stage in a woman's life. A woman who feels she's 'failed' by having a caesarean may have a very strong sense of this 'failure' when in the presence of other women who 'succeeded' in having a vaginal birth. This feeing isn't necessarily conscious and may manifest itself in many ways. What's more, many women who've had a caesarean were also having their first experience of being admitted to hospital and having surgery, so this may also be a source of stress and tension.

"I don't know what it means to bring babies into the world."

One woman I interviewed for this book, Monique de Gramont, told me about her feelings: "I don't know what it means to bring babies into the world. I won't *ever* know, even though I have two children—twins who are eleven and a half years old—because they were both born by caesarean. When a doctor came to speak to me, he said: 'Madam, stop being childish and be rational.' He just couldn't understand this aspect of the matter. He couldn't see they'd taken away my opportunity to experience something which was my right, which I'll never be able to reclaim."

Dr Brooks Ranney, who was president of ACOG in 1982 after practising as a consultant for 30 years (with a caesarean rate of 5.6%), expressed his view as follows: "Any doctor who performs a caesarean must realise that he is changing something in this woman for ever—the capacity to birth a baby, to bring a child into the world. For this reason, we shouldn't be carrying out caesareans simply because of an occasional equipment error (i.e. in the electronic fetal monitor)."[7]

One hospital-based midwife who contacted me told me about a black woman, who she'd seen at the hospital. Was this a case of discrimination, she wondered? The pregnant woman had said she wanted to have a VBAC but she was seemingly forced to have another caesarean in the end. The woman had gestational diabetes, but it was estimated that this baby would be smaller than her first baby. The consultant tried to induce her at 39 weeks, without success. He tried again at 40 weeks. After the woman had been on a syntocinon drip for 15 minutes the consultant declared, "This one's a caesarean." The midwives were shocked. The woman had the caesarean and she said to them afterwards: "I just don't understand why I had to have another caesarean."

In Brazil—a country where the nationwide caesarean rate is approaching 40%—it might seem it's the women themselves who are asking for caesareans... It might seem they actually prefer this surgery to vaginal birth. Nevertheless, according to a recent survey, Brazilian women really do prefer to give birth vaginally. It's consultants and doctors there who prefer the opposite and who claim it's the women who are demanding caesareans.[8] In 2008 a London-based study revealed that although most women who've already had a caesarean plan to have a VBAC for their next birth, many don't achieve their wish.[9] What could be the cause of that?

Very often it is in fact people *around* the pregnant woman who are negative about the prospect of a VBAC. Unfortunately, our society shows little understanding of women's disappointment with their birthing experience, whether vaginal or caesarean, as this woman's comment demonstrates: "For months everyone kept on asking me why I was so shocked. They kept on saying: 'You've got a healthy baby. You're fine yourself. You should be happy— you didn't even have to experience labour!' But that was what I wanted to experience: labour followed by a vaginal birth. It's not what I did experience in reality."[10]

Sheila Kitzinger, anthropologist and author of several books on birth, believes that people deal with masculinity and femininity quite differently. In an interview she told me that society has great empathy for a man who is incapable of having an erection or ejaculating. At the very least, she said, people understand that it's important for him and that being able to do those things is part of his identity as a male. By contrast, people have little understanding for women who are disappointed, sad and frustrated about not having achieved normal physiological functioning, i.e. for women who haven't been able to give birth.

Perhaps giving birth vaginally is a way of uniting oneself with all other women who've brought their babies into the world over the millennia. Some doctors understand the importance for women of doing this. For example, the authors of one of the first documents to have questioned certain obstetric dogmas, *Controversies in Obstetrical Management and Maternal Care,* acknowledge that when birth becomes a surgical procedure, we can legitimately expect it to trigger violent emotional reactions.[11]

In an article in *Mothering* magazine called 'The psychological effects of caesarean deliveries',[12] a woman called Ruth was quoted as saying she'd tried to convince herself that she ought to accept that she had a live, healthy baby. However, she didn't understand why she felt furious, disappointed and shocked by the caesarean. She was concerned about feeling so depressed. Nevertheless, she said that she and her partner had done everything possible to have a normal birth—they'd been well-informed, she'd been well-nourished and she'd gone walking almost every day. So she just couldn't understand why her body hadn't managed to open itself up in order to birth her baby. She'd so wanted to give birth—or at least, she'd thought she had. And she felt so ashamed she'd had a caesarean. In vain, everyone kept on telling her that nowadays it was normal to have one. "If it's normal," she thought, "then why am I so shocked?"

Elizabeth Shearer, an antenatal teacher and co-director of C/SEC, and former editor-in-chief of *C/Sec Newsletter,* said she believed the biggest difficulties a woman experiences after a caesarean aren't to do with the operation itself, but with the feeling of having been steamrollered, with not having been informed about what was happening and with not having understood this.[13] Even as early as the 1980s research was showing that women who were the least susceptible to postnatal depression were those who'd felt they'd had a positive experience of birth.[14] For a woman in labour, the feeling of being in control of the event, being able to influence certain decisions and being part of the team increase her sense of self-worth. They allow her to have a positive experience. The Canadian GP, Michael Klein, says that 'baby blues' and certain forms of depression occur in direct relation to how the second stage of labour went, particularly when there was an instrumental delivery.[15] One recent study did in fact confirm that women who have serious complications during labour are more at risk of suffering from psychological problems afterwards.[16]

There hasn't been a great deal of research into the psychological impact of a caesarean and results are inconsistent. However, the first consensus conference organised by the American government on caesareans[17] was able to confirm that caesarean mothers may experience the following reactions:

- fears about their baby's health
- relief that their labour is finally over and that the baby has been born
- feelings of impotence and loss of autonomy
- lower self-esteem, questions about their femininity and changing perceptions of body image
- the feeling that their physical integrity has been violated
- a feeling of jealousy towards other women
- difficulty coming to terms with the experience of birth
- difficulty establishing contact with their baby and even difficulty recognising it as their own baby
- a tendency to blame the baby (most of the time subconsciously)
- fear of giving birth again
- bereavement behaviour involving denial, anger, blaming and depression
- a feeling of guilt about negative feelings when everyone around is celebrating that the baby is healthy

One recent study[18] showed that some women suffer trauma after an unplanned caesarean and that health care professionals don't necessarily understand all the distress a woman can feel after this life event. Many women worry during their caesarean about what they're seeing, about the noises the surgical instruments make, and about the narrowness of the operating table. They're disturbed by the bright lights and the cold temperature in the operating theatre.[19] And if a woman's had a general anaesthetic (whether for a caesarean or a vaginal birth), it's possible that the woman will not be certain she's actually given birth to the baby she's given afterwards. Janelle Marquis, a nurse and antenatal teacher, said that women who don't expect to have a caesarean feel they've failed to give birth and that they attended antenatal classes for nothing. She says they feel disappointed about not having seen their baby being born. They often have difficulties breastfeeding because they've been separated from their baby. Women often tell her: "There's something missing in my experience of birth. Sometimes I have the impression the baby isn't mine. My experience of birth was stolen from me." She says she's often asked why their baby's birth wasn't videoed so that the mother and father can at least see the birth take place afterwards, on film.

According to Nancy Cohen, co-author of the first book about VBAC *Silent Knife* (Bergin & Garvey, 1983), nobody seems to realise that having a caesarean is more like becoming a baby oneself than becoming a mother, as experiences go. After a caesarean, women may feel as weak, powerless and frightened as a newborn baby.[20] In Cohen's view, the loss of confidence a woman experiences can affect her ability to look after her baby because some women are so preoccupied trying to understand what happened to them, they find it difficult to focus on their baby's needs. Three studies mentioned in *Cesarean Childbirth*[21] showed that parents who experienced a caesarean had more difficulty adjusting postnatally. Also, we mustn't forget that recovering after a caesarean is equivalent to recovery from any other abdominal surgery. Not only is it necessary to readjust physiologically to the hormonal changes which occur at the end of pregnancy, which are linked to breastfeeding, it's also necessary to get up during the night in the first few months and adjust to the lifestyle of being a parent.

Consider the impact on your family

According to a review in *ICEA News,*[22] a caesarean can interfere with family relationships for months or even years afterwards. According to Lynn Baptisti Richards, author of *The VBAC Experience* (Bergin & Garvey, 1987), a caesarean can affect a couple's life too,[23] particularly their sex life. She says a woman's libido may disappear and that she may experience pain during sex. She goes on to say that if a woman has really suffered on an emotional level as a result of the caesarean and if she feels she's really lost something in not having pushed out her own baby, her vagina may become constricted in places where she retains a certain emotional pain, which then transmutes into physical pain.

Women who've had a vaginal birth after a caesarean have told me how much their sex lives changed—for the better—after their VBAC. In *Transformation through Birth* (Greenwood Press 1984) author Claudia Panuthos emphasises that after a caesarean some women become very sensitive to the slightest violation of their physical integrity and may even react strongly to a simple bruise. Others feel their body 'close off' so as to prevent any subsequent violation. Even if all mothers who've had a caesarean don't experience these difficulties, at least some do. What effect did your caesarean have on you personally in terms of the way you relate to others?

Consider the impact on your partner

According to some studies and reports from couples who've had a caesarean, the only positive outcome of this intervention (apart from saving either mother or baby in some cases, of course) is that fathers often become far more involved postnatally. Many fathers develop a special relationship with their new baby, simply because they have to do this, given their partner's condition after the birth. But let's not forget that fathers also experience strong emotions during a difficult labour and birth. They are not indifferent to a painful labour which ends up being a caesarean birth. It seems their reactions also vary, just as their partner's do. They may feel relieved to see their partner and their baby safe and sound after a difficult birth; they may feel overjoyed at having been able to be present while the caesarean took place; they may feel angry towards caregivers if they were pushed out of the way and not given enough information; they may feel they were insufficiently prepared for the caesarean in antenatal classes; they may feel they were insufficiently prepared for the situation on their return home; they may feel guilty at thinking what their partner's been through; they may have feelings of impotence, deception, sadness and frustration.[24] Men—being less used to expressing their feelings—often find it more difficult to 'heal' from a caesarean, which they also experienced in their own way. Some men I spoke to admitted they'd hesitated for a long time before agreeing to have another baby. Others have difficulty understanding why their partner reacts so strongly to the caesarean.

Possible psychological effects of caesareans on mothers

According to the evidence-based organisation Childbirth Connection,[25] having a caesarean section, rather than a vaginal birth increases risks of the following:

- **Poor birth experience** A woman who's had a caesarean is very likely to rate her birth experience as being worse than a woman who's had a vaginal birth, both early on and later too. This is particularly the case when a woman's had an emergency caesarean. (Women who've had a vaginal birth, but with ventouse or forceps also tend to rate their experience worse than if they've managed to give birth without 'assistance'.) When a woman has a caesarean she is less likely to have her partner or other support people present at the birth and she's less likely to feel that she had any control over her birthing experience.

- **Less early contact with the baby** A woman who's had a caesarean is much less likely to see and hold her baby soon after the birth than a woman who's had a vaginal birth.

- **Unfavourable early reaction to the baby** Early on, a woman who's had a caesarean is more likely to have negative feelings about her baby and to evaluate her baby less favourably than a woman who's had a vaginal birth.

- **Depression** A woman who's had a caesarean may be at higher risk of depression than a woman who's had vaginal birth (although the evidence on this so far is mixed).

- **Psychological trauma** A woman who's had an unplanned caesarean during labour is more likely than other mothers to have traumatic symptoms (such as fear and anxiety) and to meet the criteria for post-traumatic stress disorder (PTSD). (Again, though, mothers who've had a vaginal birth, but with ventouse or forceps also tend to be at risk of PTSD.)

- **Poor overall mental health and self-esteem** A woman who's had a caesarean section may be at greater risk of having poorer overall mental health and lower self-esteem than a woman who's had a vaginal birth, although research carried out so far has not confirmed this.

- **Poor overall functioning** A woman who's had a caesarean may face greater challenges than a woman who's had a vaginal birth in terms of her physical and social functioning and in terms of her ability to carry out daily activities in the early weeks after the birth, although—again—there's not much research on this.

Consider the impact on your baby

Betsy MacKinnon, from the Departments of Clinical Epidemiology and Biostatistics at MacMaster University in Canada reported that paediatricians declared at the Canadian consensus conference on caesareans that this intervention affects the process of mother-baby attachment. In addition, some research which was published in 2008 showed—by means of magnetic resonance imaging carried out in the immediate postpartum period—that mothers who'd had a caesarean were less sensitive to their baby crying. This was demonstrated in terms of sensory processing, empathy, arousal, motivation, reward and habit-regulation circuits.[26] Reduced sensitivity may occur because the surgery which a caesarean involves tires the woman to the point of making her less present to her baby. Sometimes she will refuse to breastfeed, even if she'd intended to breastfeed before she went into labour. Women also sometimes have great difficulty breastfeeding after a caesarean for other reasons. In *Impact of Cesarean Childbirth* (Davis, 1981), author Dyanne Affonso emphasises the importance for parents of making peace with their caesarean in order to avoid projecting their negative feelings onto their baby. She says that if conflicting feelings are not resolved in the early days of the baby's life, it's more likely that tension and discomfort will become a feature of the relationship with the child.[27] One well-known study showed how there are sometimes difficulties in the formation of the mother-child relationship. Women—especially when they've had a general anaesthetic—were more hesitant about naming their baby.[28] I personally experienced this: my partner and I took two months to decide on a name for our son, who was born by caesarean with me under general anaesthetic, and we took just a few hours to name our daughter, who was born vaginally a few years later.

As for the babies themselves, there is very little research into long-term effects on development, after babies have been born by caesarean. Research usually looks at a period which is less than a year, and studies usually only consider a small number of babies. The document which was published after the first American conference on caesareans, which took place in 1979-80, concluded that 'generally speaking, the effects of caesareans on babies appear to be minimal and after 8 to 12 months there is no difference for the child, whether it was born vaginally or by caesarean."[29] Nevertheless, this report did mention that conclusions from research were only preliminary and that other studies should be carried out afterwards so as to confirm this conclusion. The effect of drugs administered to the mother during labour should also be the focus of other research studies, amongst other things.

According to Dr Michelle Harrisson, author of *A Woman in Residence* (Fawcett, 1993), we often forget that when a caesarean is carried out the baby has no warning that he is going to be taken out of the cosy environment of the uterus within a few minutes. If the caesarean was not preceded by several hours of labour, this may be a shock.[30] Studies which look at the area of prenatal and perinatal psychology[31] show that the fetus is not insensitive to what happens to him. For example, experiences of regression before birth under hypnosis indicate that the future baby is affected by events occurring at the time of his birth. Some authors[32] suggest that a 'body memory' exists which even goes back to uterine life. Other people suggest that how we are born may also have an impact on our personality.[33]

Even if the caesarean doesn't present any physical risk for either the woman or her baby, shouldn't the fact that it affects many women, couples and even whole families be enough to make us ensure that this surgery is only carried out when it's necessary?

Let yourself heal

As we've seen, a caesarean often leaves a scar which is not just physical. You may feel disappointed, if nothing else. Or the psychological wound may have been there for a long time and that may be the case even if the caesarean saved your life or helped your baby. A strong reaction is sometimes unconsciously linked with other losses experienced when you were young, which you have not yet mourned sufficiently. A difficult birth or a birth which ended up being a caesarean may have left you with a feeling of loss—since your dreams of giving birth naturally and seeing your baby born will have vanished. Perhaps you also regret not having shared this important life experience with your partner.

If you found your caesarean painful, it may remind you of other painful experiences you've had, or that you'll remember the experience again when similarly painful events occur in the future. These reactions can be compared to those you might have after a bereavement. You might be experiencing one or more of the following:

- Disbelief. You may be in a state of shock. You may have difficulty believing that what happened really did happen.
- Anger, frustration, irritation, envy, blame...
- Nostalgia for what you didn't experience.
- A desire to understand what happened.
- Depression. You may feel in a state of confusion. You may feel despairing.
- Acceptance. Life goes back to normal. You may be able to find a use for what you've experienced, so as to help other women.

It may take you months to go through these stages and it takes some women years. It may be a long time before you feel able to think back to what happened. As we've already noted, another pregnancy often makes feelings which have been repressed bubble up to the surface of the mind. And when women also develop post-traumatic stress disorder after a distressing birth or a caesarean it may take a while for these symptoms to emerge.[34] Nicette Jukelevics, author of the book *Understanding the Dangers of Cesarean Birth* (Praeger, 2008), does a good job of summarising how to recognise that this is happening. She says you may dream of your labour and birth; you may often think about it without being able to control these thoughts; you may want to avoid certain places, people or situations which remind you of that traumatic event. Some women have difficulty in their relationships with their children. Others have difficulty in their relationship with their partner[35] and some women even avoid sexual contact, for fear of getting pregnant again. Women who have post-traumatic stress disorder show signs of being in a hyper-vigilant state—they have difficulty sleeping and concentrating, they're irritable and they're easily startled. One woman wrote me recently, telling me how difficult it's been for her since she had a caesarean. She said that it had even affected the way she felt about her baby. She had been to see a doctor and a psychologist about her feelings, but they both reacted totally unhelpfully. They reminded her that her baby was healthy and that she should be happy about this and forget everything else. Having carried out a literature review in 2004 on childbirth and postpartum stress disorder, it seemed to me she might have post-traumatic stress disorder, so I told her this... and I gave her the name of some other psychologists. She consulted one and was very relieved when she was really listened to for the first time since her caesarean. She was also relieved when she was diagnosed as having a post-traumatic stress disorder.

One recent study[36] showed that it's normal for all women who've given birth to develop mental strategies for getting through this event, for them to experience moments during labour when they wish the experience could end, to not always be able to understand what's going on, to feel discouraged, frightened, overwhelmed. Women who develop post-traumatic stress disorder experience more moments during labour when they experience feelings of panic, anger, failure, and when they move into a state of disassociation during labour, and they more often think of death. After the birth, these women are less capable of remaining focused on the present moment. They experience a higher number of painful memories, invasive memories, moments of contemplation about birth. And we also mustn't forget that post-traumatic stress disorder can lead to depression, particularly when it's undiagnosed.[37]

Clearly, birth is not a neutral event which we need to hurry up and forget, simply reminding ourselves that we have 'a beautiful, healthy baby' (assuming that's the case). Any traumatic experience can make life particularly difficult. In the postnatal period and even over a longer period of time, women who've had a difficult experience may have several flashbacks to other previous traumatic experiences, they may have nightmares, they may become hyper-vigilant or anxious—and this all happens at a time when they have to look after a baby and, later, a child. Some women also report having a decreased desire to procreate and at the very least it usually takes these women longer to conceive another baby. Some of the women I interviewed said that nobody took care of their psychological needs during labour and birth and the attitude of their caregivers had a negative effect on them.

Nobody took care of their psychological needs during labour...

How can you heal yourself from a difficult previous birth?

So how can you heal yourself from a difficult previous birth? As I've already explained, one of the most important things you can do to help yourself 'digest' a difficult birth is to first try and understand what happened. Several authors of books about caesareans and VBACs, as well as midwives and antenatal teachers who work with women who've had a caesarean, believe that it's important—during a subsequent pregnancy or even before then—to understand what's happened. In order to do this, you may ask to see your medical records and, if you feel you need to, look through these with your consultant, talk about your records with people who won't judge you, or read up on the subject... The goal is to get to the point where you can make peace with this experience, which is often painful. This could 'liberate' the way for your next baby, particularly if the experience has left you still harbouring negative feelings. It's not easy, because it's a question of growing through the experience. You may re-experience painful feelings, but that may prove to be beneficial and it may help you prepare for a vaginal birth afterwards. The authors of *A Good Birth, A Safe Birth* (Harvard Common Press, 1992), Diana Korte and Roberta Scae, believe that negative emotions during labour increase grief, slow down labour and stop dilatation.[38] In the UK several hospitals offer women debriefing meetings. These meetings are available to any woman who wants to review her experience of birth, irrespective of how much time has passed since. (Sometimes it can be several years later.) Women meet a midwife and together they look through the woman's medical records, focusing on what happened during her labour and the woman gets the opportunity to share with the midwife how she's felt since the birth.

You may be wondering how you personally can determine whether or not you've unresolved issues relating to your caesarean... One revealing indicator may be your reactions to reading this book, or to other women's accounts of vaginal births. Perhaps you've recognised signs of trauma when reading some parts of this book. If you tend to avoid reading birth stories or even if these accounts, or births on TV, shock you, that could well indicate that you're not totally at peace with yourself. Another sign could be what you feel when you remember the caregivers who attended your previous birth. For example, you may feel angry or sad, or you may have the feeling of having been betrayed, or whatever. Yet another way of getting in touch with your emotions is to go through the process described on the next page, pausing whenever you feel it's a good idea to, and coming back to it more than one time if necessary, the same day or another day. Try to ensure you will have complete privacy and that you're not going to be disturbed when you try this. It's a good idea to begin the process right after you have done a deep body relaxation, so that more thoughts or emotions can emerge. And if it's too difficult emotionally, you may consider talking about it with a person close to you or consulting a psychologist to help you go through it.

- Think back to your caesarean(s). Consider the events which led up to the caesarean(s). (If there's more than one, think through them individually.)
- Feel the emotions you felt then again.
- Feel the emotions you've felt since then.
- Now relive the birth, seeing it as it could have happened, had circumstances been different. See how it could have been if your caregivers had known how to behave differently, if they'd been able to do so and if they'd *wished* to provide a different kind of care for you.

Reliving the pain of a 'failed' vaginal birth will not always be a painful experience. In time, wounds become scars and feelings fade away. There are ways of speeding up the process of really healing from a caesarean or from a difficult birth, even if you can't face having a vaginal birth—a VBAC.

Healing is a phenomenon which touches a person's whole being: mind, body and soul. This is what authors of one of the first articles on grieving and healing and childbirth, Deming and Comello, said on the subject: "In order to heal, the body needs rest, nourishment and exercise. The mind needs to understand what's happened. It needs facts, information. After a caesarean a woman may want to see her medical records, to discuss these with her doctor, speak to people who were present at the birth about what happened. The heart needs support and empathy from people who are around. The soul needs to make meaning out of this event in the person's life."[39]

So how can you personally heal? This is what I asked myself for a long time. I relived every stage of what happened and always had the impression I would never come to terms with it all. When I started writing this book, I still hurt a great deal inside. But in the end I understood that healing is a gradual process. I used various methods, following different people's advice, and I discovered other methods in a completely accidental way. After going through this experience myself, I've come to the conclusion that healing takes place after each layer of emotion has been reactivated and relived a sufficient number of times... Little by little you'll find you react less, you hurt less, and you'll eventually experience it all as being less dramatic. While a birth story will completely overwhelm you at first, gradually your sadness will decrease and in the end you'll only have tears in your eyes. Then you'll just be able to sigh when you hear the same kind of account and you'll be able to move on to something else. Finally, your pain will surface and diminish almost as soon as it's appeared.

Nevertheless, in order for this process to take place, you first of all need to admit that having a caesarean had an effect on you in some way. In order to become aware of this, it may be useful to write down everything you expected of your labour and birth before it took place, and all that didn't happen—what you were hoping for and expecting. Then you'll move on to the next stage, which is to express what you felt and still feel. In the realm of emotions, there is no control or logic. You'll feel what you feel—that's all. You'll feel as if you've been completely invaded by an emotion. You must try not to judge this emotion or judge yourself because of it. All your feelings are perfectly acceptable. The emotion can hurt nobody but you, if you let it fester inside you!

It's not always necessary to go and see a therapist. Talking about the caesarean, about the feelings it arouses in you, writing things down for your own sake, or writing to people who were present at the labour and birth may be helpful. Even if you don't send the letters, writing them should console you, whether you're writing to your partner, your consultant, your midwife or another member of staff. The point is to express to other people how you experienced things. Empty out your heart about what didn't work out. Also, consider speaking to people you trust, who you know will listen to you without judging you or dismissing your feelings. You can also read birth stories, cry as much as they make you cry, and watch videos or DVDs of births—believe me, that's an effective method! Reliving emotions such as sadness or anger is not easy to do, but it will liberate you. If you have too much difficulty doing any of this alone or with your partner, you may find it useful to consult a therapist after all.

Be aware, while you're doing all this, that it's not enough to just express emotions and feelings. Some people have inexhaustible 'reserves' of anger or sadness and they may feel angry about a caregiver for years and years—but that won't help much. It's you you're hurting with all this anger, especially if you do nothing about it. Get to the point where you can think about letting go, releasing your anger and sadness. For some women, this is even more difficult to do than expressing their anger or sadness. And it's not something you can do with your head. In this case, it's your heart which needs to respond, making the very difficult but liberating act of forgiveness. Forgive others for the errors they committed—that doesn't mean making excuses for them—and, above all else, forgive yourself for not having been 'on top of things', for having been so bad at enduring pain, for not having been capable of saying 'no' to one intervention or another, etc. In order to get to the point where you can forgive yourself you need to accept what happened and let go of thoughts, such as 'If only I'd done my exercises better, if only I hadn't worked so hard at the end of my pregnancy, if only I'd walked around more during my labour...' Doing all this may signal the beginning of peace inside you.

The author of *Living Through Personal Crisis* (Random House, 1992), Ann Kaiser Stearns, suggests that several questions can help you understand why you feel guilty. She suggests you think through the following questions so you can realise your innocence:

- At the moment when you gave birth, did you know what you know now?
- How could you have known or anticipated what would happen, when sometimes not even an expert can predict this?
- Do you sometimes blame yourself for what happened, as if the other people involved were not responsible in any way?
- Do you feel responsible for things which were totally beyond your control?

The final goal of healing is to arrive at a point where you can recognise that you did everything you could possibly do at that moment in time, where you can say to yourself: "I did that, I survived it and I learnt from the experience." Speaking personally, for a long time I was angry that I hadn't been able to resist a doctor who insisted on pulling my daughter out with forceps for no medical reason. In all that time—except in the few hours directly after the birth—I hadn't realised that I'd had a good labour and birth, without any medication or intervention of any kind, which had been in complete contrast to my first birth. Given the circumstances, I did everything I was capable of and that was already a great deal. Mourning after a difficult experience may be similar to what happens during labour... You can try and ignore what's happening, you can try and resist it, deny it's going on or fight it. Or you can abandon yourself to it and find within yourself strength and resources you never believed existed. These will help you to get through your pain and to give birth to a new life.

To summarise...

The emotional impact of a caesarean

- The impact of a caesarean or a vaginal birth which goes badly is under-estimated.
- Women generally tend not to speak to their doctors and other caregivers about the care they've received.
- It can take time to come to terms with a difficult experience of birth and to feel able to talk about it.
- People around the woman who's had a caesarean often show little empathy for any painful emotions she's experiencing.
- Health professionals don't necessarily understand the distress a woman can experience after a bad birthing experience.
- There is such a thing as 'post-traumatic stress disorder' after a difficult birth, which may well lead to depression if it's left untreated.
- The emotional impact of a caesarean can affect a couple's relationship and their relationship with their new baby.

Surviving a previous caesarean and creating a positive mindset

- It's possible to heal from an unpleasant experience of caesarean.
- It is necessary to mourn your loss of the experience you would have liked to have had.
- You need to try to understand what's happened.
- You may need to talk about it.
- You may need to recognise the signs that you harbour unresolved feelings.
- You may need to understand how the healing process takes place.
- You may need to try and forgive yourself and accept you did what you could.

Consider the emotional aftermath

The final goal of healing is to arrive at a point where you can recognise that you did everything you could possibly have done at that moment in time

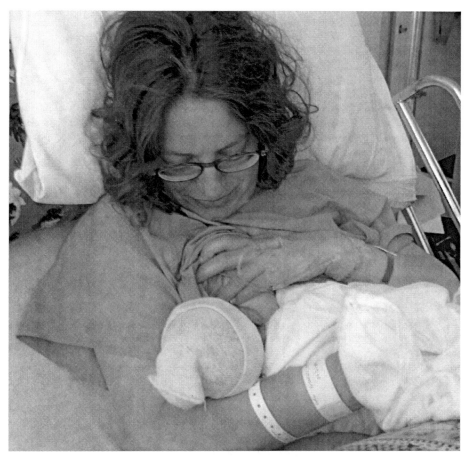

Here, Celine, who you read about in Birthframe 9, breastfeeds baby Greta, soon after she was born by caesarean

In the next chapter...

- Using the antenatal period wisely
- Finding a favourable birthplace
- Finding caregivers who are supportive of your aims
- Dealing with people around you

Birthframe 10

Dealing with the emotional aftermath

It was the year 2000. First pregnancy, first caesarean. Nobody else in my family had ever had a caesarean. I never thought it would happen to me and I wasn't prepared.

My first baby was born by caesarean because he was presenting feet first. I had a manual version a few weeks before the birth but a few days before my due date he decided to turn back again. The night before I had the caesarean I went into labour. I felt contractions, which confirmed to me that my baby was ready to arrive.

I was in a hospital which didn't facilitate things... Nevertheless, in the recovery room, I was able to have with me both the baby and its father. They left and I then had to wait ages for a midwife to finish her break and get organised so that I could be taken back into my room. The doctor had given me a massive dose of drugs, so both the baby and I were in a comatose state.

Breastfeeding was catastrophic. As far as the midwives were concerned, I was a caesarean mother so it was completely impossible for me to breastfeed. My baby only really took to breastfeeding when he was four months old. But I wasn't allowed *not* to breastfeed either so I was supported by midwives visiting from the local health centre, who gave lactation support. That was difficult. The physical pain from the operation, the comments I had from family and friends... "I see. You're both here. It's all over now. At least you're both alive. The baby's got such a beautiful round head!" For me it was not over at all. I felt bad about not feeling well and I had the impression that nobody understood the pain I was feeling about not having been able to have a normal birth.

The day I was discharged from hospital, I found a leaflet which talked about VBAC. I immediately knew that this was what I wanted for my next baby's birth. I already wanted to get pregnant again.

My baby was 11 months old when I got pregnant the second time. I got lots of information... I did my homework. I found a way of dealing with my head and my body healed. Then I chose the hospital. There was no question of returning to the first one. I asked lots of questions and went to visit several. It was 2001. I wasn't allowed to have a VBAC at a birth centre—so I chose a local hospital. During my pregnancy, my second baby was also in a transverse position. I had to resort to acupuncture and osteopathy in order to get my baby well-positioned. It was one of the doctors at the hospital I'd registered with who told me about acupuncture as a way of turning the baby. And the baby finally stayed in a good position.

My labour started late one evening. Then at 3 o'clock in the morning, my waters broke. At the hospital everything went well, despite being on a drip and having continuous electronic fetal monitoring. My labour progressed very quickly. My baby's heartbeat began to slow down and then resume its rhythm. I had to breathe all the time—I had to *think* about breathing. The midwife panicked and decided I'd need another caesarean. I didn't even think of demanding to see a consultant. I'd had all the preparation necessary for a caesarean—I'd been shaved, I'd had a catheter inserted and the midwives kept on repeating and confirming: "8cm, no 9cm..." But when the consultant arrived I already had the urge to push. And to him it was clear this was going to be a VBAC.

At 6 o'clock in the morning, after five pushes, my baby was there, in my arms, but I still felt desperately afraid they'd slit my stomach open for nothing. The moment I took my baby in my arms was the most beautiful moment of my life. He was here, in my arms. I'd succeeded! We'd succeeded. After nine months, I'd finally given birth! I was on my feet straight away—it was nothing like after the caesarean, even though I'd torn badly.

The first thing I did when I got home was to sit down on the floor and play with my toddler. I'd never have been able to do that if I'd had another caesarean. The baby's arrival was much easier than the first time because I was able to get on with everything, and breastfeeding was successful.

For the time being, I was very satisfied with my labour and birth but in retrospect I realised that quite a few things hadn't been how I would have wanted. So when I was pregnant with my third, I decided to contact a doula and, most importantly, to prepare a birth plan. This new pregnancy and labour were a fantastic experience. The midwife who was with me—Viviane—was marvellous. She respected my birth plan down to the last letter. My doula was there with me too, in case a slight problem should arise. The consultant understood my birth plan and understood what kind of birth I wanted and he even improved on it. For example, he left the cord to stop pulsating before clamping it. The baby arrived without any stress, without any worry and without me being on a drip. I felt so proud of my body. This baby was a little splash of sunshine and smiled all the time.

Our fourth little one decided to make our life a bit more complicated. I had acupuncture and osteopathy. Pregnancy was proceeding well. At my last antenatal appointment the baby was well-positioned. The next evening I went into labour. We went into the hospital. Everything was going well. The midwife examined me and found that the baby was high up, which was normal for me, since the two before had been like that too. I was 5cm dilated. She transferred me to the delivery suite. The doctor examined me. I was 7cm, but he couldn't feel the head. I started crying. I had a scan... the baby was in a transverse position but his hands, feet and umbilical cord were in the cervix. A caesarean was non-negotiable.

I cried. I'd been fine, the baby had been fine and I would have preferred to wait, change position, try and get him to move round... but it wasn't to be. For this last birth we wanted a very intimate atmosphere. That was why we hadn't hired the doula this time. Everything had gone so well the last time I'd thought we'd become experienced. I so much wanted someone to say to me: "You can say NO. Wait a bit!" Perhaps the caesarean really was inevitable, but maybe it could have been avoided. People close to me have said that I was really well taken care of, compared to my first caesarean. Me, I just cried... before, during, afterwards, then again later, and again and again... I cried! After all I'd done over seven years, to return to where I'd started... I saw my baby when he was born and for a few seconds I blamed him. I blamed myself for wanting to have him. Afterwards, I didn't see him again.

I was transferred to the recovery room without my baby. He was in intensive care. Several hours later, we learnt that he had a collapsed lung which had been caused by respiratory distress. My body hurt, my soul hurt, my heart bled. Why had all this happened? I was able to touch him with the tips of my fingers almost 12 hours later. He had tubes attached to various parts of his body and he was lying in an oxygen tent. And I felt awful too. A caesarean hurts for ages afterwards... It makes life difficult for a long time. Tiny glitches become enormous failures. Getting up, picking up your baby, breastfeeding, sleeping on your side, coughing, laughing...

That was a year ago now. The baby's absolutely fine. We've bonded very well. It didn't happen straight away, but as the days passed, as I breastfed and came into contact with him, we bonded. My scar still hurts. Adhesions drag at my body. I haven't regained all sensitivity in the skin on my stomach and, at the same time, I also still have a very sensitive abdomen. Some women see a smile in their scar, but I just see a disfigured stomach, an asymmetrical line. I hate my body. I still blame myself for not having refused the caesarean before trying to get him to move round.

I wasn't capable of announcing the good news of his birth. I had a lot of difficulties getting myself to smile again. I know very well that there are some women who can't have any children and others who never experience a VBAC. But knowing all that does nothing to relieve my suffering, the emptiness I feel inside, my pain, my grief at having missed those two opportunities to give birth.

Life goes on. The children are growing up. The days pass. But I attribute many of my current problems to my caesareans. I see a difference in attitudes between my children. First of all, a tiny change in their routines becomes an enormous problem to be overcome... With my last baby, I can't leave the room without him bursting into desperate tears. He won't tolerate any separation. My two VBAC babies are both children who are sure of themselves, who know very well how to adapt, without my help, to any kind of situation. Asthma too... From the age of six months onwards my caesarean babies have had asthma, unlike the other two who don't have it at all.

And in terms of sexuality, certain changes occurred after my first VBAC... I reassumed possession of my body. Many women are afraid of losing something when they give birth vaginally. I see it quite differently. I gained a lot... I became master of my own body. Now, my wound is still big. I need to heal and to find some confidence again. The only positive thing I can say about the caesarean is in terms of how it affects the father. I don't know if it's the obligation he felt to do more, or the fact that I just couldn't go on, but I gave him more space after the caesareans. Perhaps I wouldn't have been able to do that in other circumstances... He was very 'present' for the children, right from the beginning.

That's a bit of my history. Now, I just need to accept it. I experienced the most beautiful times of my life, and also the worst. I hope that one day I'll be able to find answers to all my questions. I hope to be able to come to terms with all my history, to appreciate every moment. I have a magnificent family and, of course, I have the most beautiful children in the whole wide world!

> Now I just need to accept it. I experienced the most
> beautiful times of my life... and also the worst.

Birthframe 11
Believing it was possible was the biggest barrier to overcome

Robert: The first baby was induced when she was 10 days overdue. After 24 hours of contractions every two minutes, the birth ended up being a caesarean because of failure to progress. Afterwards, we realised that even though we'd attended antenatal classes, we hadn't been ready psychologically. In any case, I certainly wasn't ready for Nicole's labour. We hadn't had the kind of preparation we later had for the first VBAC.

Nicole: During my first labour we were both very afraid. My sister had just lost a baby just after its birth, after 42 weeks of pregnancy. I started working to prepare myself psychologically during my second pregnancy. I did several rebirths and I realised that during my first labour I'd had a terrible fear of dying. In my second pregnancy I managed to control this fear but I still felt it when I gave birth—I was aware of it, but it didn't make me panic. In general we don't tend to realise that our own births can influence the way in which we give birth ourselves. Anyway, we did some things to allow ourselves to explore those feelings. I used to do a six-hour journey to a local centre and back, just so I could go and work through my problems while I was pregnant!

Robert: As soon as Nicole got pregnant for the second time, we talked about birth again. I felt resistant. For me it was a case of 'once a caesarean, always a caesarean'. Sometimes, it's also partners who need to reprogram themselves. You know, our children are precious, each one having been conceived after waiting for several years. Before we had our first one, we'd even started looking into adoption. I was worried about the risk of uterine rupture. I also couldn't help thinking how Nicole had been in labour for 24 hours and she hadn't opened up. I was wary of her desire to have a VBAC but in the end I didn't put up too much opposition. I said to myself: "She's got plenty of time to change her mind!" Nevertheless, I did do some psychological work alongside her. Our consultant certainly didn't want her to have a VBAC. He thought the baby's head was too big. When he was born the baby weighed 10lb 8oz (4.76kg) and he did have a big head. I was relieved. We were a bit disappointed to have a second caesarean, but since Nicole wasn't given a general anaesthetic it wasn't really too bad...

We did some of the preparation together, but what I found difficult was that the men usually didn't come along to those classes. Having children certainly makes a woman think, but it doesn't have the same effect on all men. And consultants aren't adequately prepared for birth either, in psychological terms. They're not trained to develop a good relationship with the woman they're going to be attending, with her partner or with the child who's going to be born.

Nicole: In my third pregnancy I continued to work on myself. At the beginning of my pregnancy, we moved house, Robert got a new job and he was often away. I was sorting out the house move on my own and I felt very tired. I decided to sign up for another self-development workshop which was called 'New Birth'—and I ended up bawling my eyes out all weekend. I just felt so bad! So when I was six months pregnant I decided to continue thinking about having a VBAC. I was actually determined to have a VBAC, but I somehow had trouble feeling in touch with this determination. Rebirthing helped me to make progress. Also, in the last few weeks of my pregnancy I went to see an acupuncturist and an osteopath. That did me a lot of good and my backache disappeared. In fact, during the last month of my pregnancy I felt better than I'd ever felt before.

Robert: One Friday evening I came home from work at 1 o'clock in the morning. Five minutes later, when I was giving Nicole her daily perineal massage, her contractions started.

Nicole: I'd spoken to the baby and I'd told him: "If you want your daddy to be there, sort it out! I myself have no power over him." But I was at peace with myself. It didn't matter what was going to happen—whether he was going to be there or not.

At 4 o'clock in the afternoon, my contractions started getting stronger and our doula arrived two hours later. She told Robert to go to bed and when he woke up at 7.30pm I was having a beer with her! I hadn't had one in five years. It tasted so good! That helped me to relax and I went from 2cm to 5cm in the space of an hour or an hour and a half. Then we went to the hospital.

During the first stage of labour everything was going well. Here and there I was saying, "Oh, it hurts so much!" but it was fine because I was dilating properly. I'd done a lot of visualisation during my pregnancy on dilation. I didn't have a drip or anything. Our doctor was on duty and it was the midwife who suggested to him that a drip wasn't really necessary. A few hours later I was completely dilated. I was relaxed.

Robert: We didn't want to have an epidural and in any case the consultant said it was out of the question. Personally, I knew we'd get there without one. The consultant was cool... During a few big contractions he said: "Oh, they all say it's their last baby!" That helped me to relax a bit. During this labour I felt very present to what was going on. I could see it was all very painful for Nicole but I'd realised that it didn't need to hurt me, just because Nicole was in pain. I was there to support her. That didn't stop me from crying, though!

Nicole: If you have support, you can do without any pain relief. What I found the hardest and the most surprising was pushing. I was in absolute misery and I didn't feel I was in control. At one moment a midwife said as much. She was rather harsh but I think I needed her to shake me up a bit. I pushed for 1 hour and 20 minutes. While I was pushing, if no one had been supporting me, I would have said: "Just give me a caesarean, because I'm not going to get through this!" In any case the consultant clearly wasn't bothered. He just said: "Don't get worked up. For a first baby women generally push for about an hour. You're doing your best, and that's fine." That really helped. And while I was pushing I felt as if my baby, who was upright in my abdomen, was also pushing a lot. I got the impression he was determined to be born. But at that point I still didn't believe I was going to manage to give birth. It's a good thing everyone around me thought I would! Then we saw the baby. I touched him when his head came out. When he was born, I took him and put him on my stomach. I hadn't had an episiotomy but I did tear a bit—I had three or four stitches, which I hardly felt afterwards. I controlled my pushing. The consultant let the cord keep pulsating for five minutes before cutting it. My placenta came out very quickly. All in all, my labour lasted 16 hours.

Afterwards, I felt so tired… but I still didn't believe I'd had a VBAC! It took me almost four days to realise it really was true. It really was possible for me too, to give birth just like other women. You see, up to a certain point during my second pregnancy, I had been preparing for a VBAC, but it hadn't happened. This time, I felt that even if I prepared I wouldn't succeed. That was the biggest barrier I had to overcome. After a few days, I said to myself: "Hey, listen, Nicole. Stop being stupid. Believe it's happened!"

Robert: Anyway, I believed it straight away! The doctors we'd seen antenatally and during labour had really believed that babies were supposed to come out through the vagina. That was all there was to it. And what happened for our second one—it really makes no difference whether it was a VBAC or a caesarean. For our third baby, in my opinion, we really did have a perfect birth. If we'd had another caesarean, our family would have been finished… But now, who knows?

Birthframe 12
Preparing differently and then deciding to trust the baby

My first pregnancy was completely straightforward. The same could not be said for the birth. After 30 hours of labour and after stopping at 3cm dilation, I had a pelvic exam and was told I had a narrow, funnel-shaped pelvis, which apparently sometimes means a baby has difficulty getting out. In fact, the baby never came down. The reason given for the caesarean was cephalo-pelvic disproportion, and I had it with an epidural.

Afterwards, I felt very disappointed and depressed. To me, it was a failure— perhaps the first one I'd experienced in my whole life. I told myself I should learn something from the whole experience. We never know why certain things happen in life. I thought I was going to give birth like a cat—I'd been so relaxed when I went into the hospital. I'd prepared well. I'd swum all through my pregnancy… All in all, it took me quite a while to recover from my caesarean psychologically.

The second time I got pregnant, I decided I wanted to have a VBAC. My consultant didn't agree and since I hadn't prepared or arranged support for myself, at the very last minute I got frightened and ended up having an elective caesarean. It turned out to be a big, 9lb (4.01kg) baby. I felt happy afterwards, though. I made all kinds of excuses—for example, I said: "I would never have been able to get such a big baby out through my vagina!"

The third birth was quite different. I prepared to have a normal birth but I thought, "Well, if I get frightened when I'm near my due date, I'll just have another caesarean. That's nothing to be frightened of." This time, though, I had more tools at my disposal to help me succeed and I really wanted to try. I found a different consultant who was fully in tune with me, who I really trusted. There was one condition, though, since I'd had two caesareans already: he agreed to go ahead with the VBAC as long as I gave birth before 39 and a half weeks. (According to my calculations and the scan, it was actually 40 weeks.) I told myself if I really wanted to give birth it would happen before 39 and a half weeks.

The main things I did that were different in this third pregnancy were to consult an osteopath to unblock my pelvis, do emotional work... and work to prepare like crazy! I really took care of myself and I also signed up for antenatal classes again, which I hadn't done in my second pregnancy. And two months before I was due I started having homeopathic treatments so as to make sure my labour went well. I was very determined, but I was also a bit frightened. I did trust my baby, though. I told him: "If you're supposed to be born that way, you'll get through somehow." I really communicated with him. Anyway, all my preparation didn't go to waste, it actually helped me. And even if the VBAC hadn't worked out it was good that the pregnancy had given me so many excuses to focus on myself.

Even if the VBAC hadn't worked out it was good that the pregnancy had given me so many excuses to focus on myself

During the last two months of my pregnancy I did a lot of visualisation. I visualised the hospital entrance, my room there, the early part of my labour. I visualised how I would feel when it started to hurt. I was afraid the pain would stop me from going ahead because it had really hurt in my first labour and the intensity of the pain had really surprised me. (I'd even yelled at the midwife who'd run my antenatal classes in that first pregnancy: "Why didn't you tell us it was going to hurt?") I visualised how I would feel all through. In my imagination I tried to get through the pain—to diffuse it, make it melt away—and I abandoned myself to it. I did all this with a cassette I'd made to help me do the visualisations.

The week before I went into hospital I was already 2cm dilated. (This was something which hadn't happened in my two previous pregnancies.) The previous Thursday, I'd had a session with my osteopath to help prepare me to go into labour.

It was Sunday when I went into the hospital—the date for my caesarean had arrived! In the evening, I went back home to have dinner with my husband, we went to the cinema, then off for a long walk and I even went to bed for a while before we went back into the hospital. By the time we got there, I realised I was having contractions... but I didn't say a word. My husband stayed with me at the hospital. Then at 2 o'clock in the morning, my waters broke.

They wanted to prep me for my caesarean but I immediately said: "I'm in labour. That's out of the question." At 5 o'clock in the morning I asked them to call my consultant. He arrived, looking a bit annoyed. Fortunately, he was pretty free that morning. My labour carried on progressing and, along with my husband, one midwife really helped me all through the day. She was a *real* midwife! My husband wanted me to have a VBAC even more than I did. He'd even told me to give birth at home. He helped me so much I could almost say he half gave birth for me. It really hurt, though! My relaxation cassette was virtually useless—it still hurt whether I listened to it or not! And I felt frightened too. I'd put on 50lb (23kg) during that pregnancy!

A few hours later I demanded another caesarean. I just couldn't go on. This time, it was the consultant who refused, because by that time I was already 5cm or 6cm dilated. He said: "You've been going on and on about having a VBAC—so don't bank on me giving you a caesarean."

My cervix was dilating 1cm an hour. The consultant gave me something to help me relax a bit and the midwife and my husband somehow gave me strength from outside, which I then lost again. Then at last I was 10cm... although the baby's head hadn't descended at all. The consultant said: "Now we're going to see whether or not it'll come through." I thought: "Don't tell me I've done all that work, only to be told now that I've got to have another caesarean."

I pushed for two hours, but it no longer hurt. At a certain point the consultant said: "You know, if you don't push better than that, it'll be a forceps birth." Finally, to my delight, the baby came out, 12 hours after my waters had broken. The consultant was happy and so was I! I flung my arms round his neck.

That birth was the most joyful thing I've ever experienced. In the photos I'm absolutely radiant. Giving birth gave me incredible energy. Two years later, that energy still hasn't left me. I hope all women will be able to experience that. We should all labour like that. The communication I had with my baby inside me had been very important. It was my son who gave me so much energy. When my fear washed over me again, I just trusted my baby. Of all my children he's the one I communicate with best.

That birth was the most joyful thing I've ever experienced

I don't know what happened... why I succeeded. Everything was on my side—from the consultant being free... the one I trusted. At one point during my labour I turned to him and said: "I hope you know what you're doing here!" The midwife also played an important part. She'd had a quick dinner so that she could get back to me. My husband too... Everything was perfect around me. And I was very determined. My consultant said: " You know, if you really want to do it, you'll be able to."

So how was this birth different? I accepted that I needed help. The first time it was me who was going to give birth. I was supposed to be capable of doing that! It was *my* pregnancy, *my* birth, and *my* daughter. I controlled so much. I didn't let my husband lift a finger until she was 2 years old! I was subconsciously on some kind of trip where I wanted to be completely independent—to control everything. I wanted to give birth vaginally but I wasn't focused on doing that (so perhaps that's why it didn't work out). I didn't realise it's also important to know how to let yourself go.

If I had to do it all over again, I would be attended by a midwife because midwives create a particular atmosphere during pregnancy and birth. I would also advise other women to have treatments in osteopathy. It's very physical and I really believe it's effective. I think those treatments I had really contributed to my VBAC success.

Nevertheless, they need to think of something to make labour hurt less! During my very first labour I realised that I'd never really experienced pain before. I didn't know what it was to experience suffering. I was healthy, though, and it had been a good pregnancy. I was sure I was going to give birth just as my mother had.

Basically, what I'm saying is that you have to *want* a VBAC in order for it to actually happen. Many women who'd also had two caesareans contacted me afterwards. I even met up with them. They'd chosen not to try for a VBAC so they experienced their pregnancies on another level. When it came down to it, they just couldn't change during their pregnancy.

138 birthing normally after a caesarean or two

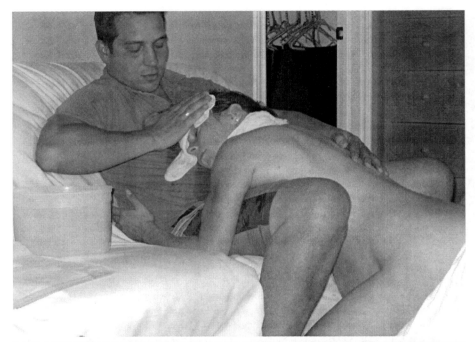

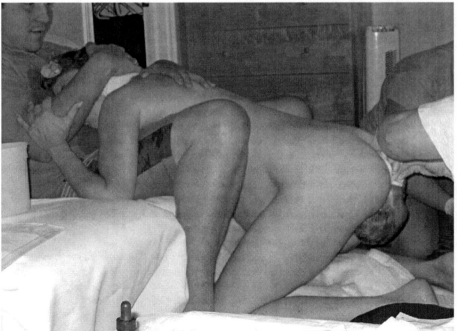

Above and right: Marie-Josée, from Birthframe 17, having a completely normal birth!

Consider the emotional aftermath

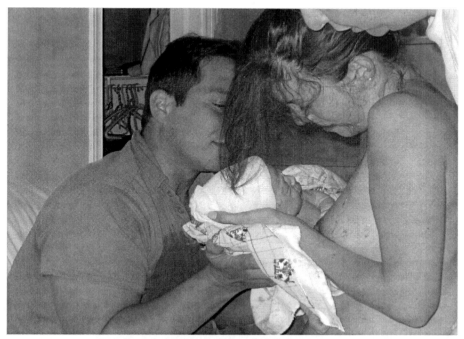

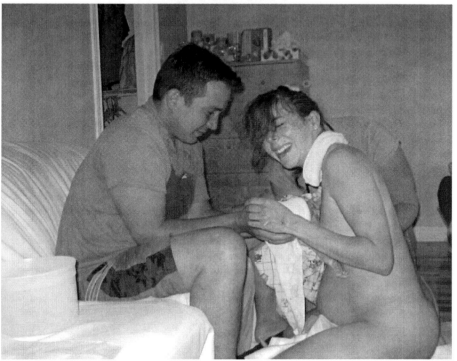

Birthframe 13

Experiencing a new kind of emotional landscape

A family of five turkeys crossed our hillside on the day of my second VBAC. I picked up a turkey feather from the roadside this afternoon, the third day of Sonja's life. A long, dark grey feather barred with brown. This has been a summer of wild turkeys, dozens of them, rushing through the treetops or disappearing into the woods as a car passed. This was my first outing since the morning of her birthday. The milk has come in, throbbing in my chest and drenching my shirt every time Sonja suckles at the other breast.

According to Native American belief, the wild turkey symbolises both gift and sacrifice: the bird that gives its body to feed the people. The animal medicine felt very fitting on that morning: a group of five on the day our fifth family member was born. And isn't birth always both a gift and a sacrifice?

The obvious metaphors are child as a gift and the mother's suffering as sacrifice. But giving birth is itself a gift so huge one longs to do it all over again, for this child or many more, the same way or a dozen different ways. Perhaps the sacrifice is to relinquish the babe that has become so much a part of my life and body, so close I know its every movement. And the gift: to hold her in my arms, to have her with me in a new way. Thank goodness caring for a new baby is so intense, so sensual—holding, feeding, changing, sleeping next to her. Otherwise the end of a pregnancy would be too big a loss, losing half of oneself.

The biggest lesson of this labour was the leap into the void, the moment when I let go completely. In the space of one contraction, my cervix went from 7cm to pushing. A few minutes later, she was born.

My labour began after an acupuncture treatment. The baby was already 12 days late. "Acupuncture won't start labour off unless the baby is really ready to come," my midwife Melissa told me. It was the most gruelling acupuncture treatment I've ever received. Axel used six pairs of needles: in the webbing between my thumb and forefinger, a point in my ears, in the big toe, in the shins, and two pairs in my belly. In previous acupuncture treatments I have never felt more than a light vibration at the needle site. This time, some of the needles caused a dull ache; others felt like an electric shock. The needles just below my navel didn't hurt, but the baby reacted to them with violent kicks.

"We need to make it uncomfortable for the baby," Axel said.

It wasn't so much the pain of it — I can stand quite a lot — but somehow the emotional energy from the treatment was very disturbing. I found myself in floods of tears halfway through. Perhaps this signalled the hormones of birth building up.

We were spending the summer in Vermont, a place full of family and memories for me. We stayed in my mother's summer house, where I spent many of my childhood summers. My grandmother, now 91 years old, still lives nearby. Two of my mother's three siblings also live not far away.

My husband and I had spent a lot of time debating the living arrangements, and the pros and cons of being far from our home in London for this birth. I had been pining for Vermont and family for years and at a certain point in the pregnancy it came to me that it was the place I wanted to spend the summer and bring this child into the world. The baby was due in mid-August. In order to travel while the airline would still allow it, I took my maternity leave from the financial firm where I work six weeks before the due date. My husband couldn't take so much time off from work, so I travelled on my own with the children. Our son Nikita, who was 7, and his sister Asya, 5, left school in London three weeks early.

Arriving in early July, we spent a few weeks visiting my dad's family farm in upstate New York, then stayed at my grandmother's house in North Pomfret visiting other relatives. But by the end of July I was eager to settle where I planned to give birth. I needed to feel at home there. I hadn't lived in the white clapboard house on Barber Hill Road since I was 14, the year we came back from Russia. My father had taken a sabbatical from *The Washington Post*, and was writing a book about his four years as Moscow correspondent. I have fond memories of that time, and still feel connected to the house through helping to renovate it. I still point proudly to the pegs I helped put in the floorboards, and the wallpaper I chose and helped to hang in my bedroom. It didn't take long for me to feel comfortable here.

My husband had arranged to take a whole month off from his London law firm — part holiday, part paternity leave. His parents wanted to spend time with their grandchildren, so we found a place for them to stay nearby. We considered having them stay with us, but we didn't want them underfoot, especially around the time of the birth.

I had hired a midwife sight-unseen following a thorough search via Internet, email and a number of telephone interviews. I chose Melissa Deas for the gentle and loving way she spoke about pregnancy and birth, as well as her self-sufficient approach. Before I arrived in Vermont in July, we had monthly phone 'check-ups' which I scheduled after each of the check-ups with the independent midwife I had originally hired in London.

I finally met Melissa a month before my due date. She works out of her house in Bristol, Vermont, nearly two hours' drive north from Pomfret. The only closer homebirth midwife I really liked, Ruth Richardson, was already booked up by the time I found her. She agreed to be our backup midwife. (Under Vermont regulation, a homebirth VBAC must be attended by two licensed midwives. Even though I had already had a successful vaginal birth following the caesarean, Ruth still needed to be there too.)

When I walked into Melissa's house for the first time, I was surprised to find not one but three women waiting for me. Melissa introduced herself and her two assistants, Heather and Olympia.

"One of my assistants will attend your birth with me," Melissa said. "Heather will probably come with me on the day. But I wanted to make sure you got to meet Olympia, too."

Heather was about my age, with two young children. Like me, she came from a previous career in the financial industry, but had recently enrolled in a midwifery degree program. Olympia was in her early 20s, grew up in California, and had been volunteering with Mexican migrant workers before apprenticing with Melissa.

More people I didn't know? And someone else had invited them to my labour? Shortly after this introduction, I burst into tears. I liked Melissa, but I was uneasy about the idea of extra people at the birth. After I got home that evening, I phoned her back and said I wasn't comfortable with Heather coming to my birth, but that it would be OK if Olympia came. Something about Heather made me nervous — I felt she had the same over-educated, over-articulate vibe I have myself. Too left-brain a person to have at my birth. Olympia felt calm and sunny to me. She exuded warmth.

During the following month I saw Melissa every week. I loved that one-and-a-quarter-hour drive across the state, over a mountain pass and into the little hippie town of Bristol. One week, both Melissa and Ruth visited us in Pomfret to make sure they could find the way when they came for the birth.

Pregnancy in the US was a completely new adventure! I decided for my own peace of mind to check out all my hospital options, in the unlikely event that I had to transfer. I felt I would be more easily able to lay aside any worries if I knew where to go if necessary. At a certain stage in the pregnancy I had been concerned that the baby was breech. I fully expected it to turn before the birth, but I felt that before I left for the US I needed to be sure I knew where I would have the baby if for some reason it hadn't turned. My London midwife was comfortable attending a breech at home. But under Vermont regulation, homebirth midwives are not permitted to attend a breech homebirth. I did actually locate a small hospital where the midwives and doctors said they would accept a vaginal breech birth in their birth centre, so I felt I could confidently travel to the US knowing I had all the bases covered. I also contacted Dartmouth Medical Center, the largest local hospital, where I planned to transfer in case of an unexpected emergency. I made an appointment to register with a consultant just in case. The visit was amusing. The new Dartmouth Medical Center is an enormous citadel a few miles outside of Hanover, New Hampshire. I found my way through a labyrinth of elevators and passages, and was duly shown into the consultant's office. I explained my complicated story: that I lived in London, was planning a homebirth in Vermont, but had come to see him to make sure I was registered at Dartmouth 'just in case.' After asking for a few vital statistics, the consultant asked me to lie down on the bed so he could check the baby. Without even asking my permission, he began to squirt conductive jelly on my middle. Apparently it never occurred to him that anyone would object to a Sonicaid. Fortunately, I could see it coming, having had a number of ultrasound tests before.

"Is that jelly for the Sonicaid?" I asked. "Please would you use a Pinard or fetoscope instead? I don't want to expose the baby to high-frequency Doppler ultrasound."

"What's a Pinard?" asked the pimply young medical student who was observing the appointment. The consultant explained to him, but had to confess that he had neither a Pinard nor a fetoscope available, but that if I didn't mind skipping it, that was fine with him. He advised me that it would be far preferable to have the baby in hospital, and said he was sure I would find the birth suite to my liking.

"Could I take a look?" I asked, so he gave me a personal tour.

"I hope we'll see you back here for the birth," he said as I left.

"I'll send you a postcard to let you know how it goes!"

Consider the emotional aftermath   143

Earlier, I had spoken to another Dartmouth consultant by phone, a woman who attended 'high-risk' births. I wanted to know the hospital's policy on breech birth. This doctor had told me that, although no one could absolutely force a woman to have a caesarean for a breech presentation, that it was hospital policy, and that they considered a managed breech delivery to be very dangerous. (So do I! 'Hands off the breech' is the safest way.) By the time I managed to reach her on the phone, the baby had actually turned head down, so it felt to me like a fairly moot point.

Her response pretty much summarised the American hospital approach.

"No, you're absolutely right to ask," said the doctor encouragingly. "It may be head down now. But you can't trust those babies!"

It was probably acupuncture that brought things on, since my labour began 14 hours later. Perhaps the baby would have come then anyway. The night after the treatment, I woke up at 2.30am feeling something wet between my legs.

"Oh no, my waters have gone and I'm not in labour," I thought. It turned out to be more of the mucus plug, which had begun to come out over the last several days. An hour later I began to feel cramps. By 4am I was having contractions. They came every 3 to 10 minutes, and lasted 20 to 30 seconds at first. By the time the rest of the family started waking up around 7.30, they were lasting 30-40 seconds, and still coming at about the same intervals.

My husband got the children dressed, and they all drove up the road to buy the paper. I put on my new hiking boots and went for a short hike up the hill to see if the light of day would end the contractions so I could get some sleep, as I had during my labour with Asya, my second baby and first VBAC.

It was an exquisite morning. I walked up the road a few hundred yards. At the edge of our property, I turned off the road and up the hill, backtracking towards the house. It felt good to go up such a steep hill. I paused to breathe through contractions when they came. They already felt fairly intense. The grass was heavy with dew, and my feet were soon soaked. I tried to remember every detail. Spider webs in the grass sparkled with dewdrops. The trees in the old orchard held a few dozen green apples. The last dairy cows left our pastures 10 years ago, and the barbed wire has all but disappeared among the old stone walls bordering the neighbours' property.

The contractions continued. I counted through each one: "One-one-thousand, two-one-thousand..." I climbed over the top of the first rise and looked down at the white clapboard house, the old garage, flowerbeds, green lawns, the swing I hung for the children the week we arrived. "This is going to be a daytime labour," I thought. "Maybe we'll meet this new person before tomorrow."

A new experience. With Nikita, my first baby, I had intermittent contractions all day, but never experienced strong labour at all. He was born by caesarean, leaving many unanswered questions. I laboured in the dark with Asya, two nights in a row, with a day's rest in between. She was born around 4.00am on the second morning. I had expected this labour to be similar.

I laboured in the dark with Asya, two nights in a row, with a day's rest in between. I'd expected this to be similar...

At the treeline I came upon a prickly bush covered with bright oval-shaped orange berries. I picked three sprigs. All the plants I encountered that morning made me think of autumn. I brought home an autumnal bouquet: twisty, dark stems of dried seeds from the rhubarb bed, purple burrs ripening on a leafy stem, crab apples, green, orange and red berries. "I thought this would be a summer baby. It's not—it's going to be a autumn baby."

I set my bouquet in an earthenware jug and took a picture of them to remember the day. Then I called Melissa.

"I took a walk to see if the contractions were going to stop, and they haven't," I reported.

"The other thing you can do is take a half-hour bath. If it's going to stop, that will sometimes do it," she said. (I was half-expecting this pre-labour to stop, as it had in my previous labour, and didn't want to make Melissa drive the two hours to Pomfret if nothing was happening.)

"OK, I'll report back after the bath," I said, somewhat reluctantly.

The contractions melted away in the hot water. I climbed into bed, hoping to fall asleep again after my sleepless night. As soon as I began to drift off, a new contraction began rolling in like gathering surf. After a few more, I got up again. No use.

My husband had got breakfast for the children. I ate what was left of the porridge. Mum picked up the kids to take them up to their Russian grandparents, who had rented a cottage a few miles up the road from us for the month of August.

"Call me if you need anything," Mum said. I had talked with her about supporting me during the birth. But in the event, I didn't really want her there. It had been the same with my other labours — in theory, I liked the idea of her being there. But she managed to miss all three of my births. I think I must have wanted it that way!

I called a few friends during the morning.

"Something's happening," I reported to my sister-in-law. She and my younger brother had their first baby in June. They tried everything in the book to bring on the labour. Long walks, hot sex, acupuncture—nothing worked. Castor oil finally brought him on, 14 days late, only hours before the hospital had threatened drastic measures to induce. Mum called me after their labour began, and we all waited breathlessly for news. My sister-in-law then called me early in the morning in London, just after Koa was born. I wanted to share this labour with them.

I also called my best friend Melissa in London. "I'm in labour!" I reported. I got to meet her third baby, Toby, the morning he was born at home last May. Melissa wouldn't get to meet this baby until weeks after the birth. Both of us were disappointed. I wanted to share the birth with her, too.

"Olympia and I are going to come on down to you in a few hours," Melissa told me when I called her next. "Seems like things are moving along."

After the children left, my husband and I took a walk up the road to the gate of Evergreen Glen. He talked on and on about trips we might go on someday, something he'd read in the paper, what a colleague told him. All I can remember is that I had even less to add than usual. "I wish he'd stop talking," I thought as I paused behind him on the road to breathe through a contraction. Walking up the road, the pain in the small of my back seemed not to let up even between contractions. Sometimes I held his hand through them, mostly just went through them on my own, counting to 30 or 40 over the peak. They seemed to be getting gradually longer and stronger. Probably I should have asked him to be quiet, but at the time I was too absorbed by what was happening in my own body to give directions.

On the way home, we sat down on a huge quartz boulder at the turn onto our road. It was such a relief to feel something solid under my bottom. Finally, a break from the pain in my back. We must have sat for 5 or 10 minutes. I had a few contractions, but they felt gentler.

I had a few contractions, but they felt gentler

Around 2.30, soon after we got home, Melissa and Olympia arrived, sooner than I had expected them. As soon as they arrived, my contractions ceased. "It's because I have an audience," I laughed sheepishly.

'Don't worry, that often happens," Melissa said.

My husband drove off for lunch with his parents and the kids, to give me time to settle with the midwives. Melissa checked my dilation at 3.08pm. I was only 3.5cm. I was a bit disappointed—the contractions had felt plenty strong to me.

We sat out on the steps in the sun. I wept with Melissa about my sadness at Nikita's caesarean birth, how I wished I'd been able to give him a better birth. I felt it was because I was so upset that he cried incessantly for two days after he was born. She said it was healthy that he cried, he was releasing the upset he felt, which meant he wouldn't carry it with him. It felt right to acknowledge my sadness about the caesarean during this labour.

The contractions still hadn't come back, so I went upstairs to try to take a nap, since I'd been up since 2.30am. Melissa and Olympia tactfully went outside to wait.

Almost as soon as I lay down, the contractions started up again. I lay down through a few, but it soon became too uncomfortable to lie still. I felt hungry, and got myself a bowl of cottage cheese and peaches, and a large glass of iced rooibos tea.

Melissa and Olympia were sitting on the lawn in the sun, reading the paper and talking. It was too hot in the sun, so we moved the garden chairs into the shade. I wanted to walk and move through contractions, but Melissa advised me not to if it made them seem more bearable. I should do whatever made the contractions more intense, even if it hurt more. If staying still did that, then it would make them more effective. (I'm not sure I agree with this advice. If contractions are more bearable, it seems to me it might make them more effective, because I would have to expend less energy trying not to panic, and might be able to go into the energy of opening more.) Melissa suggested I try to squat during contractions. She and Olympia took turns holding me up in a supported squat through rushes.

I threw up all the cottage cheese and iced tea on the grass near the swing. That afternoon the grass was strewn with early yellow leaves. "The vomit will blend in with the leaves," I thought.

My husband drove up. He held me through some contractions, and I leaned over him sitting in a chair for some.

Ruth, the backup midwife, arrived. She and my husband went upstairs to begin filling the pool. Looking back on it, I wish I hadn't let him walk away so soon. In the end, that was the only time that he was really supporting me during the labour, and it wasn't necessarily his fault that he wasn't there more. Maybe I should have let him be with me. I liked being able to hug him during contractions, he's so solid. Later, when I was pushing Sonja out, he asked if I wanted him nearer (he was sitting in a chair in the corner), and I said no. I don't regret his not being next to me at that point, because pushing was so overpowering, I didn't want any distractions. And I don't think he would have wanted to get too close. But I could have used his solidness near me earlier. But that's just where I was at that time in myself — resenting him and pushing him away most of the time. Who knows, perhaps there will be a next time. Or perhaps I will find other ways to be closer to him now, after the birth.

The birthing pool started leaking. My husband came out asking where to find the water pump. "In the room downstairs," I told him. He and Ruth bailed out the pool and started over again just around the time the sun sank below the edge of the hill. That's when the air always feels cooler and mosquitoes appear. We moved inside, around 7.00pm according to Melissa's notes. I needed the toilet, so she and I went into the downstairs bathroom. She suggested I try taking a shower while the others filled the pool again. I went to the toilet, but I felt almost afraid to get undressed and try something new. The contractions were so strong, the prospect of any change was frightening. It felt such a struggle to get through each new rush. "Can I really do it? How can I bear this?" I thought during each one. I felt panicky each time a new one came roaring in. They began with a strengthening ache in my lower back that reminded me of the early rushing of the surf around the ankles as a wave starts building up. "This one's going to drown me!"

'That's one contraction less that you need to get through," Melissa said after one finished.

'Thanks a whole lot!" I thought. "Infinity minus one is still infinity!"

I got into the shower, and for a little while it felt good, though the water was only lukewarm. All the hot had been used up and pumped out the window, when they'd been trying to fill the pool the first time. I dried off and put my dress on again, shivering after the cool shower. Melissa helped me climb the stairs, a frightening prospect in the middle of contractions.

"Let's check you out," she said. I clambered onto the bed. Only 7cm. Only 7? After all that pain?

"You'll be in transition soon," Melissa said.

"You smiled when I said that," she told me the next day.

"That means I'm almost there!" I was thinking. I pulled off my dress and, with Melissa supporting my elbow, climbed into the pool. It wasn't that deep, but it still felt good. I expected it to take the pain away completely, as it had during Asya's birth, but I still felt the intense pain in my lower back. Olympia was leaning over the pool. I grabbed her hand and pressed it to my back as hard as I could. I needed help, I couldn't get enough leverage on my own back.

"Want me to come closer?" My husband asked.

"No, it's OK," I said.

"Visualise your cervix fully open, passing back over the baby's head," Melissa said.

I was stepping into the birth pool.

"Visualise the baby's head entering the birth canal."

For the first time during this labour, I let go into the next contraction in spite of the pain. Up till then I was struggling to keep it together, to stay on the edge of the cliff, not to panic, not to scream, not to let the pain take me over. This time I leapt into the void. Transition happened in the space of that one contraction. By the end of it, I was pushing. Unlike the hour I spent pushing Asya out, this time pushing still hurt. It was acutely painful in a different way from the stabbing in my sacrum. I had to let it happen.

"Yes!" I shouted with the next push. It felt as though my whole body would turn inside out. A new wave of pushing rushed through me. "No," I whimpered. I was afraid. Then corrected myself as it came on stronger. "Yes!" I knew I had to affirm and accept this powerful process. With a pop and a bit of a sting, like a balloon bursting, I felt the waters breaking, and felt the whoosh as the fluid flowed out into the pool. I was on hands and knees in the pool, which was only about a third full. I pushed a few more times.

"I'm not going to miss feeling the head come out this time," I thought. I put my hands down, and as I pushed, there came a soft, bulging curve out between my legs. It felt too soft to be the head, all slippery. It slipped back in as the rush ended. Another rush came on, stronger and stronger. It was irresistible. I felt the burning stretch in my perineum as the head pushed against it. I did my best to think 'soft', to think 'gentle', as Melissa had told me I needed to, in order to prevent tearing. I pushed again. Oh! This time the bulge didn't go back in.

"The head's out!" I said in surprise.

"Lift your bottom up!" Melissa said. "I've got to check for a cord."

"You surprised us!" Melissa told me afterwards. "I thought, 'Well, I guess she wanted to catch this one herself.'"

The next push went on and on and on—shoulders, belly, long legs. The baby swam out into Melissa's hands behind me, and immediately began to cry. Who had just been born? I turned and awkwardly raised my leg over the baby and cord, and took it in my arms.

"I love you," I said to the small, surprised face with wide open eyes. The little body felt soft.

"I wonder who this person is," I thought to myself. "How wonderful to meet the baby as itself, before anyone defines it as 'boy' or 'girl.'" We all had decided this was going to be a boy.

I wanted to be sure to find out this baby's sex myself. That was a small regret I had about Asya's birth—our midwife announced she was a girl before I'd had a chance to find out for myself. "This time when the baby comes out, I don't want anyone to tell me what it is!" I told all the midwives, my husband and the children.

"This time when the baby comes out,
I don't want anyone to tell me what it is!"

I felt between the legs. I felt a soft little bottom, and two little bulges—more like a vulva than a scrotum. I wasn't totally sure, but it felt like a girl. I held the baby to my breast for her to suckle.

"The breathing sounds a little wet," Melissa said. "I think we need to suction her a little."

I looked at the baby's bottom. It was a girl.

"You promised not to tell me the sex!" I complained the next day.

"I usually refer to babies as 'she'," Melissa said. "And then it turned out it was a girl, and I thought, "Oh shoot, Nina will think I gave it away!'"

"It didn't matter, I already knew," I said.

I held the baby in the pool for a while

I held the baby in the pool for a while. I think Melissa suctioned some mucous out of her mouth and nose while I held her, but I didn't really notice. Someone put a hat on her to keep her warm. Melissa was concerned about the baby being warm enough, so she asked me to get out of the pool. It was only part full and the water wasn't very warm. Supported by the midwives and still holding the baby, I climbed up onto the bed.

Then my husband called the rest of the family. The two older kids and three of their four grandparents were a few miles up the road in North Pomfret, having dinner together and waiting for news. A little earlier my husband had called to say it would probably be a while yet — and here she was already. 10 minutes later the whole family arrived downstairs. My husband went down to see them. He planned to shoo his parents away until the next morning, but I asked him to let them wait downstairs while the children came up to meet their new sibling.

The children tiptoed in, their faces lit up with joy. Each carried a bouquet of wild flowers. "We picked them when Papa called," Nikita said.

They gazed in awe at their baby sister.

"So soft!" breathed Asya, gently stroking the baby's arm.

The placenta hadn't been born yet.

"Try giving a really good push and see what happens," Melissa suggested. I didn't feel any contractions, but I gave a push. Out slid the placenta onto a pie plate. Once no more blood seemed to be flowing through it, the children helped to clamp and cut the cord. I pulled off and ate a small piece of placenta to help my uterus clamp down, and we kept the rest for later.

(Nikita and I examined it in great detail a few days later, sitting on the step in the sun. Fascinating to see all those membranes and blood vessels that had protected and fed the baby all those months. Later I fried up a piece of it for my supper. Before I ate it, I thanked Sonja for nourishing me as I had nourished her. I offered my mother some of this ritual meal, but she politely declined. The rest of it I planted under three baby rose bushes.)

Melissa examined my perineum. "Yes, you've had a bit of a tear," she said. "She came out with her hand next to her face. That usually causes a tear, when the elbow comes through. That was the first thing I saw. Then I saw that the baby has dimples."

(I recently reread my story of Asya's birth. I had forgotten that my perineum tore in the same place when she was born. Perhaps she came out with her hand up, too?)

I put on a T-shirt and pulled up the bedclothes for the grandparents' visit. Grandpa was the most astounded of all. When his two sons were born in Moscow in the late 60s and early 70s, no fathers were allowed at births. Often fathers didn't even see their babies until several days or a week later. He got to see his new grandchild less than two hours after she was born. The two grandmothers were delighted, too. After a brief visit, they all tactfully left.

Once the grandparents had left, the midwives weighed the baby. 8lb 16oz. Because it was a second degree tear towards my anus, Melissa and Ruth decided to give me a few stitches. My husband held the baby and Nikita watched intently while the midwives worked on me. Asya felt sleepy and went off to bed.

By 11.00pm, everyone had gone. Nikita and Asya were sleeping in their room across the hall, and my husband was downstairs in the guest room. I gave the baby a change—my first time using the new cotton nappies I'd ordered earlier that month. Then the two of us settled into the big double bed. I left a night light on so I'd be able to see to check her and change her during the night. I kept opening my eyes to look at her and listen to her breathing. When she woke during the night, I breastfed her and we both went to sleep again.

The bed is a big, handmade platform bed, higher than most I've slept in. I had been tossing and turning in it all summer with only my belly for company. (I had banished my husband to the guest room downstairs early on, because I was sleeping so badly and the weather was terribly hot.) I would wake every few hours in the last weeks of the pregnancy and look out the window as the moon crossed the sky and the sun slowly rose over the woods. Two full moons had crossed that window while I carried her, and now here she was in my arms. A very peaceful feeling.

The next morning, the children came in early to visit their new baby sister. So little and perfect. Of course they squabbled over who got to hold her first. I reminded them that she wasn't going anywhere, so they'd have plenty more years to play with her.

Later that morning, my husband and I discussed her name. We'd been so certain the baby would be a boy, we hadn't even made a short list of girls' names. But just as with Asya's name, we both had the same idea: Sophia, in honour of my husband's paternal grandmother, who had died in the Siege of Leningrad when my husband's father was 6 years old. The baby's nickname would be the same as her namesake's: Sonja.

Afterthoughts...

It was a beautiful, joyous birth. I love Melissa and Olympia, and I loved the warm and protective atmosphere they created around me. I was happy that my husband wasn't that close to me at the time of the birth. I didn't feel he was in the way—I didn't particularly notice his presence. I also have no idea what Ruth was doing. I think she was in the room, but I wasn't aware of her at all. She is always lovely and quiet. Melissa is more proactive than someone like Michel would have been. For me, the main thing is I didn't feel intruded on. I didn't feel that I wanted anyone to leave the room. I had talked with my mother about having her be with me at the birth. In theory I also really wanted the children to be there, to share it with them but in the end it didn't happen.

Some people would probably say that's how it was meant to be. And I expect they'd be right!

The idea of 'going into the pain' seems to be a particularly American idea. You see that with some other women's birth stories—I assume they're told the most painful position will make the contractions more intense and therefore more effective. My midwife friend Sarinah also mentioned this idea with the birth of her first child a few years ago in Washington, DC—that her midwife asked her to go into the pain to help birth her son more effectively. This is quite the opposite of what many midwives and consultants would say, I think. If I had it to do over again, I would have walked around more instead of staying still. That may be part of why it was so painful. Possibly the fact that the baby had her hand by her face could have made it more painful—a non-standard presentation?

It's quite difficult to know what might have happened

Perhaps it was an unnecessary induction, but the acupuncture didn't cause the kind of problems that nipple-twiddling caused me with Nikita's birth. With Nikita, again, it's quite difficult to know what might have happened. From what I understand, it's supposed to take at least an hour of very steady nipple-twiddling to make enough oxytocin to do anything much. I only did it for 10 minutes before the waters went, so possibly it was going to happen anyway... Hard to say. He passed meconium about 12 hours later.

At the suggestion of my London midwife, I wrote to the hospital for a copy of my birth notes last year and went over them with her. I had always believed that the meconium was very light, no cause for alarm and that if I'd been at home with an independent midwife no transfer would have been necessary. (Of course, it would ALL have been different from start to finish if I'd had an independent midwife. I never would have felt time pressure if I'd been cared for by someone who knew me!) At any rate, Mal showed me from the notes that the meconium was a lot denser than I had thought, at least by the time I got to hospital, and according to the consultant on duty. So perhaps by that point he was distressed, and needed to come out. (Although his heart tones were fine as long as my contractions weren't being artificially induced, so perhaps he wasn't distressed...) At any rate, it was useful to me to go back over the caesarean as preparation for this birth. I seem to need to keep on working through the first birth in a new way with each subsequent one. I have also discussed it a lot with Nikita himself and now I feel less that I'll be saddling him with a lot of heavy baggage.

it was useful to me to go back over the caesarean as preparation for this birth. I seem to need to keep on working through the first birth in a new way with each subsequent one

So much to ponder with any birth!

Nina Klose

CHAPTER 5:

Create a supportive environment

This chapter is about preparing for your labour, so that you have the best possible circumstances in which to give birth. Nevertheless, if you're reading this very late on in your pregnancy and you feel it's too late to prepare, please remain optimistic... You may well find a caregiver who accepts your requests and an appropriate setting in which to give birth—you just need to persevere. If you're really far on in your pregnancy, it's still not too late to decide to have a vaginal birth, even when you arrive at the hospital, so be prepared to assert your rights, if you've decided you want to have a VBAC. Of course, some women have also succeeded in having a VBAC without any preparation, when they went into labour before the date the caesarean was booked for.

If you do have a lot or even only a little time to prepare, the more you do, the better. Many women have benefited from an atmosphere and conditions of labour which were very favourable... This chapter will give you some idea of what you can do and, of course, what you use from these suggestions will depend on your own personal situation.

Use the antenatal period wisely

If you want to optimise your chances of success—especially if any previous caesarean was performed as a result of 'failure to progress' or cephalo-pelvic disproportion—it's widely believed that the best approach is to prepare yourself well and have good support.[1] After all, giving birth vaginally after a caesarean is like climbing a mountain... and who would attempt that without a basic level of preparation?

Why, when and how can you prepare? Although I know—if you're reading this book—that you had a caesarean in the past, I don't know whether or not you have any experience of giving birth vaginally. Do you only have the experience of giving birth by caesarean? Whether or not your answer is yes, whether or not you found the experience of having a caesarean painful (either physically or emotionally), whether or not you accepted your caesarean(s) easily and whatever the reason for the caesarean(s), there's a high chance you don't have much confidence in your ability to give birth 'like other women', i.e. vaginally. Of this I'm quite sure. I've heard women who've already had a VBAC say: "If you've never done it that way, you don't know if you're capable of giving birth." Even if you believe that the baby was the reason for the caesarean(s), and not you, (e.g. because he or she was in a difficult position), there might still be a doubt in your mind right up to the last minute. Almost all women I interviewed confirmed this to me. Personally, I was actually in the process of pushing my baby out when I wondered out loud if I'd end up having another caesarean. Everyone laughed and said: "Just look what you're doing now! A caesarean's no longer a possibility."

Another reason to prepare earlier, rather than later is because finding a consultant and a hospital which supports VBAC may be difficult, so it's best to use all the time and opportunities available to you. Even though—during the 1990s—it looked like the climate was turning back towards favouring VBACs, the lowering of the VBAC rate since then in many hospitals (with many consultants) suggests the opposite is actually the case. This means you need to research your own local situation carefully while you're pregnant, even though this is even more tiring and stressful to do when you're pregnant than at other times. The current shortage of midwives no doubt makes this situation even worse... Ideally, in order to experience a calm and harmonious pregnancy you should have prepared before even getting pregnant! Nevertheless, finding a suitable birthplace and birth attendant always takes determination and sometimes it's necessary to be tough in the face of the refusals you're almost bound to face from some medical staff. Don't let yourself be discouraged by the horror stories you may hear illustrating the dangers of uterine rupture or the stories you hear about caregivers who are willing to let you have a trial of labour but want to impose numerous conditions.

Fortunately, particularly in large cities, the situation as regards VBAC is changing and more caregivers are up-to-date with the research. Nevertheless, some maternity hospitals still refuse to support VBACs and some women still have difficulty finding a consultant who will take them on. If you live in a rural area you're not necessarily at a disadvantage because a small local hospital may be more open to VBAC, because it represents a more humane option. However, if you don't fulfil your local hospital's conditions to be a VBAC candidate, you'll need to be as determined as women were a few years ago, when they encountered a complete refusal to contemplate any type of VBAC. Like those early pioneering women, you'll have to be well-informed... Perhaps you'll need to show your GP or consultant a copy of the NICE guidelines (which you can find at www.nice.org.uk by clicking on the 'Find Guidance' tab) or the guidelines from RCOG.[2] As long as your medical history doesn't put you firmly in one of the categories where a VBAC is clearly contraindicated, showing a potential caregiver the guidelines should provide them with some reassurance. (Also see pages 84—95 to see how easily you personally will be accepted for a VBAC.) It may also be helpful to find other women locally who've had a VBAC themselves because they'll be able to tell you the names of midwives, GPs or consultants who've supported VBACs in the past and they'll be able to provide you with contact details. To sum up, you need to be prepared for a search which isn't necessarily going to be easy!

Be prepared for a search which isn't necessarily going to be easy

Overall, when considering how you can prepare yourself during your pregnancy. there are as many ways of preparing for the adventure of birth as there are women on the planet. With this in mind, focus particularly on the following questions so as to establish what's important for you and your partner personally:

- Is it important to you to labour and give birth in a supportive environment?
- Do you both feel the need to prepare yourselves physically?
- Do you feel the need to prepare yourselves psychologically?
- How much do you need to familiarise yourselves with the processes of childbirth?
- How much do you feel you need to find out about ways of facilitating labour and birth effectively?
- Where would you prefer to give birth?
- What kind of support do you need to anticipate, so that you have help, if it's needed?
- What kind of caregiver would you prefer to have?

Consider finding some antenatal classes

To begin to help you consider these questions, it might be very helpful to attend antenatal classes, particularly if you didn't have any experience of labour before you had your previous caesarean(s). Having said that, if you're planning a VBAC I would suggest you choose a different type of course from the hospital-based ones which first-time mothers often attend, if at all possible. This is because many classes are, in fact, a kind of apprenticeship for submitting to the 'control' of labour which often takes place in a hospital environment, where intervention is the norm. You may also want to avoid classes which focus mainly on encouraging you to practise breathing exercises or intensive 'coaching' during the pushing phase.

In *Pregnant Feelings* (Celestial Arts, 1986), the author Rahima Baldwin explains how in our society women giving birth are often put on their backs and effectively cut off from their bodies, as well as from other women who've given birth already. She explains that since the world began birth has been seen under a male model of perception, as a phenomenon which needs to be controlled. This control, she explains, is accepted by women out of fear and a desire to be taken care of. According to this author, and many others, women submit themselves to machines, timetables and technology and even if they're conscious, they are only spectators at the birth of their own babies.[3]

Antenatal classes which are not based on coaching or controlling are usually run by midwives working in birth centres or midwifery-led units (attached to hospitals), or by independent doulas or antenatal teachers, many of whom are working within organisations which aim to promote normal birth, e.g. the NCT (National Childbirth Trust) and the Active Birth Centre. In these classes, not only is birth seen differently, the atmosphere is also different...

Women and couples are encouraged to talk about their feelings about their previous caesarean(s) and about any fears they're dealing with in their current pregnancy. Emphasis is also often put on making labour and birth an event for all the family to share—including the baby! In these classes you'll learn how to facilitate both the first and second stages of labour (the second stage being the pushing stage, of course). For example, you may be taught how to protect your perineum, how to push your baby out without forcing him out—without holding your breath and while letting yourself go completely.

Unfortunately, it's rarely possible to find antenatal classes which are specifically designed for the needs of women or couples preparing for a VBAC, but you may be able to find a course, or some other support of a similar nature in your area. Some therapists working with women have often confirmed the following similarities amongst women who've had a caesarean—and I must admit I recognise myself in this description! Frequently, these women are not very fit and they have a poor self-image in terms of their physique. They are not very in touch with their bodies, and they're usually are critical about their physical characteristics. They often show—in their life in general—a need to control things, as well as a certain resistance to change. Since these women are often over-educated, they've usually read a lot, but they have difficulty letting themselves go during labour, given the intensity of the experience.[4] If this description fits you too at all, it's perhaps easy to see why classes of some kind might be helpful.

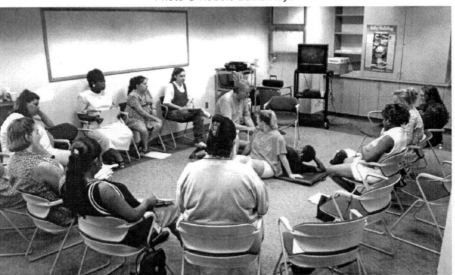

All kinds of women attend antenatal classes and they often help women to explore emotional and physical aspects of the birthing process

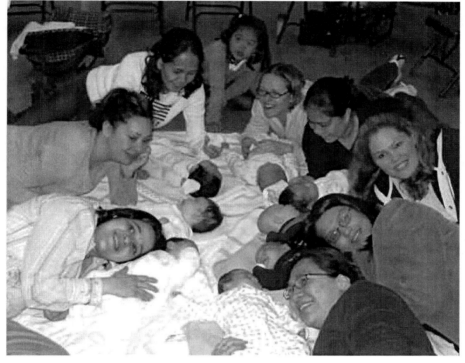

Women who prepare together antenatally often develop strong bonds of friendship. Here a group of women have a class reunion with their new babies.

Prepare physically

Pregnancy is a special time in your life for taking care of yourself... for the sake of your baby-to-be. You need to eat better, stop smoking (if you smoke), stop drinking alcohol (if you drink), take regular exercise and try to rest more often. There are plenty of books which will tell you how to have a beautiful baby and give birth to a healthy baby. You'll find them in any bookshop—so I won't spend too long on this subject. One which might help you prepare in all ways, not just physically, is *Birth: Countdown to Optimal* (2nd ed) (Fresh Heart, 2011).

Staying fit is particularly important if you're planning to have a VBAC because being fit and healthy will maximise your chance of giving birth normally. If your caesarean took place because you were overdue and didn't go into labour spontaneously, or if it was because of a difficult labour—e.g. failure to progress, involving irregular or ineffective contractions, or because your labour slowed down—eating as healthily as possible and doing regular exercise certainly won't do any harm... in fact, quite the opposite. You can also help nature along by familiarising yourself with techniques which help you stay relaxed and fit, for example following antenatal yoga classes, relaxation or gentle gymnastics, meditation, singing, dance... or even something unusual such as belly dancing. (Experts generally feel that belly dancing is perfectly healthy during pregnancy, although you're advised to move more gently during the third trimester when the hormone 'relaxin'—which is produced in higher quantitites then—may make your joints more susceptible to dislocation. Usually, there isn't a problem, though.) The most important thing is to learn how to relax and breathe more freely, without tension. Courses of different types are available in most areas and sometimes they're even adapted to the needs of pregnant women.

Caesarean women often lack confidence in their ability to give birth naturally afterwards, and our society—with its biomedical model of birth—does nothing to restore confidence to women

As I've said before, after a caesarean women often lack confidence in their ability to give birth naturally afterwards and our society—with its biomedical model of birth—does nothing to restore women's confidence.[5] Bearing this in mind, you might find it helpful to do something during your pregnancy which will help you to regain confidence in your body. This might involve taking up a form of physical exercise to strengthen your body, so that you have an experience of physical 'success' before you go into labour. Ideally, you need to take this up before even getting pregnant (because then you can choose any kind of physical activity whatever—because you can't do anything too athletic while you're pregnant.) Nevertheless, it's never too late to start, so consider what form(s) of exercise you can add to your weekly routine.

Certain types of therapy which focus on the muscular, skeletal aspect of physicality might also help to prepare you for a VBAC. I'm thinking here, for example, of something like osteopathy. A 'physically' oriented therapy like this might be particularly helpful if you had a caesarean because of failure to progress (with labour stopping or slowing down substantially, or because of malpresentation of the baby). In *Vaginal Birth After Caesarean* (Middlesex University Press, 2008) there's an account by a woman who finally had a VBAC after *four* caesareans—two of which were failed VBACs. She apparently went to an osteopath during her fifth pregnancy and he found that her pelvis was out of alignment, probably due to a skating accident years before. This seemed to explain why the baby had become malpositioned after previous good engagement at the beginning of labour. Following treatment by the osteopath, this woman's fifth labour ended in a successful VBAC. As well as osteopathy, there are also other physical methods, such as Bonapace[6]—see www.bonapace.com/en/—which may help you deal with the pain of contractions, or Janet Balaskas and other accredited Active Birth teachers teach antenatal yoga exercises, which may also help you prepare physically.[7]

Create a supportive environment

Photo © Regroupement Les Sages-Femmes du Québec, Canada

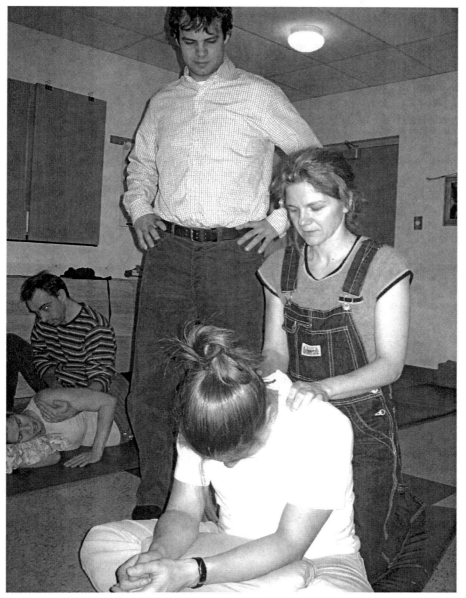

You may be able to find a suitable class in your local area for antenatal yoga, or even just massage—to help you relax!

Explore different options to help you prepare physically

Prepare mentally

Other psychological techniques, such as self-hypnosis, visualisation or meditation, may also be useful when preparing for a VBAC. It's a well-known fact that more and more athletes use 'mental conditioning' with the help of psychotherapists so as to prepare themselves for the challenges they subject themselves to. The technique of biofeedback is based on the idea that we're capable of influencing certain bodily functions or physiological events using our own minds. For example, using biofeedback it's possible to increase one's own temperature or even block painful sensations. Recently, self-hypnosis has been used more and more often to cope with the pain of contractions. Techniques taught by hypnobirthing teachers around the UK (and indeed around the world) have reportedly helped many women to have unmedicated vaginal births. (Check out www.hypnobirthing.co.uk for information about local teachers and classes.) Hypnosis during labour can have the following proven benefits:

- It can reduce the need for drug-based pain relief.
- It can make women feel they're experiencing less pain.
- It can shorten the length of labour.
- It can reduce or eliminate the need for induction or augmentation of labour using synthetic oxytocin (syntocinon).
- It can increase the number of spontaneous births, which take place without recourse to forceps or ventouse.[8]

> Psychological techniques, such as self-hypnosis, visualisation or meditation, may be useful when preparing for a VBAC

Visualisation is based both on auto-suggestion, the power of positive thought and on guided meditation. The related technique of using affirmations aims to increase a woman's confidence in her own ability to give birth, after negative beliefs which could inhibit her have been identified. It may be that some of our thoughts are sustained by emotional baggage (which we carry as a result of past experiences), which can influence us and even take control over certain aspects of our lives.

If you're interested in trying out visualisation, note first of all that this is very different from fantasising. While fantasising is about impossible dreams, visualisation implies a determination to obtain what is desired, as well as a desire to cultivate the belief that you'll be able to attain your wish. It's a useful technique because when an image becomes imprinted in our hearts and minds, it makes the subconscious sensitive to elements or situations which will help us reach our goal. According to Dr Maxwell Maltz, our nervous system cannot differentiate between an experience which is imagined and one that is real.[9] He has said that "When you see a thing clearly in your mind, the creative *success mechanism* within you takes over and does the job much better than if you'd done the same thing by conscious effort or *willpower.*"

Create a supportive environment   159

Alternate days of visualisation with days of positive affirmations

I've created the guided visualisation on the next two pages for you, in the hope that this will help you create an appropriate mindset. (Of course, this visualisation can be adapted to your own personal needs.) The approach I'm recommending was inspired by my own personal experience, as well as by work done on visualisation by Marie Lise Labonté, Gayle Paterson and Claudia Panuthos.[10] By the way, I suggest you don't try this visualisation until a few weeks before your due date. (You can spend the early weeks of your pregnancy coming to terms with your previous caesarean(s), if you like, in the ways I suggested in the last chapter.) When you're in the middle of your pregnancy, I suggest you repeat affirmations frequently, so as to change your deep-down negative beliefs. Then, a few weeks before you give birth, I suggest you use the visualisation overleaf, and perhaps alternate days of visualisation with days of positive affirmations, not mixing up the two because each type of mental work requires intense concentration. (I'll explain about affirmations soon.)

When you're ready to do a visualisation, make sure you have about 20 minutes of uninterrupted time. Do the visualisation once a day, or even twice each day, if you can. Sit in a quiet room on your own, where you know you won't be disturbed. Take the phone off the hook and turn off your mobile phone and mute any other computerised messaging services (e.g. incoming email alerts). Sit comfortably in an armchair or on a mat (e.g. a yoga mat). If possible, pre-record the text(s) overleaf so you can just be guided by your own voice. And when you read the texts out to record them, read slowly and softly, adjusting the intensity of your voice to the intensity of the work you feel will be required of you at each part of the visualisation. Pause whenever you feel a natural pause occurs in the text—so as to give yourself time to focus on the content. Use the present tense (and other immediate verb forms) as I have overleaf, so as to make everything seem more real. However, don't make the visualisation so powerful that it makes you go into premature labour! Beyond all this, note that each visualisation should consist of three stages:

- a period of relaxation which makes your body more receptive to what's suggested and which facilitates the work of the right side of the brain (which controls the imagination, sensations, etc)
- a period of careful visualisation, in which you see a scenario, as if you're watching a film on a large screen in front of your eyes
- a period of transition when you allow yourself to gradually come back to reality, to the room in which you find yourself

If thoughts go through your mind as you're doing the visualisation, just let them pass. (The more visualisation you do, the less you'll have a problem with invasive thoughts.) Some people find it easier to do this kind of exercise than others, but persistence is always helpful. If you have difficulty 'seeing' what's suggested, focus on making it real, on feeling it deep inside your being. If the visualisation triggers an emotion of any kind, don't block it... Just be aware of it and continue to breathe and to focus on the visualisation.

A visualisation to help you prepare for a birth which will go well...

First, let me relax...

I'm observing my breath. I'm breathing quietly and with each out breath I'm letting go of any tension I feel... I'm letting go of any stress. I'm going to take three separate slow breaths and after each successive out-breath I'm going to let go of a bit more tension... One... two... three...

Now I'm going to begin a journey into my body, so as to help each part of my body relax. My feet are relaxing. They're becoming heavier. They're becoming warm... Now I'm focusing on my calves... now my knees, now my thighs... my abdomen... my torso... my hands... my arms... my shoulders... I'm continuing to breathe gently.

Now I'm relaxing my head, releasing the tensions in my neck... I'm releasing any tension in my forehead... my eyes... my cheeks... my lips... my jaw... Next I'm relaxing my throat and breathing in, letting the air relax each organ in my torso: my lungs... my heart... my digestive system... my stomach... my pelvis... my genitals... my buttocks... I'm relaxing my neck... and my spine...

All my muscles are relaxing. I know my baby gets more oxygen when I breathe deeply and when I'm as relaxed as I am now. I'm feeling heavier and heavier... I'm sinking into a state of complete well-being. It's as if I'm floating on a cloud.

Now I'm going to focus on a positive scenario...

I can see myself at the end of my pregnancy. My baby is ready to be born. I'm going into labour. I'm in a place where I feel safe. I have the support I need so as to get through what's coming. Calmly, my contractions are becoming more and more regular. Each contraction feels more urgent than the one before. The contractions feel like menstrual cramps which are getting stronger and stronger. Each one is making my cervix draw up more and more. Now my contractions are making my cervix open up. Between each contraction, I'm relaxing and resting... My baby's head is pressing against my cervix. I can feel it. Now I can feel another contraction and this one, like the others, is also helping the cervix open up a bit more. It hurts but thanks to this work I'm doing my cervix is opening up more with each contraction... My body knows how to give birth. My contractions are coming one after another, like waves in the sea... getting stronger and stronger and they're still intense. They're invading my whole being, one after another... One... two... three... four... and they're becoming more and more intense.

Now my cervix is open—I'm fully dilated. My baby is moving down... More contractions are coming. They're helping the baby move through my vagina.

I'm relaxing between each contraction. When I feel it helps I get down on my knees, I make groaning sounds, I cry out... I vocalise in whatever way I want and my birth attendants and caregivers can hear me. These sounds tell them my labour is progressing well. I'm safe here and everything's going well. It hurts but the pain is normal and it means that my labour is progressing and my baby is getting himself born. The contractions are becoming stronger and stronger. It's as if my body's going to explode, the pressure is so great! I open myself up to my baby, who is now right near the opening into the outside world. After each contraction the baby pauses and rests. The contractions are massaging him and preparing him to breathe soon, outside my womb. My baby is now pressing against my perineum and that's beginning to stretch out, as it needs to. I feel an irresistible urge to push this baby out of my body. I breathe exactly as I want to, also panting if I want to, so as to give my perineum time to gently stretch out... Now I can feel a burning sensation so I know that in a few minutes my baby will be here. His hair is already visible. I'm helping my baby to come out, pushing as each contraction passes through me... One... two... three... There we are, he's arriving. I can see his hair in the mirror. I'm making another effort and his head comes out! Another contraction comes and his body slips out too. He's so beautiful! He looks up at me... He's lying on my stomach now. We did it! I feel so happy!

But, hang on—it's not all over yet. My womb is contracting again so as to release the placenta. Now it's contracting again to close itself up again over the next few days so as to go back to its usual size.

My baby is now lying on my chest, resting on my breasts. I feel so happy! Everyone around me is happy and everyone's congratulating me. I've done it! I've given birth to this baby vaginally. This baby has come out the way it was supposed to come. And it all went well.

Now I'm slowly going to return to the present moment...

I'm letting these last visual images fade away, as they do at the end of a film. I'm slowing coming back to the place where I started. I'm becoming aware of my breathing again—observing my breath as it comes in, then goes out again and I'm aware of noises around me. My baby isn't yet ready to be born. He'll know when it's time to come out.

Now I'm gently moving my hands and feet and when I feel ready I'm going to open my eyes.

I'm taking a few minutes to rest before I gently stand up and go back to my normal activities.

When you get to the end of the visualisation, you should feel relaxed and at peace. If you feel stressed out, there may be some kind of psychological block. Consider getting the help of a therapist so as to work out what is causing the block and so as to successfully work through it.

Even if you feel sceptical about the success of this visualisation process, take this beautiful journey every day (or every other day, with affirmations in the days in between). If you feel you need to, make changes to this visualisation, you could try, for example, imagining giving birth in a place which pleases you enormously, which makes you happy! And don't let any voices in your head discourage you. At least continue for a few days, even if only to find out how you feel afterwards.

Another approach, which is related to visualisation, is to use images to help you believe in positive scenarios. A woman called Nicole (who you can read about in Birthframe 11) drew a series of circles, which got bigger and bigger (going from 1cm to 10cm) and which represented the dilation of her cervix. She stuck these images on the wall of the room in which she was labouring. She also drew a series of illustrations which showed the progression of the baby from the womb, down through her body and out into the outside world… and Nicole had a VBAC after two previous caesareans. If you'd like to use some similar images, here they are in print—in case you're not an artist yourself. (Feel free to make copies and enlarge them too, if you want to.)

Dilation of the cervix, from 1cm to 10cm…

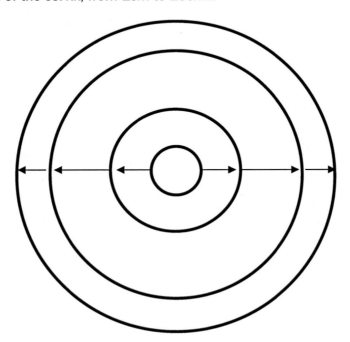

Create a supportive environment 163

The baby's descent down and out through your body

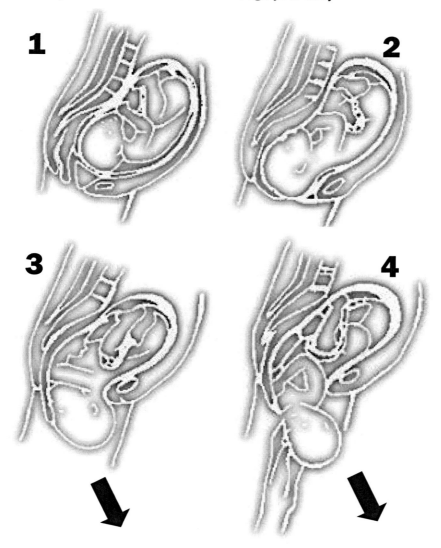

    Finally, meditation is another method of mental preparation you may want to consider. It may be a good way of calming your mind and coming to terms with some difficult emotions. You can get some information on meditation at www.dipa.dhamma.org, www.wccm.org and www.meditationexpert.co.uk.

Find the right birthplace

Although your choice of birthplace may go hand-in-hand with your choice of caregiver (because the two are often linked) you may prefer to start by choosing where you're going to give birth. If you do find an institution which is supportive of VBAC, where the staff are not worried by this prospect, you should then easily be able to locate a consultant or midwife who works in the same place, who will offer you support. Other women start by looking for a consultant or midwife who they feel in tune with, telling themselves that this person, and not the hospital where they work, will have the last word in their particular case. If all caregivers within that institution agree to respect your wishes, even if you're not their 'patient' or 'client', so much the better... but this isn't always the case. Personally, I'd prefer to choose an institution first of all, where VBAC is viewed positively, instead of finding a caregiver who supports it, who is alone in the conviction that it's an appropriate choice, and not always on duty—if I had the choice, of course. In 2010, the NIH Consensus Development Conference on VBAC emphasised among the factors influencing women's access to VBAC the caregivers and their attitudes towards VBAC.[11]

To get some initial information on options available to you, check out the Birth Choice UK website at www.birthchoiceuk.com When you have some possible places in mind, it's then helpful to find out about a hospital or birth centre's protocols as regards labour and birth in general, as well as the protocols relating to VBAC specifically. (In case you don't already know, a protocol is a rule or guideline which dictates the practices and requirements of a particular institution.) Your caregiver should be able to tell you about these—or, failing this, your doula or antenatal teacher may be able to help, if they're familiar with the practices of local institutions and the views of the management in each one. Here are some questions you can ask people, to find out more about protocols or guidelines which might affect you personally:

- What are your general protocols for a woman giving birth? What are they in the case of a planned VBAC? (Read Chapter 6 to get an idea of what kind of protocols you might need to find out about.)
- Are individual women's differences taken into account or are all women treated the same, irrespective of their wishes and personal situation? (In this respect, you need to be aware that you legally have the right for any kind of care and a midwife is supposed to act as your advocate. If you have trouble asserting your wishes when you're under the care of a midwife, ask to see the Supervisor of Midwives, who should be able to offer you support. If you're under the care of a consultant, you'll need to seek out another consultant who is happy to support you in your choices.)
- What's the caesarean rate at your institution?
- How many VBACs take place here each year?
- What percentage of vaginal births involve episiotomies, forceps or ventouse?

Create a supportive environment 165

- What's the perinatal mortality rate? (Here, you're asking how many babies die within 28 days of their birth. The current rate for the UK—according to the most recently available statistics—is 3.2 deaths per thousand live births. The postneonatal mortality rate, i.e. deaths between 28 days and one year, was 1.5 babies per thousand live births. 5.1 per thousand babies were stillborn, i.e. the rate was approximately 0.5%—that's 1 in every 200).

So as to get a better perspective for any statistics you hear, you can also consult the Birth Choice UK website (www.birthchoiceuk.com), as well as the Office for National Statistics website (at http://www.statistics.gov.uk/statbase/Product.asp?vlnk=6305) and the World Health Organization website (at http://www.who.int/reproductivehealth/en/). When you hear any statistics, also take into account the type of institution you're finding out about. After all, an institution which specialises in providing care for high risk cases will clearly have a higher caesarean rate than an ordinary hospital and it's also likely to have a higher perinatal mortality rate. (In 2001/2002 22% of births nationwide were caesarean deliveries,[12] which is high given the WHO recommendation that no more than 10—15% of all births should be caesareans.[13]) A low caesarean rate accompanied by acceptable statistics for perinatal mortality is a good sign. In any case, when considering statistics you need to bear in mind that the best results for both mother and baby could involve statistics which include a caesarean rate which is between 5% and 10%.[14] Caesarean rates higher than 15% are problematic...[15] According to the organisation Childbirth Connection, studies such as the one carried out by Johnson and Daviss, or the one conducted by Rooks, et al,[16] on healthy women experiencing low-risk pregnancies revealed low caesarean rates, and births which were generally without complications.[17]

Whatever response you get when you ask questions, do remember that you have a right to know what's going on in the field of obstetrics. In certain US states as a result of work by pressure groups who are promoting what they call the 'humanisation of childbirth', women expect to be informed of statistics for institutions where they register for care. In Massachusetts a law called the Maternity Information Act was even brought in. This stipulates that every hospital has to provide its pregnant clients with a leaflet including statistics about rates of obstetric interventions, as well as percentages of births in birth centres, and the number of women who breastfeed, etc. In the USA in 2007, another group was formed to collate information on all practices in maternity hospitals. The project (which was called 'Transparency in Maternity Care') also involved surveying women about their experience of giving birth. The objective was to collect data on all maternity facilities. This project was piloted in New York in 2007, the ultimate goal being to extend the survey to the whole of the USA.[18] Apart from these projects, more and more websites are appearing to allow patients to rate their doctors by filling out a questionnaire. (The Rate Your Doctor website at www.ratemds.com includes medical staff rated in the UK.)

166 birthing normally after a caesarean or two

As well as exploring statistics associated with a particular institution, you may also want to consider giving birth at a birth centre, or even in your own home. Many midwives in the UK are prepared to support homebirths, if that's what women prefer, and while they'll inform you of the risks involved—as they would in any other case—they should also provide you with good support. (See www.homebirth.org.uk for more information on homebirths and click on 'The VBAC Pages' to read about issues relevant to VBAC homebirth.).

As far as having a VBAC at home is concerned, only one small study has been carried out so far.[19] This looked at 57 women who'd had a VBAC in their own homes. Amongst these women there were no cases or uterine rupture, but given the small number of women considered and the absence of other studies, the authors of this study preferred not to recommend this option. Personally, I would hesitate to take this path. After all, although a homebirth VBAC presents fewer risks of iatrogenic uterine rupture (i.e. rupture caused by the behaviour of medical staff—e.g. as a result of interventions such as induction of labour), when rupture does occur there is a higher chance that outcomes will be poor—simply because a fast emergency caesarean can only be carried out in a hospital environment.

I have come across only one study about VBACs which take place in birth centres. The rate of uterine rupture was not high, but the authors of this study preferred not to encourage women to give birth in birth centres. In any case, some other academics criticised the conclusions of this study because they claimed the authors did not take sufficient account of the cumulative risks associated with having more than one caesarean. Other academics are of the opinion that women shouldn't be discouraged from having a VBAC at a birth centre in cases when they want more than one additional baby because the success rate in birth centres is higher than in maternity hospitals and the cumulative risks associated with having more than one caesarean (hysterectomy, breathing difficulties for the baby, serious placental problems, etc.) strongly suggest repeat caesareans should be discouraged. Quite apart from all this, birth centres generally also have much lower rates for all other kinds of interventions too.[20] Giving birth in a birth centre therefore seems to be a good option for most women wanting a VBAC. The study suggests that it's perhaps only inadvisable for women who've had two or more caesareans previously or whose labour is post-term (i.e. beginning after the woman's due date). Beyond that, any birth which takes place in a birth centre (or at home) needs to involve an agreement with a nearby maternity hospital—where emergency care can be provided, if necessary—and there needs to be excellent communication between the two places (i.e. phones and roads, or a flying squad which uses helicopters).

Always obtain the agreement of a nearby hospital

If you're interested in giving birth at home or in a birth centre, the most favourable situation is one which involves minimal risk of uterine rupture.

This means having had only one previous caesarean, an interval between this labour and the caesarean of at least 18 to 24 months, two-layer suturing technique used for the caesarean, a cross-sectional uterine segment measuring more than 2.3mm or 2.5mm and labour which is not post-dates (i.e. which doesn't take place beyond 40 weeks of pregnancy). In addition to these ideal preconditions, as we've already seen in previous chapters ideal in-labour conditions involve not having labour induced or augmented—so that the uterus is not put under undue pressure during ineffective contractions. Also, wherever you are, as I've already said, it's essential to make sure your caregivers have good back-up arrangements with a local hospital, in case there is a need for transfer. This also means that a consultant at the hospital will need to know when you're in labour so that he or she can be ready to welcome you and offer you care, if necessary, if ever a transfer to hospital became necessary.

Find a supportive caregiver

Whether you begin by finding a birthplace or focus on finding a caregiver first, it really is essential to find a GP, midwife or consultant who will agree to discuss the possibility of a VBAC with you, and who will encourage you to work towards this goal. Even if you're sure you want a VBAC, you may prefer to begin by finding a supportive caregiver. If you don't know any caregivers (and you're not sure where they're based), you can contact the following organisations to get some ideas:

- NCT—www.nct.org.uk
- AIMS—www.aims.org.uk
- Birth Choice UK—www.birthchoiceuk.com
- International Cesarean Awareness Netwework (ICAN)—www.ican-online.org
- Independent Midwives Association—www.independentmidwives.org.uk
- Doula UK—www.doula.org.uk

Another, less easy route is simply to phone around local hospitals and birthing facilities to check what their policies are on VBAC and to ask who usually attends VBACs. (You can obtain precise statistics on every hospital in the UK at Birth Choice UK (see above).) In the same way, you could phone around or visit local GP surgeries or community midwifery practices to see what response you get at other places locally, or simply ask around.

If any of the professionals you approach refuses to take you on, ask him or her to at least suggest another professional who is supportive of VBAC. According to Dr Walter Hannah, who used to be president of the SOGC, every caregiver should do that, at the very least. If this fails, approach midwives, instead of consultants or doctors, because they may well have a different attitude (as well as a good familiarity with local options for you)—since they're generally more focused on promoting normality in birth. In the unlikely event that no midwives, GPs or consultants in your area within a 300-mile radius will support you in your wish to have a VBAC, you can obviously not choose to have a vaginal birth unless you're prepared to travel further afield, as described in Birthframe 25. If there is no support locally and it is possible for you to travel further distances, it would be preferable because a caregiver who has experience of attending VBACs will believe in your objective, he or she will respond properly to all your questions and will think you have a good chance of achieving your goal.

In short, the ideal is to find a caregiver who considers birth a normal process, who has no *fear* of VBAC, who will only intervene when it is really necessary, and with whom you can have a good relationship. Finding out about any prospective caregiver's previous success rate with VBACs will do no harm and may give you an idea of whether or not a potential caregiver fits this description—but be aware that statistics are not always a reliable indicator, especially if the caregiver is a consultant whose clientele is mostly 'high risk'.

You need to take your search seriously because one factor which could prove to be very important in terms of your VBAC is the presence of a supportive caregiver, particularly if you're afraid of giving birth.[21] If you realise—even late on in pregnancy—that your relationship with your caregiver is deteriorating and your consultant or midwife is getting more and more nervous about the prospect of your VBAC, don't hesitate to go elsewhere to find someone else, if at all humanly possible. If you don't act on your intuition, even at a late stage in pregnancy, you may regret it afterwards, as I did about my caregiver for my VBAC. The caregiver you have can sometimes determine whether or not you'll have a vaginal birth or a caesarean at the end of your labour. If you're worried about transferring from GP care, remember that most women nowadays give birth with a caregiver who is not their usual GP. Also understand that care is rarely given by one person under a 'caseload' model (which involves a single, continuous caregiver)... In other words, you're likely to have a number of caregivers during your labour and birth, who are working on shifts. Nevertheless, be assured that your desire to have a VBAC will be written in your medical notes and that your main caregiver (whether a midwife, GP or consultant) will be supporting you in this choice if he or she has agreed to take you on. Any other caregiver who comes to attend you while you're in labour and giving birth is also obliged to support you in your choice to have a VBAC—so remind them of this, if necessary. It's a tragedy that some women who fervently want to have a vaginal birth are refused care which will help them do that right in the middle of their labours, simply because the consultant on duty is against VBAC... Remember you have the right to assert your wishes.

Many organisations, including the RCM (the Royal College of Midwives) and the NMC (the Nursing & Midwifery Council, which regulates midwives) have done a lot of work so as to protect women's right to give birth as they want to. However, the situation is far from ideal. I will not expand on this point, except to say that whatever type of birth you choose, you and your partner have the right to insist that it takes place according to your wishes (except, of course, in the case of an emergency, in which case it's necessary for action to be taken very quickly). Even when you have a VBAC you have the right to negotiate the birth you want. But it's far preferable to do this *before* you go into labour.

More than anything else, remember that giving birth is a family event and that a caregiver who sees birth as a normal, non-medical event will be helpful. If your caregiver sees birth in this way (which is increasingly the case), your chances of success will be much higher. This is simply because your caregiver will have confidence in your ability to give birth. He or she will know ways of helping nature along, when necessary, and will be unlikely to intervene impetuously. According to Nicolette Jukelevics, some medical experts believe that a large proportion of caesareans could have been avoided. One of the ways of preventing unnecessary caesareans is to ask questions about caesareans and VBAC. Here are some questions you can ask caregivers:[22]

- What are the immediate risks for both myself and my baby of having another caesarean?
- If I have another caesarean, how will this affect my future pregnancies and births?
- If the hospital where you work will not allow me to have a caesarean there, can you refer me to another hospital where a caregiver is likely to approve my request for a VBAC?
- What does your hospital do so as to help women avoid having unnecessary caesareans?

Photo © Robbie Davis-Floyd

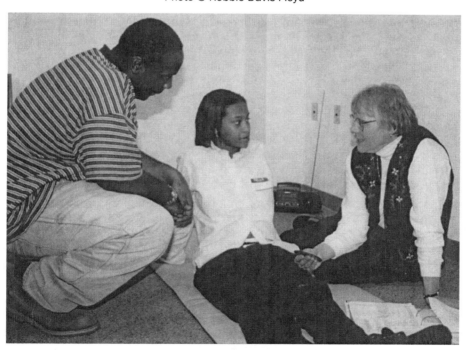

Discuss key issues with your potential caregivers and explore all your options

170 birthing normally after a caesarean or two

If ever you find yourself faced with caregivers who are clearly not supportive, remember you have the right to seek out new ones. Even though it's not easy to do, you can even change hospital in the middle of your labour. This is what one woman did... She told me that when she arrived at the hospital in active labour she was faced with staff who were refusing to let her have a vaginal birth. She left the hospital and travelled by car for one and a half hours so she could check herself into an institution which would agree to her request. Remember that it really is your right by law to refuse to have another caesarean—something it's not easy to do and which can trigger dramatic reactions from medical staff. Nevertheless, as I said, it is your legal right to refuse any treatment, including another caesarean.

Beyond all this, wherever you choose to give birth and whoever your main caregiver is, you may find it helpful to use the services of a doula. It was Dr John Kennell, co-author of the first studies on labour support, who pointed out the enormous benefit a doula can provide. If anyone said that a new drug or electronic device could reduce problems associated with fetal distress and labour progress to a third, or even that it would shorten labour by half and facilitate mother-baby interaction after the birth, there would be a stampede to make sure this new drug or equipment was available in every maternity unit in the country, whatever the cost involved. As Dr Kennell pointed out, this is exactly the benefit a doula can provide... Co-authors of one of the first books on VBAC, *Silent Knife* (Bergin and Garvey, 1983), Cohen and Estner, said they believed that when a woman begs for pain relief during labour, what she's really asking for is support. In fact, support during labour is a very important factor in determining the success (or otherwise) of a VBAC. Even more so than for an ordinary labour (when the woman has not had a previous caesarean), a woman who has chosen to have a vaginal birth after a caesarean generally needs to have at her side someone she can trust, who believes in her, and who will support her during her labour. For some women, a partner is the ideal person, but in the field of birth more and more people are beginning to question this. After all, it's a lot to put on a man's shoulders, particularly since he's also experienced a 'failure' in the past (when the previous caesarean was carried out). Besides, how can a man be an expert at birth? What about the fact that he'll need to rest from time to time and have something to eat...?

According to one report[23] about women and maternity, men have been assigned the role of bodyguard, supporter, lover, protector, masseur, etc... without even being asked if they really wanted to do all this during the birth of their child. These men, whose women want them to occupy a less traditional male role in other areas of their lives, are in fact assigned the very traditional role of being the 'strong' one. They're supposed to be insensitive to the pain their woman endures and they're supposed to help her 'be a good girl' and 'do it well'. This report points out that, confronted with a woman who is shocked by the intensity of contractions and who is overwhelmed by pain, it is the attitude of *availability* which gives the woman support, whatever happens. What helps is not pushing the woman to perform, but just being present... being *with* her, during her labour. They conclude that it's this that makes all the difference.

Create a supportive environment 171

Many people nowadays also question the value of 'coaching' during labour, which was traditionally also considered to be the man's task. In fact, even though labour might seem similar to a sporting event, best results in childbirth are not necessarily obtained by applying the methods which are appropriate in the world of sport. My first labour—which ended with a caesarean after 30 hours of labour—was fantastically well 'coached' by my partner. At that time we had a feeling of togetherness which I shall never forget, which remains my only good memory of this painful experience. Strangely, the second time, my most pressing need during labour was to have a woman at my side—a friend who was also a midwife. She knew I was capable of giving birth. She knew what giving birth was like and she held my hand for all the hours that we spent at the hospital. Contraction after contraction, she supported me and encouraged me—I had little courage and I often complained—but her constant support and encouragement meant I could continue without any drugs and get through to the end of my labour. My partner was there, of course, and if I gave birth again I'm sure we would experience another labour differently again. We would feel even more united because I know now—and he does too—that I'm capable of giving birth and that it won't kill me to do so!

According to the systematic review by Ellen Hodnett, a perinatal researcher, continuous support during labour and birth should be the norm, not the exception[24]—but think carefully about who will best be able to provide this support. Apart from your partner or a female friend, it could also be a doula, because—as I've already suggested this may offer you numerous advantages which have an important effect on the outcome of your next labouring and birthing experience.

Appreciate the benefits of getting the support you need

The question of support during labour has been extensively studied by researchers. Only *beneficial* effects have been found for mothers, babies and couples in terms of both short- and long-term outcomes when women have a doula around them while they're in labour and giving birth. All the research started when the paediatrician John Kennell and the neonatologist Marshall Klaus were carrying out research into bonding (i.e. mother-baby attachment) in Guatemala.[25] They noticed that the presence of a woman offering continuous support during labour had a significant impact on the mother, the birth itself and on the interaction between the mother and her baby. The effects of continuous support which have been most often studied relate to labour and the baby. Other positive effects relating to caregivers have been noted, even though these have been less of a focus of the research. Benefits include a decrease in amniotomy rates (i.e. women have their waters broken less often by caregivers), a lowering in the use of electronic fetal monitoring, less recourse to ventouse, higher rates of spontaneous births, less perinatal trauma (i.e. less tearing), more positive behaviour, increased maternal satisfaction, higher rates of breastfeeding and less postnatal depression.

To give you an idea of the scope of the research, in 2007 about 15 randomised controlled trials had been reviewed by the Cochrane Library. This covered more than 13,000 women.[26] (As you may know, a randomised controlled trail—also known as an RCT—compares two groups of randomly selected subjects, one group having one experience and the other not having this experience. This type of research is considered to be the most reliable of all scientific approaches.) It again confirmed the beneficial effects of continuous support, particularly when the doula was not part of the hospital staff, when the doula was present early on in labour and when her support was continuous, rather than intermittent. These results were the same in different countries (either developed or developing), with all types of women—in terms of their socio-economic status—with first-time mothers as well as with women who'd already had several babies.

Research has confirmed the beneficial effects of continuous support during labour by an independent doula

Let's look at the various benefits of continuous support in a little more detail...

- **The impact on labour...** As we've already noted, there are numerous important effects on labour. When a woman has continuous support from a doula her labour tends to be shorter and fewer interventions are usually involved, than when a woman labours alone.[27] The women's experience is more positive.[28] Women expressing their levels of satisfaction say that they feel they have accomplished something important, that they felt in control and that they felt taken care of.[29] This feeling of having been in control has also been confirmed by others, as well as a lower rate of postnatal depression.[30] Women who are accompanied during labour experience fewer feelings of anxiety and they feel less pain—and they also say they feel empowered.[31] In addition, they retain excellent memories of their experience of labour and birth.[32]
- **The impact on the baby...** Although a Cochrane systematic review does not conclude that continuous support makes a difference to Apgar scores, some research has shown that it does.[33] Continuous support during labour is followed by higher rates of exclusive breastfeeding,[34] and women also have fewer difficulties breastfeeding.[35]
- **The impact on the mother-baby relationship...** Improved bonding has been observed and there is increased incidence of behaviour which is considered 'maternal'. A woman who's had a doula seems to find it easier to mother her baby and she spends more time doing so. She also takes fewer days (2.9 days) developing an intimate relationship with her baby than a woman who had no continuous support (who typically takes 9.8 days).[36] The doula therefore serves to reinforce bonding behaviour between the new mother and her baby.[37]

- **The impact on the father...** When his partner has a doula during labour the father typically feels more comfortable and he also forms a better relationship with his new baby. Although men and their partners are sometimes afraid of having a doula at first,[38] the doula is usually later seen as being a real asset by the new father. In one randomised controlled trial all the fathers in the group who'd had the services of a doula found the doula's help extremely important. Several felt they wouldn't have survived the labour and birth without her presence.[39] Another study[40] also reported a positive impact of the presence of a doula on the father-baby relationship.

In our society we often forget that having a woman around when another woman is giving birth is a common phenomenon in non-industrialised societies. This kind of support reduces the anxiety the labouring woman feels.[41] This makes sense because in general it's widely accepted that at a time of stress the need for support from another human being increases in proportion to the amount of anxiety experienced...

If a woman in labour doesn't have this kind of support, she will need to depend on her own resources to face the situation she's in and her sense of reality may be affected. Being able to talk to another woman, look at her, be touched by loving hands and being kept company usually minimises any fear the labouring woman feels, it reinforces her sense of hope that the labour and birth will proceed well and it helps her to stay positive.

One study concluded that all women in a group of women who'd given birth vaginally had a support person of some kind during their labours and births, while 25% of the women who ended up having a caesarean had been alone in labour, and 33% had been alone during the pushing stage.[42] Perhaps the growing trend to have an epidural was also relevant because when a woman has an epidural midwives are less able to provide emotional support, simply because they are forced to focus on medical aspects of the labour.

When you arrange support for your own labour, ask to have at your side people who you've personally chosen. You don't need to choose between having either a doula or your partner. A doula—a friend who's already given birth and who feels confident that you can succeed in giving birth yourself, an antenatal teacher or a woman who has been trained to offer labour support—can ensure that your needs and requests are respected during your labour, although—by law—you need to make these clear yourself too. (This can, of course, be done before you go into labour through the use of a birth plan.) A competent person will increase your confidence in your ability to give birth because for her, the pain and intensity of contractions are normal, positive and necessary. The doula's presence and experience of birth, her knowledge of massage techniques which will console you and her awareness of positions which might be more comfortable for you and facilitate labour will help you to have a better experience overall and help you to work through your labour and birth successfully, right through to the birth.

Dealing with people around you effectively

When a woman starts saying she wants to have a VBAC people can react in very different ways. Even though VBACs have started to become well-known, many people still believe in the old maxim 'once a caesarean, always a caesarean'. They may worry about your decision and even try and talk you out of it. You can choose how you respond...

> ### When a woman starts saying she wants to have a VBAC people can react in very different ways

First of all, when dealing with other people's reactions it's essential not to allow yourself to be influenced by these reactions, which are no doubt caused by ignorance and prejudice, if not by other irrational causes. Next, you can choose either to ignore what other people say or to teach them about VBAC— particularly if the people are very dear to you. The International Childbirth Education Association (an American organisation) drew up a letter for people around the pregnant woman, which was called 'Yes, I'm having a VBAC'. You may want to write your own. This is a creative way of letting people close to you know your intentions. It will allow you to give them a little information but also you can ask them to respect your decision, even if they're not in agreement with your little adventure. Another approach is to say nothing to people around you about your intentions. This approach may help you avoid difficult situations. Alternatively, you can choose not to inform certain people.

> ### Ask people to respect your decision, even if they're not in agreement with your little adventure

For any labour and birth creating a favourable, supportive environment can only be a helpful thing to do. In the case of a VBAC it's particularly important— I would even say fundamentally important. Nevertheless, if for whatever reason you're unable to arrange 'ideal' conditions for your labour your own determination will help you to overcome any obstacles which may appear in your path. As one doctor I spoke to emphasised, what's important in the end is not your consultant, your midwife or other medical staff, but you—the woman who's giving birth. In his view, if a woman has confidence in herself she won't need her caregiver, or anybody else for that matter. Medical staff are only there to help... to reinforce your confidence. This might be particularly true if you've done all the other kinds of preparation mentioned before, so as to build your confidence in preparation for your upcoming VBAC.

> ### For any labour and birth, creating a favourable, supportive environment can only be a helpful thing to do. For a VBAC it's very important—I would even say fundamentally important.

Create a supportive environment 175

In conclusion...

When you're having a VBAC it's particularly important to take responsibility yourself and get all the information you need. One study, unsurprisingly, showed that women who like to be well-informed during their pregnancy and labour ask questions.[43] The study concluded that asking questions allows women to reassure themselves and take part in any decisions made which affect them. As a result, the study concluded, there is much less chance that these women's labours will end up as caesareans (when compared with women who put themselves passively into the hands of their caregivers). A passive attitude—when a woman keeps quiet about her needs and her intuitions, when she wants to be 'saved', when she gives herself up to others entirely—doesn't help women to have a fulfilling birthing experience. Taking responsibility for yourself means you need to do the following...

- Take care of yourself. Eat healthily. Stay fit. Find ways of relaxing which will help you give birth more easily. Perhaps focus on maintaining elasticity in your perineum by having your partner give you a daily perineal massage for the few weeks leading up to your labour. Research has shown it reduces the risk of damage to the perineum during the birth (i.e. tears).[44]
- Plan what kind of birthing experience you want to have, without forgetting that a caesarean may be necessary. Communicate your wishes clearly, firmly, and as many times as is necessary to get your preferences across to your caregivers. It might be helpful to write a birth plan.[45] You will find examples of birth plans in *Birth: Countdown to Optimal* (Fresh Heart, 2011)—where they're called 'care guides', and also online. Since the birth you're going to experience needs to be *your* birth, make sure you request whatever you want so that it proceeds according to your own tastes, except, of course, in the case of a real emergency. (In your birth plan you'll also be able to include what you would like to have happen if ever you have to have a caesarean.) Writing a birth plan will help you to clarify what you want and it'll also help you to establish agreement with your consultant or midwife in advance of your labour. It'll help you decide on the atmosphere you want and the kind of labour you want to experience, as well as the people who will support you during your labour and birth (midwives, other consultants if your personal consultant is not on duty)—and it'll help you to communicate all details clearly. Nevertheless, bear in mind that although the first birth plans appeared back in the 1970s, birth plans are not always well received by some caregivers or by certain hospitals. For this reason, amongst others, you might be advised to call yours a 'care guide', instead of a 'birth plan'.
- Ask as many questions as you need to, in order to feel satisfied. You may find the following webpage helpful when thinking of relevant questions: http://www.motherfriendly.org/pdf/Having_a_Baby-English.pdf
- Insist on being treated as an individual. Be prepared to change consultants or hospitals, if necessary.
- As well as doing so in writing, also communicate your wishes to your birth attendants verbally before your labour, as well as while it's going on.

To summarise...

Use the antenatal period wisely
- Consider attending some appropriate antenatal classes
- Prepare yourself physically
- Prepare yourself mentally

Find a favourable birthplace
- Find a hospital and find out what generally happens within hospital environments and in that one in particular.
- Consider also finding a birth centre. Arranging a VBAC in a birth centre increases the probability that you will, in fact, have a VBAC. This, in turn, will help you to avoid future caesareans and their complications. It's a particularly good idea to register at a birth centre if you want to have more than one additional child. However, a birth centre is not advisable if you have already had two or more caesareans, if you're overdue or in any of the situations which increase the risks of a VBAC (including induction).
- If you're considering a homebirth, take your circumstances into account.
- If you give birth at home or at a birth centre, make sure you have good back-up arrangements with a local hospital and/or emergency services.

Find caregivers who are supportive of your aims
- Find a consultant or midwife who is encouraging and ask him or her some good questions.
- Find a doula, because having a doula during labour and birth has been shown to be beneficial.

Deal with people around you
- Decide whether or not you're going to talk to people about your plan to have a VBAC.
- If you do decide to talk to other people, inform people you're close to about your planned VBAC.
- Consider writing a letter for use with people who ask about your plans, so as to save yourself repeating the same things with numerous people.

In the next chapter...

- Things to avoid, ideally, if you want to optimise your chances of avoiding another caesarean
- Things to do to facilitate a vaginal birth
- Frequently asked questions about labour and birth

Create a supportive environment   177

Birthframe 14
Getting different treatment from different caregivers

I had my first baby by caesarean. I knew in advance the baby was breech, but my consultant wanted me to experience a few hours of labour in case the baby turned round. He told me I had a very good pelvis.

The consultant gave me an appointment to have a contraction stress test (a CST), but without any warning he raised the level of syntocinon in the drip and my contractions continued. I didn't realise what he was doing and it took me completely by surprise. My sister stayed with me... After four hours my cervix had dilated to 7cm. Half an hour later, I was given a caesarean under general anaesthetic. I'd refused to have an epidural because that kind of anaesthesia had given my sister terrible headaches, which had kept her in bed and kept her out of action for several days.

I had to wait four hours before I could see my baby

I had to wait four hours before I could see my baby—a daughter. I felt 'disconnected' from her. She was a stranger to me. I felt as if I was in a different world. I think that was because of the anaesthetic. Unlike my later births (which were vaginal), for weeks afterwards I had enormous difficulty staying awake at night so as to be able to feed my new daughter.

Postnatally, I recovered fairly well. For two months I stayed at my mother's. Of course, because of the incision I had to take it easy for a few weeks. Since my daughter was mostly unresponsive in those early weeks, I asked the hospital what her Apgar score had been. They didn't want to tell me. After six months, though, they said the first score had been 1. Apparently, at birth, her pulse had been very low and she'd had to be stimulated. That worried me a lot, even though I have to say she's fine now.

Two years later, I found I was expecting my second baby. Around that time I heard some women talking about giving birth vaginally after a previous caesarean. I thought, "Why not?" I started looking for a doula so I'd have some support before and during labour. She gave me lots of information about birth and told me about a herb which is supposed to help labour along—raspberry leaf, which is infused in water and drunk as a tea. I also did Kegel exercises, went swimming and attended some antenatal classes.

My contractions started at around 10 o'clock one evening. At midnight I had a hot bath, then at 2 o'clock in the morning I went to the hospital—the same one as before—armed with a pot of tea and some honey. My contractions were coming every 5 minutes and I vomited a few times—but by 6 o'clock in the morning I was completely dilated.

Suzanne, my doula, helped me a lot. She massaged me and stopped me from panicking. She encouraged me to try different positions, helped me to visualise what was going to happen—she told me the cervix was opening up, etc. Finally, I got taken down to the delivery suite, where I was left, lying on my back. It was a while before I felt the urge to push. I felt like going to sleep. The consultant said: "If you don't hurry up, we'll have to give you a caesarean!"

"If you don't hurry up, we'll have to give you a caesarean!"

178 birthing normally after a caesarean or two

After an hour and a half they used forceps because the baby wasn't completely engaged. Then I had the urge to push and after a few long pushes, I managed to get my baby out—she was a big girl and in wonderful shape. I kept her on my body for a while, while I was given a few stitches (because of the episiotomy). They were in a hurry though when they'd finished sewing me up and they didn't want me to breastfeed her straight away—so they took her into the nursery for a few hours.

While I'd stayed in hospital for six days after the caesarean, this time I was able to leave after just two days. It was a good experience giving birth like that. I felt very proud of myself and I appreciated the presence of the doula enormously. That's support I would recommend to anybody! After the birth I felt much more agile and alert. Everything was easier. I had help for two or three weeks, but it was still hectic because having a 3-year-old and a baby is not restful!

The third time, I got pregnant unexpectedly when the baby was 13 months old. I decided to change to another consultant because the first one had been difficult to get hold of and he hadn't given me enough time at appointments. A friend recommended a consultant at another hospital. This consultant's clients always had vaginal births, he gave them plenty of time and attention and he also let them talk about any worries or difficulties when they were pregnant—or even about life in general… It was so much better! Apart from that, I did nothing to prepare, except perhaps eat well. With two children on my hands, I didn't have time!

Since I was almost 37, the consultant gave me a scan when I was four or five months' pregnant. It showed that everything was perfect. Two weeks before my due date my labour started with some vague cramps, which were rather like period pains. I took a hot bath, went back to bed and then at 5 o'clock in the morning my contractions got stronger. I couldn't get hold of my doula—the phones weren't working—so I called my brother-in-law, who took me along to the hospital.

As usual, I had my pot of tea with me. Labouring on my own at the hospital, my contractions became very intense. A junior doctor came along wanting to break my waters. I didn't let him do it. I was constantly experiencing low backache (I seemed to have a trapped nerve), so I asked for a sedative. He wouldn't let me have one, though, because I was nearly fully dilated. A midwife just popped in to give me a few words of encouragement every now and then. After all, it was my second vaginal birth!

At 7 o'clock in the morning my consultant arrived and I was fully dilated. Then, quite unexpectedly, my mother turned up. She was with me during the 20 to 25 minutes I was in the delivery room and she saw the baby arrive, after the consultant had massaged my perineum. That gave me the urge to push—I was still holding back a bit because of all the pain in my back—and the baby came out very quickly. I didn't even have an episiotomy.

My mother was impressed by this consultant—by the way he behaved, by his confidence. I loved having him look after me.

My mother was impressed by this consultant—by the way he behaved, by his confidence. (She'd had five children and had seen all sorts!) As for me, I loved having him look after me.

Create a supportive environment 179

Birthframe 15

Resentment because of the way in which decisions were made

On 2 July 2008, when I was 37 weeks' pregnant plus a few days, I attended an appointment with the consultant who was looking after me during this second pregnancy. I felt confident because everything had gone well from the beginning, and I had prepared well for my VBAC. So I asked the questions that came into my head... Mostly, I wanted to know if she thought it'd be possible for me to have my longed-for VBAC all the same, if another consultant was on duty on the day. I had even taken the trouble to arrange for a doula to be with us. I'd done a lot of work on myself during this pregnancy, I often talked to my baby and I'd been impatiently waiting for this particular appointment because it was sure to be one of my last ones. But when I was at the appointment, my blood pressure was a bit high. The most important one in terms of diagnosing pre-eclampsia is the lower figure and that was about 90. But since there was a bit of protein in my urine, my consultant decided to run me through an assessment for pre-eclampsia. So the next day I started off a 24-hour urine culture, as instructed, and returned to the hospital to have a blood sample taken, to have my blood pressure checked and to have the baby monitored. The baby was fine (the readout was perfect), my blood pressure was high at first, but the two other times it was a little lower. My blood samples tested fine. So I didn't have the well-known signs of pre-eclampsia which were present during my first pregnancy... no flashing lights before the eyes, no headaches, no feeling of pressure in my chest.

When I'd taken the 24-hour urine culture back in, early in the morning, I soon had the results... Around 10.15am a woman phoned from me at home, telling me I had to go back into the hospital again straight away and that I had to take my suitcase with me. Apparently, Dr X, who was standing in for my own consultant, wanted to see me because she'd seen my records. I was told my protein levels were so high they required immediate admission. The woman who phoned told me that she didn't know if Dr X would put me on complete bed rest or if she would get me to see a urologist (to check for a kidney infection), or if she would do something else. I woke up my husband, who was asleep—he was working nights—we finished packing my suitcase and went into the hospital, confident that we'd see Dr X there.

When we arrived at the maternity unit, I told a midwife that we were expected by Dr X. She immediately told another midwife to settle me into the recovery room and told us that Dr Y, a gynaecologist, was going to give me a caesarean straight away. She also said she didn't want any trouble from us... Those were her precise words! I also heard her say that they were waiting for another patient, which Dr X would see as soon as she arrived. My first reaction was to reply that Dr X needed to see *us* and that she needed to examine *me*. The midwife told me that because of my records and my test results I was going to have a caesarean. I just couldn't believe it! After all we'd done, someone *else* had decided that I was going to have a caesarean? Without even explaining why?

Someone else had decided I was going to have a caesarean? Without even explaining why?

My husband called our doula, who came in straight away. While we were waiting for her to arrive I saw the gynaecologist and asked her several questions. I wanted to know about the risks of having a uterine rupture, which she claimed were 1 in a 1000. Then I asked what the risks were of having a repeat caesarean, compared to the risk of having a uterine rupture. All she said was that it was for my health, that nowadays fewer and fewer people were having VBACs because the risks were too high. Although I was upset and angry at being treated like this, I told her that I'd been preparing for a VBAC with my consultant and that two days earlier she'd told me my cervix was favourable and that, because of the test results, we could try an induction. I asked if Dr Y could at least examine my cervix. She did but said it was well and truly closed and that induction was impossible. Once more, she said the caesarean was for my own health. Even my doula, who'd arrived while this was going on, tried to get some answers to our questions, but without success.

> Even my doula, who'd arrived while this was going on, tried to get some answers to our questions, but without success

What makes me angry is the fact that their decision was taken before I'd even arrived. They simply didn't leave me any choice. For sure, for a moment I thought about getting a second opinion at another hospital, but when she said my health was at risk, that they wanted to save both me and the baby, it was difficult to think clearly. Now I keep telling myself, "I have a beautiful baby, who is healthy." But why do I have the feeling they stole my labour from me? Why do I feel they ought to have done a better job of answering my questions, that they should have given me some statistics and reasons for this intervention? Why didn't I feel I had the right to refuse this caesarean? Why hadn't I been able to see my consultant or her stand-in?

I was promised I'd be able to have skin-to-skin contact with my baby and that my husband would be able to too. They also said my baby would be with me in the recovery room. Instead of all that, I only saw my baby again several hours after the birth, but I decided not to let it get to me. I just clutched this baby, who'd been such a wanted child. I rocked him lots and gave him all my love so that I wouldn't have to relive what I'd experienced with my daughter. For me, this birth was meant to be wonderful... It was supposed to turn me into a real mother through the first mother-baby contact, because that had been impossible when I'd given birth the first time by caesarean. I'd been waiting for this contact between me and my son for months and even though it hadn't been possible for it to take place in the first few minutes or hours after his birth, I certainly caught up for lost time afterwards.

Now that he's 10 days old, my son only stops crying when he's pressed up against me and that's my biggest achievement. Today, I've resolved to talk to as many mothers as possible about VBAC, so as to give them information about it and make them understand that it is possible to have one. I'm going to urge them to be better informed than I was... I don't want them to have the birth they've so wanted stolen away from them.

> I'm going to urge other women to be better informed than I was so they don't have their birth stolen away from them

Birthframe 16
Having trouble finding support, but getting there in the end

I had my first baby by caesarean after 12 hours of labour. The baby was a face presentation. According to the consultant who attended me, the caesarean might not have been necessary...

During my second pregnancy I made contact with about 20 consultants by telephone and I also met four of them personally. I wanted to know not only if they supported VBAC, but also if they'd already had clients who'd had one. I found this whole process very difficult. Quite a few of the consultants couldn't see me for several months because they were simply too busy. Often, I was told: "Yes, it's possible"—but there was no conviction in their voices. In the end, it was my physiotherapist who found me a consultant! I'd thought it was essential to actually visit hospitals and even meet the staff at each one. I also contacted local birth groups, who helped a lot, and I read a lot about VBAC. So in the end I found a hospital I liked because the consultant we'd found worked there, and two other consultants at that hospital were also positive about VBAC. I liked the way I was welcomed and the sensitivity of the team. Nevertheless, I got the impression, judging from everyone's reactions, that even if they did do VBAC in theory, they certainly didn't do them very often in practice. Also, the consultant I'd registered with told me that if I wanted to have a VBAC he'd prefer me to give birth during the daytime and not at a weekend!

Fortunately, after 2 hours 40 minutes of active labour, I did give birth vaginally one Friday at 3.50pm... When I'd arrived at the hospital, the staff hadn't believed I was in labour—I was in such a good mood and so relaxed. They were really worried because I was 'The VBAC', but my consultant was fine—he was 65 years old and very laid back. The only thing I didn't like about him was the way he spoke when I was pushing. He said: "Push, or you'll have to have another caesarean!" Another thing I didn't like was that I was put on a drip (even though I'd asked not to have one in my birth plan). Also, against my wishes, I had a shot of anaesthetic in my vagina which didn't wear off until four hours after the birth... Nevertheless, by that time I had my baby on my stomach. It's funny, but I got his name mixed up and used his sister's name. It was as if I'd finally completed her birth in having this one. It was as if this birth had a dual purpose. And I felt fine—happy.

Afterwards, there were moments when I couldn't believe it had really happened. My husband thought it was all wonderful. (He'd also suffered during the first birth.) When I'd had my caesarean (which I had under general anaesthetic) he'd been told to leave the room. We'd both had to go into therapy afterwards to help us heal from the experience, because it had been so painful. My husband was happy to see that I was fine after this birth. And to think at first he'd thought I was being silly when I'd said I wanted to have a VBAC!

But I would never have thought it'd be so difficult to find a consultant who would take me on for a VBAC. After all, the only reason I had to have a caesarean the first time round was malpositioning—that's all.

Birthframe 17

Developing increasing confidence in supportive environments

When I was at university, I took several courses relating to the medicalisation of women's bodies. This meant I developed a fairly strong view about medicalised labour. At that time, I didn't yet want to have any children, but I already knew that I would never want to give birth in a hospital.

When we were expecting our first baby in 2001, Sebastian and I decided to use the services of a midwife who was well-recognised within the community. At that time it wasn't legally possible to use the services of a birth centre if a woman was planning a home birth.

We prepared for this birth in a very innocent way, having wonderful confidence in life. Then, when I was 34 weeks' pregnant, my GP said our baby was presenting bottom first and he allowed us to confirm this with the help of a scan. When I was 35 weeks' pregnant, it was confirmed: the baby was breech! All the same, I continued to have confidence in my baby. After all, the birth itself was still a long way away!

Our midwife suggested acupuncture and osteopathy, so I went along for several appointments over a period of six days. Unfortunately, though, my labour started spontaneously a week later, at 36 weeks, and the baby was still breech. We chose to go into the hospital, because we thought it was possible that my wish for a vaginal birth would be respected there. In the end, the baby didn't have her chin flexed on the sternum so we were told it was possible her chin would get stuck in the cervix. So we decided to opt for a caesarean.

Even after this disappointment and the grief we felt about a birth which hadn't taken place, I never had a single doubt about my ability to give birth, to have a baby. My first meeting with Maxine hadn't taken place in the way I would have wanted but I knew that meeting me was only part of the process.

In 2003, when we were expecting our second baby, the law didn't allow midwives to attend VBACs taking place at home. Homebirth was therefore not an option. Since I'd really appreciated being received with respect at the hospital, I decided to return there for this birth, which I had no doubt would be a VBAC.

Our little Lia was born on 15 December. Contractions started at around 2.00am, in the middle of the night. Sebastian had to get up at 5 o'clock to go to work. He suggested staying with me, but I refused. Completely naïvely, I was convinced we wouldn't have this baby for a few hours because the contractions really were very bearable and spaced out. What's more, since this labour was considered my first, it would no doubt be very long.

At 7.00am I felt more and more certain that this wasn't a false alarm because the pain got worse and I was no longer capable of talking during contractions. I wasn't even capable of preparing some toast for my 2-year-old daughter, who was very impatient. I called Sebastian's father, Michel, so that he could come and look after Maxine.

I felt more and more certain that this wasn't a false alarm.
I wasn't even capable of preparing toast for my daughter.

Create a supportive environment   183

I had another bath, walked around a bit… It was already almost 9.30am. As far as I was concerned, it was going to take a long time, so I didn't count anything—neither spaces between contractions, nor the length of the contractions themselves. I virtually lost my grip on things! Michel, who was a policeman, had seen a few women give birth, right from the beginning, because policemen are also ambulance men, after all. He told me to call Sebastian so he could take me to the hospital. I refused, telling him we had plenty of time… but that day, 15 December 2003, we'd had our first snowstorm of the year. It was still snowing heavily and there was a great deal of traffic on the motorways. We were 30 minutes away from the hospital, driving in good weather, with no traffic. Michel left me in peace for a while, but not long afterwards he again asked me to call Sebastian, which I *again* refused to do. I got a black look from him and—in a serious voice—he said: "You listen to me. You're having contractions every three minutes, each one lasting a minute. There's a storm outside. Sebastian's not here and you're nowhere near to arriving at the hospital. It's fine with me if you don't call him… but I'm going to call him myself." So I phoned Sebastian! (I admit I'd had no idea I was having contractions every three minutes.)

When Sebastian got home, my contractions, which I was tracking a bit now, were coming every two minutes and they were still pretty long. I hesitated… we were only five minutes away from another hospital and, because of the temperature, more than an hour away from the one I was booked into. For a while Sebastian insisted on going to the hospital we'd chosed but I admitted I didn't know if the baby would be able to wait until we got there. Then I made up my mind… We'd set off for completely irrational, vague reasons—I simply didn't want to give birth at the local hospital. I would make sure the baby waited! I would stop doing the visualisations I'd been doing, which involved thinking 'I'm opening up a passage for my baby" and "My cervix is a flower." Instead, I would visualise my cervix waiting and I would imagine my baby high up inside me. That all seemed to work very well and contractions became spaced out, three or four minutes apart.

We arrived at the hospital at about 12.30, at lunchtime. I let myself go completely and then things started to happen quickly—contractions starting coming closer together and they were also becoming more powerful. We went to the assessment room, after needing to stop and lean against the wall several times, with me clutching the railing. The midwife saw no need to attach me to the monitor so as to confirm I was in labour. She gave me a vaginal examination but said nothing about what she found. In fact, that didn't matter to me because I would have been disappointed if I'd been 3cm, and in any case I didn't see any reason to know. She wanted me to give her a urine sample before I was taken to my room. I was incapable of taking two steps without having a contraction so it took ages for me to return a full pot to her. Then the midwife suggested I use a wheelchair to get to my room. I refused—I wanted to walk so as to speed up the labour. She insisted, saying that I could walk around as much as I wanted when I was there, but that we'd get there quicker in the wheelchair. Since I was having a contraction every time I took two steps she was probably right—it would have taken forever—because my room really was a long way away!

As soon as we got to the room another midwife asked me if I wanted an epidural and I very politely replied: "No, thank you." Another midwife added that if I wanted one, I should have it now because I was already 8cm dilated. That was how I found out that it was almost over! "That's not possible. That's too fast..." I was surprised and a little disappointed. I'd been waiting for this moment for so long and it was already almost over.

> That's not possible. That's too fast..." I was surprised and a little disappointed. I'd been waiting so long for this moment.

The midwife who was assigned to us was middle-aged and seemed quite cold and a bit dry in her manner. Several times she insisted that Sebastian should go to Reception but I told her in no uncertain terms that he was going nowhere. He was staying with me!

When I felt myself pushing the midwife examined me again and told me I was almost 9cm. I decided to lie on my side for a few minutes so I could rest a bit. (It was more because everything was going so fast than because of the pain.) The midwife went out and I had another contraction. On the next one I put my hand down to my vulva and touched the baby. "Sebastian!" I said, "The baby's here." He came up to me, pulled my legs apart and confirmed that it really was. He stepped back slowly and turned towards the door so as to let the midwife know. They met in the doorway and Sebastian told her that we could see the baby. She replied in a tone I shall remember all my life: "Really, sir. Just two minutes ago she wasn't even fully dilated!" I had another contraction, opened my legs and showed her. I admit in retrospect I was rather pleased when I saw her literally pounce on the intercom switch, to ask the consultant to get there straight away.

Less than a minute later the consultant and a student came running in. The only phrase I kept on repeating, over and over again, was: "It's going too fast. I'm not ready." Sebastian tried to convince me I was ready by saying: "Marie, you haven't got any choice. The baby's here!" (It was almost crowning.) I held my arm out to Sebastian because I wanted him to help me get up again, so I could get into a squatting position... get up on my feet. I didn't want to give birth lying on my back. "Marie, the baby's here!" (She was definitely crowning now.) I learnt that it's not possible to move without someone else's help when the baby's so close to being born! I pushed when I had two more contractions and the consultant said: "Take your baby." My first reaction was to feel I wasn't capable, that I didn't want to hold it... but at the same time I knew that if I didn't, I would regret it bitterly later. So I summoned all my remaining energy and took hold my daughter. It did me so much good to feel her on me. It was 2.09pm.

> It did me so much good to feel my baby on me

Lia's birth allowed me to confirm something I've known for a long time: I am capable. Nevertheless, deep inside me—so as to finish things off—there remained the desire to experience a home birth, not only because I knew I was capable of having one but also because it's a normal way of giving birth!

Our little Tommy was born on 21 July last year in the comfort of our own home, in the presence of our two daughters. The law relating to midwives had changed in 2005, so midwives were now allowed to attend women who'd previously had a caesarean. The question of insurance for home birth had also been sorted out, so it was now possible for me to use the services of my local birth centre. At appointments with my midwife, Sebastian and I clearly explained what we needed because we knew we could cope just fine on our own—we just needed her in case something didn't go so well. In other words, we wanted to be at home because we wanted some peace! And we wanted to fully experience the birth.

> Sebastian and I clearly explained what we needed because we knew we could cope just fine on our own— we just needed her in case something didn't go so well

Four days before the birth my eldest daughter Maxine spoke to the baby inside me, saying: "You'll arrive in four days' time." And every day, she counted down... and she was right. All through the week I had several bouts of 'practice' contractions, which were quite strong. I was getting so used to this that on the night of the 21st, when contractions began, I got up, took a bath and had something to eat, all of which would have more or less had the effect of stopping contractions on previous days. By around 5 o'clock in the morning I was making so much noise and breathing so heavily that Sebastian woke up. Contractions were coming every three minutes, each one lasting about a minute. They really hurt, so I had no doubt that today would be the day. At 7 o'clock, I called our midwife to ask her to come over, in her own time. I also phoned Sonia, a friend from way back and she agreed to come and look after the girls, who were going to be present at the birth.

Both my friend and the midwife arrived at around 9.30am. I was in the bath, with water up to my ears and with my nose hardly showing. (Human physiology was forcing me to behave like that!) Our midwife was indescribably discrete. She'd probably been in the bathroom for several minutes without me even realising before she asked me if she could listen to the baby's heartbeat. It was all beautiful. She asked me if I wanted to have a vaginal examination. As far as she was concerned, it wasn't necessary so as to confirm that I really was in active labour—so I decided not to have the internal just then.

I got out of the bath and walked around. Out of the window I watched my daughters bouncing on the trampoline. It was beautiful and so calm! Sebastian was with me... I would have loved my stepfather to have been there (who Tommy will sadly only know from our memories), but I nevertheless like giving birth with my hubby around!

I so appreciated the incredible respect our midwife had for our intimacy. The only thing she did was ask me twice if everything was going as I wanted it to. She understood very well what I wanted and her presence and her discretion allowed me to experience the birth fully.

> I so appreciated the incredible respect our midwife had for our intimacy. She understood very well what I wanted...

Towards the end of the afternoon, she asked me if I would be happy to have a vaginal examination. She found I was more than 9cm dilated. This time, I was happy it was almost over. I knew I'd never worked as hard and laboured as strongly as I had when I'd had Lia, but still... The second midwife arrived just before my waters broke. Sonia prepared the girls—she told them the baby was going to come really soon.

This time, I knew I would no longer be able to move when the baby was almost out. So as soon as the vaginal examination was over I leant on Sebastian, who was sitting on the sofa. This time, I wouldn't give birth lying on my back—I would stay on my knees, leaning forwards. (We suspected that the baby wasn't perfectly positioned, that his nose was pointing towards my back, so I wanted to help him finish rotating by leaning forward all the time.)

When the baby's hair first became visible, the girls came in to join us. I knew they were there, I *felt* they were there, but I didn't see them and they'd never been as quiet in their whole life! I was so happy they were with us. We'd prepared for this birth together. I knew they wanted to be present and, at the same time, I knew that it was even more important for me to have them there, than it was for them.

Pushing was gentle and I followed our rhythm—the rhythm set by me and the baby. Nobody told me what to do or how to do it. It was me who decided and as far as I'm concerned that was absolutely priceless. Sebastian had wanted to catch the baby himself, from the moment we had our first experience of labour. That's what we'd planned for this time. But a few moments away from the birth, I just couldn't manage to crouch down so he could catch the baby. I knew at this precise moment that I would be disappointed (and that he would be too), but I just didn't feel capable of taking the initiative to move.

Just before the birth, when I felt a real 'ring of fire', I wasn't sure the head was really coming out. My instinct told me that a good part of it had emerged, but at the same time, it was as if I couldn't feel it. I asked if it had come out a bit and it was my little Lia who quickly replied that the whole head was out. That gave me the courage to confirm it by feeling with my hand. I found it very special touching the baby's whole head while—for a few seconds—nothing moved. Everything seemed straightforward and it didn't hurt as much as all that at that particular moment. The baby was born 15 to 20 minutes after the girls had rejoined us in the room.

We didn't know the baby's sex and we were very surprised to see it was a baby boy. We'd all—Sebastian, me and our daughters—been convinced it would be a girl! Maxine, who was then $5\frac{1}{2}$, quickly decided she'd rather go and play with her friends. She thought the baby was beautiful, but also a bit disgusting. I admit I'd forgotten to tell them the baby might be covered in something, and to show them babies covered in vernix—so they were expecting to see a nice clean baby! Lia, who was then $3\frac{1}{2}$, didn't even consider the baby dirty and she immediately gave him lots of kisses. She very proudly told anyone who would listen: "It was me who cut the cord!"

During our antenatal appointments, when we'd said we wanted to have some peace and quiet for this birth, that seemed a rude thing to say. But it really had been what we wanted. We wanted to be at the heart of the event. We didn't want to have to ask for things. We didn't want to have to justify ourselves. We didn't want to have to argue for what we wanted.

Tommy's birth taught me that I was much more instinctual than I'd believed (apart from the business of not knowing the baby's sex!) and that gave me even more confidence. There's always something to learn when we give birth—good things and bad. Giving birth is a rite of passage for the baby, but also for the mother, the father and the whole family. A rite of passage serves to teach us about ourselves. As far as I'm concerned, these three births significantly moulded the woman I am today.

Tommy's birth taught me that I was much more instinctual than I'd believed and that gave me even more confidence

Photo © Noa Mohlabane

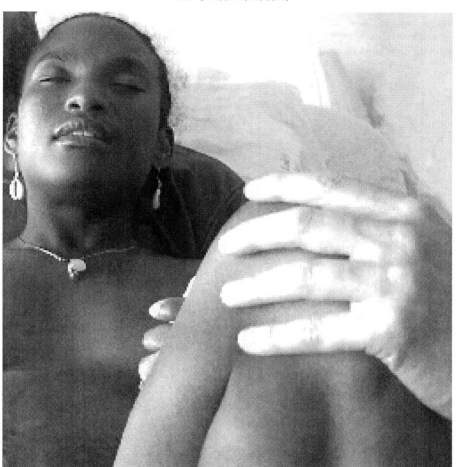

Here a woman tunes into the feelings going on within her body as she prepares to push her baby out into the world

CHAPTER 6:
Make wise decisions during labour

As we've already seen, for anyone who is supportive of VBACs, the most important things are the conditions under which the birth takes place. Above all else, a VBAC is a birth, and since an 'unfinished' VBAC is associated with more complications, it's important to facilitate any VBAC attempt by making the environment appropriate and having caregivers who are supportive and who believe that women can give birth to their babies themselves. According to health care professionals I consulted, for a few generations pregnant women have had less and less confidence in their own ability to bring their babies into the world. This explains why it's so important for a pregnant woman to prepare herself well and to try and increase her awareness of what is helpful and what is not helpful during labour.

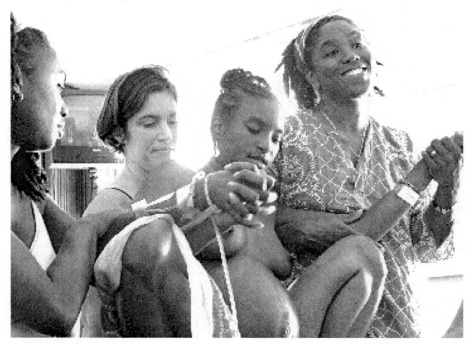

In this situation the labouring woman clearly has an excellent relationship with her caregivers and birth attendants, so decision-making is likely to be collaborative
Photo © Noa Mohlabane

What's it helpful to do? What's it helpful to avoid?

Things to avoid ideally!

In order to make your labour and birth flow well, you need to remember to avoid certain situations, if at all possible.[1] The following notes relate to protocols or procedures which are likely to increase the likelihood of another caesarean being considered necessary. When these protocols or procedures are applied routinely they have no positive effect on either mothers or babies, according to scientific studies or recommendations by health authorities like WHO[2] and Lamaze International.[3]

When these protocols or procedures are used routinely, they have no positive effect on either mothers or babies

- Not allowing low risk women access to midwifery services
- Not allowing low risk women access to birth centre facilities
- Consultation of third trimester scans to estimate the size and weight of the baby at birth (ostensibly to determine the probability of a vaginal birth)
- The use of drugs so as to soften (or 'prepare') the woman's cervix before induction. (This is, in fact, already part of the induction process.)
- Induction before the end of 41 weeks of pregnancy
- Amniotomy (i.e. the breaking of a woman's waters)—which is another form of induction or augmentation of labour
- Keeping a labouring woman in hospital before she has gone into active labour
- The use of continuous electronic fetal monitoring. (Intermittent monitoring of the baby's heartbeat—i.e. auscultation—is better for low risk women during labour.)
- The use of an intravenous drip
- The use of an epidural for pain relief, particularly before 4cm of dilation, when the baby's head is not yet engaged in the mother's pelvis
- Being restricted to labouring in bed and/or not being allowed to move around freely
- Not allowing labouring women access to continuous physical and emotional support (e.g. in the form of the presence of a friend or relative, or the woman's partner)
- The requirement for a woman to push while she's lying on her back, with feet in stirrups (i.e. in the lithotomy position)

If you can, avoid having your cervix 'softened' before your labour begins, avoid having your waters broken, and avoid continuous EFM. Later on, avoid labouring in bed and remember, it's best if you're not lying on your back when you're giving birth!

Things to do to facilitate a vaginal birth

On a more positive note, it's good to know what will actually make a VBAC more likely, rather than another caesarean. In a minority of labours, it is indeed sometimes necessary to intervene judiciously so as to 'help nature along'. However, so as to prevent this arsenal of weapons being brought into play from the beginning of your labour why not try the following, which are used more and more often in maternity units around the country and around the world? Research has already shown that they can be effective. If you need to make reference to any of this research in order persuade your caregivers to 'allow' you to use them, simply refer to the systematic review produced by the Coalition for Improving Maternity Services.[4] All the items in the following list will help you to labour effectively. They can also be used when labour *isn't* progressing well, when things are moving forward very slowly or when the baby is poorly positioned during the first stage of labour. As this list shows, there are many things you can do during labour, before resorting to an epidural or instead of having one at all, or instead of having your labour augmented. Here, then, are the things which will help you while you're in labour and giving birth...

STAY MOBILE

The World Health Organization (WHO) encourages mobility during labour. It's important not to stay lying down. Get up, go for a walk, move around and stay upright, so as to help the baby descend. Being upright will make contractions more effective and it'll therefore also shorten your labour, help your cervix dilate more quickly, reduce any discomfort and pain you feel, reduce moulding of the baby's head, lower the incidence of abnormal variations in fetal heart rhythms (a sign of fetal distress) and help the baby to remain in good condition during labour. Moving around freely will also make you feel better. It'll make it less likely that your caregivers will suggest a drip of synthetic oxytocin (so as to augment labour) or an episiotomy during the pushing stage. Moving around freely will also make tearing less likely. Most importantly, freedom of movement will decrease the chance that ventouse, forceps or a caesarean will be thought necessary. And you don't need to fear any negative consequences because there's absolutely no evidence to suggest that it's harmful to move around. On the contrary, lying down would slow down the circulation of blood between you and your baby and this is likely to cause fetal distress. Lying down would also increase your levels of stress hormones and make it more difficult for your womb to contract, both of which would inhibit the progress of your labour.

Whenever you feel you need to, if you have any difficulty staying upright lean on your partner, your doula or on both of them—or against any items of furniture or a wall. You can also sit on a birthing ball—many are now available in maternity units—or lean the top part of your body on a hospital bed. A birthing ball will help you to keep your pelvis mobile because you'll constantly have to readjust your position in order to keep your balance. Another possibility is to use a massage chair, in a fairly upright position (so that you're not leaning back), whether or not you use it for massage purposes. While you're pushing (during the second stage of labour), ask to have a horizontal bar, if one's available. (You'll be able to use it to push on and hang from while you're kneeling down.) You may also be able to use a birthing chair or birthing stool, or you can ask your partner or a midwife to support you from behind, under the armpits, in a semi-squat—or you can just use whatever furniture is around, or the floor! As I said, whatever you use, the important thing is to move around as you feel you need to because quite apart from all the advantages for the baby, you'll probably also find contractions less painful that way—compared to lying down.

TRY OUT DIFFERENT POSITIONS—e.g. AN ALL-FOURS POSITION

Some positions—such as going down on all fours—can help to move the baby round into a better position for the birth. This is particularly the case if the baby is in a posterior position because kneeling on all fours will help him or her to turn round. (Posterior labours are known to be more difficult from the point of view of pain experienced and also from the point of actually getting the baby out in the second stage.) Being on all fours is also preferable for some women, who say that they experience less pain in that position, compared to when they're sitting down.

STAY NOURISHED

Giving birth takes energy, so while you're in labour it may be important to have drinks and semi-solids or even light meals, which are easy to digest. WHO recommends that labouring women eat and drink, as they wish, all through labour and a recent Cochrane review of research also concluded that this practice is not harmful for low risk women. The review concludes: "Given these findings, women should be free to eat and drink in labour, or not, as they wish."[5]

Research has actually shown that total fasting may be dangerous because there is a risk of inhaling gastric juices under general anaesthesia—if an emergency caesarean is needed later. (Note that this is in contrast to what was originally believed.)[6] Going without food and drink completely weakens the whole organism, which is in the process of doing some extremely strenuous work, but—even more importantly—it increases the quantity and acidity of gastric juices. Staff now accept that the possibility of aspiration of stomach contents is remote and they usually recognise that an enforced fast is stressful for a woman in labour. According to Dr Murray Enkin, professor of obstetrics at McMaster University in Hamilton (Canada), eating or drinking semi-solids (smoothies, soup, yogurt, etc) can be a good compromise to eating full meals. Some maternity units are indeed happy to let women eat while they're in labour.[7]

USE WARM WATER OR MASSAGE

Both warm water and massage can be used to help you relax. If you don't have access to a bath or a hot shower, hot compresses may be useful. (These can simply be towels which have been made wet, then wrung out. They can be applied to your body by your partner, doula or midwife.) Getting yourself a massage (from anyone who's prepared to give you one) may also help you while you're in labour. If you want them to, your birth attendants could massage your neck, head, back, buttocks, thighs and feet. According to research, massage reduces the perception of pain, lowers maternal stress and anxiety levels, and helps the woman cope with pain. It also reassures and comforts her and encourages her to persevere.[8] Taking a bath can also lower arterial blood pressure, decrease anxiety, reduce pain perceived in the first stage of labour, and decrease the need for pain relief or augmentation of labour (using synthetic oxytocin, i.e. syntocinon).[9] (However, be aware that some experts warn against using warm or hot water in the very early stages of labour because they have observed that it can slow labour down, or even stop it completely. RCOG and the RCM recommend that "early labour could be managed by mobilisation and other activities within a labour room rather than water immersion," so it may be better to wait until you're in active labour before immersing yourself in warm water.)[10] In the second stage of labour, being in warm water helps the baby to become well-positioned and many women say it gives them the feeling of freedom of movement and intimacy.

CHECK OUT YOUR EMOTIONS

If something or someone in the room you're labouring in is bothering you, or if you're afraid of something, make sure you say this to whoever is around. If necessary, ask—or even insist—that a particular person leave the room. After all, fear is an emotion which may slow down or stop labour altogether.[11] This is because we produce the hormone adrenaline when we're fearful or stressed out and this hormone actually stops production of the hormone oxytocin, the hormone which orchestrates contractions.

TAKE ENOUGH REST

If your labour seems to be going on for a long time, stop for a while and take a rest—perhaps sitting, leaning forward, or lying down on your left-hand side. (This way, you'll avoid the disadvantages of lying on your back.)

URINATE FREQUENTLY

A full bladder can obstruct the baby's descent, so it's important to go to the toilet often, even if you don't notice the need to do a wee.

It's important to go to the toilet often while you're in labour

STAY COOL—DON'T PUSH IN A PANIC!

When you're fully dilated, it's not necessary to push straight away. Some women feel a strong urge to push, while others don't at all. Some women need help pushing their baby out, while others don't. And some babies stay high up in the pelvis (or even higher up) until the point when their mother starts pushing. Just take it easy and follow your body's signals to push or relax.

USE UPRIGHT POSITIONS

When you're completely dilated, you can help yourself through the pushing stage by remaining upright, perhaps sitting on a toilet seat or squatting—but only squat when the baby's head is engaged. According to research,[12] squatting significantly expands pelvic dimensions, it lowers the possibility of having to use forceps or ventouse, it means a lower risk of perineal tears,[13] and upright positions generally make pushing more effective and therefore they also shorten the length of time this stage of labour takes. (If you're unable to stay upright, lying on your left-hand side is the best idea.) WHO recommend an upright position for pushing because they say that the second stage will be shorter and less painful. It'll also make fetal distress less likely. Pushing in an upright position, they say, is also likely to result in less perineal damage (i.e. tearing), cause less swelling in the vulva and result in less blood loss.[14] And don't forget that it's *you* giving birth so it's up to you to choose positions which you prefer for pushing (as at any other stage of labour)—not your caregiver. One woman told me how when she'd been on all fours pushing, her consultant had asked her to turn over onto her back for her baby's birth. As he said this, he lifted up one end of the pillow she was leaning on to encourage her to move. Shouting out, "No, I won't, you bastard! I'm the one giving birth!" she snatched back the pillow and plunged her head into it... just as she gave birth, still on all fours, of course. Remind your caregivers, if necessary, of your right to give birth in whatever position you choose... If necessary, also feel free to remind them that you're the one giving birth, not them!

The best approach is to push gently during contractions, relaxing your buttocks as much as possible and the perineum, keeping your mouth partially open and letting yourself follow your body's signals as much as possible—groaning as you need to. This kind of pushing is 'physiological' and contrasts with what's called 'commanded pushing'—the kind of pushing that often takes place in hospital environments. Commanded pushing can be damaging for the baby because it can lead to fetal distress[15] and it can perhaps also lead to transverse arrest when the baby is descending in a posterior position.[16] In fact, it seems that no research supports the practice of commanded pushing. Research is beginning to show that directed pushing—as opposed to pushing according to one's own body reflexes—can be damaging for the perineum, while it also offers no benefits to the baby.[17] Focusing on opening up so that your baby can emerge safely will help you get through this phase of labour.

Push as your body tells you to

Pushing as your body tells you to may make this stage proceed more quickly, it makes interventions less likely and it leaves the baby in a better condition at birth.[18] Having said all that, a woman who's had an epidural may well require commanded pushing in order to get her baby born. (This is why most caregivers in the UK prefer an epidural to have worn off by the time a woman reaches the pushing stage.)

Overall, caregivers generally don't want the second stage of labour—the pushing stage—to go on for too long because they're worried about the possibility of fetal distress. This perhaps explains why women trying for a VBAC often (and other women having vaginal births) had forceps deliveries in the past. However, in the view of one doctor I interviewed, Dr Lirette, this view is not at all evidence-based because women have pushed for two or three hours without any problems occurring. Although pushing for a long time increases the possibility that forceps or ventouse will be seen as necessary, understandably, it does not seem to hurt the baby. As long as the baby seems to be doing OK, why should caregivers panic? The woman will feel cheated if she has a forceps birth (and will be highly inconvenienced by her episiotomy for weeks, if not months, afterwards).

AVOID HAVING FUNDAL PRESSURE

Fundal pressure is when a caregiver uses his or her hands to push on the woman's abdomen, over the upper part of the uterus and down towards the birth canal during the second stage of labour. It is carried out with the intention of shortening labour and assisting a vaginal birth, but it presents significant risks.[19] This practice is carried out by many caregivers, even though there is a lack of good research on this practice. It should therefore not be used without a valid medical reason.[20]

The following guidelines for avoiding fundal pressure are based on recommendations made by the American perinatal nurse, Kathleen Rice Simpson and Eric Knox:[21]

- Caregivers of all kinds need to be more patient. They need to avoid imposing arbitrary time limits on the second stage of labour. They need to allow women to let their baby descend in its own time, even if this means a delayed pushing stage.
- The balance of drugs in an epidural (if an epidural is used) needs to emphasise analgesia, rather than anaesthesia.
- If it's used at all, directed coaching should only ever be used to support a woman's spontaneous urge to push.

Potential risks and benefits of fundal pressure should be carefully analysed, remembering the medical principle, "First, do no harm." In short, you should refuse to allow fundal pressure to be applied unless you're told there's a very good clinical reason to do so and it's explained to you what this is.

Make wise decisions during labour

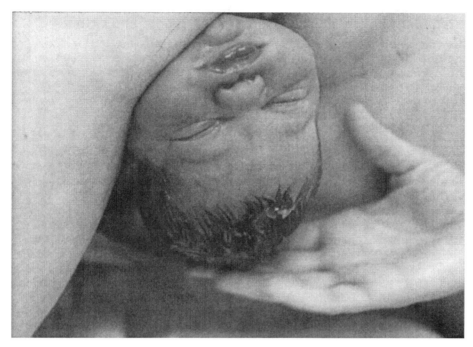

Follow your body's signals as much as possible, groaning as you need to... Open up so your baby can emerge in his or her own time—then you'll be able to say 'hello'!

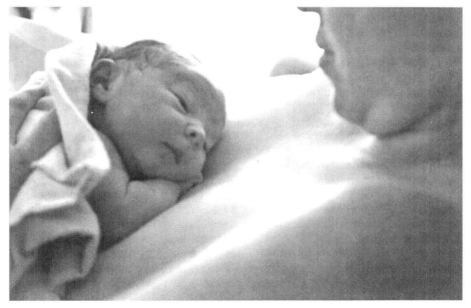

Photos © Regroupement Les Sages-Femmes du Québec, Canada

Frequently asked questions about VBAC labour and birth...

Beyond these basic guidelines, we'll now also consider a few common questions, which will help us to review certain key issues and also cover some new points too. All of the questions below are often asked by women who've previously had a caesarean... and many are surprised by the answers!

DO I HAVE TO GO INTO HOSPITAL AS SOON AS MY LABOUR STARTS?

When women request a vaginal birth after a previous caesarean the list of conditions they are presented with often includes the stipulation that they must go into hospital as soon as their labour starts. Why? Where's the urgency? Many doctors I interviewed felt that continuing to potter around at home, as normal, in a familiar environment was not dangerous. According to Dr Enkin, consultant obstetrician and professor of obstetrics, it's a decision which each woman needs to make for herself. In another doctor's view (a certain Dr King) it's preferable for labour to proceed at home until the woman is 4—5cm dilated, for most women, but when a woman's already had a caesarean he feels it's better to go into hospital earlier on; after two (or more) caesareans he feels that it's best to go into hospital as soon as possible after labour begins. Another doctor, Dr Shea, said that if you arrive at the hospital too early, hospital staff will have more time to worry about you and too many opportunities to intervene![22]

DOES A CONSULTANT NEED TO BE AT THE HOSPITAL WHILE I'M IN LABOUR?

When hospitals started allowing VBACs in the 1980s a consultant was often at the hospital while a VBAC client was in labour. (VBACs had effectively not been allowed in the USA since 1916, when a certain Dr Craig said "Once a caesarean, always a caesarean" at a conference in New York.) Following 1999 and 2004 ACOG recommendations, the practice of having a consultant in the hospital has again become customary even though there is no evidence (from research) to suggest that it's absolutely necessary to have a consultant immediately available. It would certainly be wise for a consultant and an anaesthetist to be informed that you're in labour, so that they're on call, outside the hospital somewhere—but it's perhaps not necessary for them to be in the same building, waiting, especially if your VBAC is a 'low-risk' VBAC (i.e. if there are no particular risk factors). However, RCOG specifies that VBAC "should be conducted in a suitably staffed and equipped delivery suite, with continuous intrapartum care and monitoring and available resources for immediate caesarean section and advanced neonatal resuscitation, Obstetric, midwifery, anaesthetic, operating theatre, neonatal and haematological support should be continuously available throughout planned VBAC and ERCS (elective repeat caeseareans)..."[23] but no scientific study supports this assertion. Actually, when considering this issue, we're actually touching on the question of how quickly a caesarean needs to be carried out if signs appear indicating that a uterine rupture is occurring. It's generally agreed (based on

ACOG and SOGC recommendations) that a caesarean needs to be performed within 30 minutes. One study does, in fact, suggest that the delay should be no longer than 17 minutes.[24] Some hospitals which don't have specialists on duty 24 hours a day, refuse to allow women to have a VBAC for this reason. However, I wonder why the same hospitals allow other women to have a 'vaginal birth' in their institution, given that any labour involves the risk of serious complications, and the fact that many other risks are higher than the risk of uterine rupture... Interestingly, in the report of the recent NIH Consensus Development Conference on VBAC there is, in fact, a request for ACOG to reconsider its guideline relating to the need to have a fully staffed operating theatre ready just in case. Sadly, ACOG did not accept this requirement in its July 2010 new guidelines on VBAC. However, it did add in its guidelines that this requirement was not based on a high level of evidence.[25] In any case, it's not always the case that a maternity unit which has all the staff and equipment necessary to proceed with an emergency caesarean manages to do this within the 17 or 30 minutes which is considered necessary.

IS IT REALLY NECESSARY TO BE ON AN INTRAVENOUS DRIP?

Often, when a woman arrives at a hospital a drip is suggested. In fact, a heparin lock would be less inconvenient. (This is where a small needle is inserted into a vein, but not attached to a drip.) A heparin lock could mean the fast set-up of a drip, if ever it urgently became necessary. In any case, it's preferable to have an intravenous drip set up only when labour is very advanced, if you agree to it. One nurse with experience of cardiology and surgery told me she felt that setting up a drip 'in case it's needed later' was a useless procedure. She said a drip can quickly be set up if it's needed and, in any case, emergencies are usually signalled well before they become urgent. If the drip is intended for the administration of a glucose solution, this nurse feels that this is not a good substitute for drinking and eating, and she says it can upset the electrolyte balance of a woman in labour. In one publication it was noted that there is no evidence to support the routine setting up of an intravenous drip.[26] Quite apart from all this, if labouring women are allowed to eat and drink, there's no need for a drip to keep them hydrated and supplied with calories.[27] In any case, not a single study has shown that the administration of a glucose solution (or any other kind of solution) improves outcomes for either mother or baby. On the other hand, many people have observed that a drip can cause discomfort and stress, it can interfere with mobility and administering too much liquid solution can cause anaemia and a reduction in osmotility (which affects how well hydrated the woman is). What's more, the use of an intravenous solution without electrolytes can lead to problems for both mother and baby—and the problems which affect the newborn baby include a higher risk of hyponatraemia (an electrolyte disorder, which relates to the amount of salt in the baby's blood), and jaundice (which means there's too much bilirubin in the blood). A glucose solution can also cause hyperglycaemia (low blood glucose) in the newborn baby.[28]

IS CONTINUOUS FETAL MONITORING NECESSARY?

In the last few years many VBAC protocols have changed in most hospitals. Perhaps this is because while some medical groups are recommending electronic fetal monitoring (EFM)—a continuous form of monitoring—there is actually no research on VBAC which confirms that it's necessary. It's even possible that EFM could inhibit the progress of a VBAC because it forces the woman to remain lying down, so it doesn't facilitate labour (in the ways that moving around does, as I've already explained)—and the supine position can even *cause* fetal distress!

A systematic review of the scientific literature carried out by CIMS in 2007 concluded that when compared with intermittent monitoring (carried out with a fetal stethoscope or Sonicaid), EFM did not reduce perinatal mortality rates, improve Apgar scores, prevent babies from being admitted to intensive care or prevent cerebral palsy. EFM actually increases the chance that a woman will need to have an instrumental delivery (ventouse or forceps) or a caesarean—the latter being precisely what a woman trying for a VBAC wants to prevent. What's more, when electronic fetal monitors are linked to a central midwifery station, which is the case in some hospitals, there is a reduction in interaction between hospital staff and labouring women—and consequently a reduction in the human support women need. Finally, EFM does not in any way help to prevent the death of the baby.

Having said all that, it is important to monitor the baby, but intermittent monitoring should be sufficient. A Sonicaid (which uses ultrasound) can be used without the labouring women needing to lie down. WHO recommend that the fetal heart be checked once an hour during the latent phase of labour (i.e. during the early hours of labour) and that it be checked every half an hour during active labour (when contractions are coming thick and fast), then every five minutes during the second stage, i.e. when the woman is pushing her baby out. Increasingly, hospitals are using telemetry to check the fetal heartbeat. For this to be possible, the labouring woman needs to carry a bag around, which contains the surveillance equipment—but this doesn't prevent her from moving around. Readings are automatically relayed to the midwifery station. This is therefore one method which allows medical staff to track the fetal heartbeat continuously (in line with some recommendations), which doesn't limit the woman's freedom of movement.

In defense of EFM, it must be said that a small number of studies have suggested that EFM reduces the incidence of convulsions in newborns, but most studies reviewed in the Cochrane review did not note this effect. (In any case, the few studies which suggested that EFM could lower the incidence of convulsions in newborns had too few subjects for their results to be conclusive.)[29] In fact, the only significant effect associated with EFM by all studies was an increase in the caesarean rate and an increase in the number of instrumental deliveries.[30] Even in the case of high risk pregnancies, there is little convincing evidence to suggest that the use of EFM is any better than intermittent auscultation (checking) of the fetal heart.[31]

ARE VAGINAL EXAMINATIONS A GOOD IDEA?

WHO recommend that cervical dilation should be checked once every four hours during both the latent phase of labour and the active phase. Some caregivers believe that the method of carrying out vaginal examinations should be changed.[32] NICE guidelines emphasise that healthcare professionals who conduct vaginal examinations should ensure that any one vaginal examination is really necessary and will add important information to the decision-making process. The guidelines also advise caregivers to be aware that for many women who may already be in pain, highly anxious and in an unfamiliar environment, vaginal examinations can be very distressing, to ensure that women give their consent before the examination, to ensure women's consent, privacy, dignity and comfort. They also stipulate that the reason for the examination and what will be involved should be explained, and that the impact of the findings should be explained sensitively to the woman.[33] Finally, some researchers have concluded that vaginal examinations may be a ritual which invades a woman's personal space.[34]

IS IT OK TO HAVE MY WATERS BROKEN?

Caregivers often want to speed up the progress of a woman's labour by breaking her waters. Is this always desirable? And is it absolutely necessary to speed up labour? One of the reasons caregivers give is to determine the colour of the amniotic fluid because tainted fluid is one indicator of fetal distress. Dr Michel Odent prefers to use an amnioscope to do this, i.e. a metal tube with a light at the end, which can be inserted into the vagina to look at the colour of the fluid, without breaking the amniotic membranes (a woman's 'waters').[35] Another reason why caregivers sometimes want to break a woman's waters is because they want to attach a fetal monitor to the baby's scalp (either by inserting a clip or attaching a suction cup) to verify the reading of external monitoring. Except for cases where there's good cause to double check there's no fetal distress, this is certainly not necessary. One doula attending a woman who wanted to have a VBAC told me the woman was told the head clip was necessary 'just in case'...

Beyond all this, when a woman has her waters broken this increases the risk of infection, particularly when the woman is lying on her back (since the amniotic fluid flows around less freely and can flow back into the woman's body, after coming out). Also, if a woman's waters are broken too early on in labour, this intervention is less effective (in terms of what it's intended to achieve) and it can also increase the risk of infection in both mother and baby, even when she's not lying down. Amniotomy also increases the risk of cord prolapse, where the umbilical cord drops down before the baby. This would be very dangerous because the cord would then be highly likely to become compressed, which would cut off the baby's oxygen supply.[36] In addition, when a woman's waters have been broken the baby's head is no longer 'cushioned' in any way. For all these reasons, amniotomy should not be performed routinely, but only in cases where the situation really requires it. Apart from

Photos © Regroupement Les Sages-Femmes du Québec, Canada

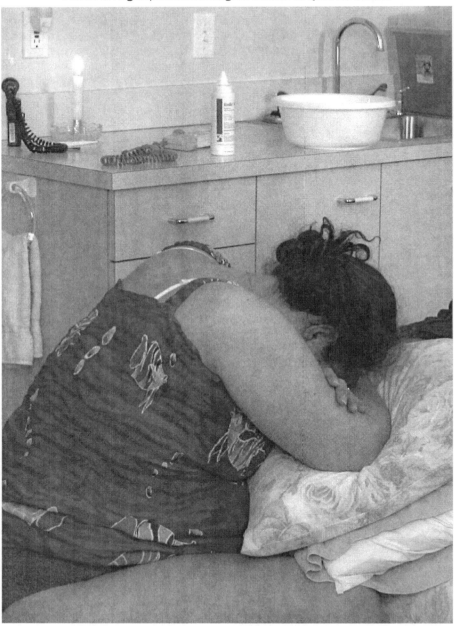

It's possible that EFM could inhibit the progress of a VBAC because it forces the woman to remain lying down, so it doesn't facilitate labour (in the ways that moving around does, as I've already explained)—and the supine position can even cause fetal distress!

anything else, having your waters broken will make contractions more painful and intense even though this intervention is only likely to shorten labour by one or two hours. The systematic review of research carried out by CIMS[37] concluded that as well as bringing no advantage to the baby, amniotomy may also increase the risk of fetal distress—i.e. the risk of non-reassuring heart rhythms occurring, which is an indication that distress might be taking place.

IS IT OK TO HAVE MY LABOUR INDUCED OR 'HELPED ALONG' WITH SYNTOCINON?

You might well wonder why modern women have such inadequate or ineffective contractions that it's often necessary to stimulate them with artificial hormones. Actually, it seems that consultants and midwives (and other maternity caregivers) are so used to seeing contractions stimulated artificially, they no longer recognise natural contractions.[38] Many caregivers seem to have forgotten how labour can progress normally, without any medical intervention. Increasingly, caregivers are using synthetic oxytocin (syntocinon)—which they often simply call 'oxytocin'—during women's labours. In the USA a national survey revealed that more than half of women are having their labours induced or augmented in this way. In the chapter about the risks associated with VBAC, I explained how the use of prostaglandins and syntocinon can increase the risk of uterine rupture, particularly when labour is induced. Nevertheless, with augmentation, the situation is less clear-cut... Stimulating labour in a well-controlled, carefully monitored way, using low doses of syntocinon could sometimes make the difference between having or not having a vaginal birth. In this case, it is also not problematic to use analgesic pain relief. Often, however, as Dr Michelle Harrison notes, analgesia does not make the pain of augmented contractions disappear and it makes the labouring woman less capable of facing the pain and of remaining in control of her labour.[39] In the view of associations which support VBAC, groups which offer information on caesareans and people who are aware of the disadvantages of interventions during labour, it's preferable to do without syntocinon, if you can, because there's the problem that it's likely to lead to a cascade of interventions, which may culminate in a caesarean. (See the diagram on page 203, overleaf).

HOW LONG IS LABOUR SUPPOSED TO LAST?

Very often, time limits are put on a woman's VBAC labour. In these cases, caregivers are forgetting to consider the woman trying to have a vaginal birth as a 'first-time mother', which she effectively is, since in most cases her body has never really been through a full labour before. Most women attempting a VBAC are therefore more likely to take longer than the 12-hour limit usually imposed. But is it possible to remain confident and relaxed when it's necessary to 'perform'? Is it possible to go through an uncontrollable process against the clock? In Dr Enkin's view, it's important not to be rigid about time limits, but if labour isn't progressing this fact can't be ignored indefinitely. What counts, he told me, is how the mother and baby are faring.[40] According to the VBAC researcher Dr Bujold, imposing a time limit in advance is not helpful in the case of a VBAC. Nevertheless, one study which he led did lead him to conclude that a labour which isn't progressing should not be allowed to continue indefinitely, if the cervix is already well dilated.[41] In the book *The Vaginal Birth After Cesarean Experience—Birth Stories by Parents and Professionals* (Greenwood, 1987), the author Lynn Baptisti Richards mentions that one woman attempting a VBAC decided not to allow her caregivers to give her a vaginal examination every two hours—because her labour appeared to be going well. (It was 'failure to progress' in her first labour which had led to her previous caesarean.) She reasoned that if she wasn't constantly reminded of how much (or how little) progress she'd made, she wouldn't get discouraged, so would be more likely to avoid having another caesarean. (She did at least allow her caregivers to regularly listen in to the baby's heartbeat.) She also refused to have her labour augmented with syntocinon... and a few hours after her labour started her baby did descend and she was completely dilated. She had a vaginal birth.

WHAT SHOULD I SAY IF I'M TOLD SOMETHING IS ROUTINE FOR A VBAC?

As I've already explained, it's useful to find out about protocols at the hospital or birth centre where you're registered to give birth (if you're planning to give birth in a hospital or birth centre)—particularly if these protocols relate to VBACs specifically. It's also a good idea to find out about protocols which apply to *all* vaginal births. In the 1980s, many consultants—such as the Phelans (a husband and wife team in Los Angeles), Dr Shulman (in New York) and Dr Enkin (in Hamilton, Canada)—believed that women having a VBAC should not be treated differently from any other women having vaginal births. Even if these doctors' attitudes were motivated by a desire to normalise VBAC, this belief unfortunately had the consequence of exposing more and more VBAC women to induction and augmentation in labour. Although these procedures were (perhaps unhelpfully in any case) becoming more and more common for births generally, they also increased the main risk associated with a VBAC, i.e. uterine rupture, as we saw before. For this reason—and because other interventions might also increase risks, even if they might also involve certain benefits—it's a good idea to ask some questions before you agree to any intervention. Here are a few questions you might use:[42]

- Is this intervention really necessary at the moment?
- Is this an emergency or do we have time to talk about this?
- What would be the advantages of carrying out a caesarean right now, instead of using this intervention?
- What would be the risks involved in carrying out a caesarean, for both me and my baby?
- What else would be necessary if we decided to go ahead with a caesarean—i.e. what other procedures or preparation would be necessary?
- What are the alternatives to this intervention?
- What would happen if we were to wait for an hour or two before deciding?
- Would my baby or I be in danger if I decided not to have this intervention?
- Would either my baby or I be in danger if I decided not to have a caesarean?

These questions are necessary for two other reasons, as well as the fact that the risks of having a VBAC may increase as a result of having certain interventions. Firstly, some interventions may not be necessary (i.e. they will not be medically indicated) and, as I've already pointed out, many interventions are likely to trigger a cascade of interventions (which may culminate in a caesarean). Secondly, the current medical climate (involving mistrust in the physiological processes of birth) has led to an increasing use of interventions for all women and these haven't necessarily improved outcomes, i.e. there has been no significant improvement in the rates of maternal or neonatal mortality or morbidity. For instance, a study conducted in the USA on VBAC and repeat caesareans showed that neonatal and maternal mortality rates did not improve despite increasing rates of repeat caesareans during the years after ACOG changed its guidelines for VBAC in 1999. The table below aims to portray how certain interventions can make other interventions more likely:

A cascade of interventions[43]

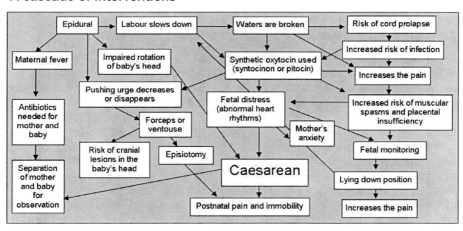

Note: Arrows indicate where risks exist of subsequent interventions occurring.

It's also worth coming back to the point that unnecessary interventions increase the likelihood that a woman will end up having a caesarean because one intervention often leads to many more. One recent study which looked at 800,000 women's labours and births did in fact confirm the tendency for a cascade of interventions.[44] For example, when a woman's waters are broken, since many hospitals stipulate that the birth must occur within 24 hours afterwards (because they are concerned the woman may become infected), augmentation of labour with syntocinon soon seems necessary. This intervention makes contractions more painful, so analgesia is offered (pethidine, diamorphine, etc) or an epidural. This pain relief then increases the risk that forceps will be needed, which can mean the newborn baby then needs to have various procedures carried out after the birth—all of which disturb early mother-baby contact and bonding.

The trend towards the over-use of interventions does not mean you should refuse all interventions offered to you. As GP Yolande Leduc put it, you need to judge on a case-by-case basis, which isn't easy, and accept interventions when they're needed. In any case, you also need to be aware that interventions are too often undertaken without the woman being informed of the risks they involve for herself and her baby, even though this is in contravention of the NMC Code (the code of practice issued by the Nursing & Midwifery Council, which regulates all midwives in the UK) and all other official guidelines (e.g. those of the RCM and RCOG). Restrictive conditions (which often ensue when interventions are used) reduce women's chances of having a successful VBAC, because they medicalise birth and may reduce women's confidence in their ability to succeed in what they and their partner have set out to do.

Interventions are too often undertaken without the woman being informed of the risks they involve for herself and her baby, even though this is in contravention of the NMC Code

AM I ALLOWED TO REFUSE AN INTERVENTION IF I DON'T WANT TO HAVE IT?

Often women giving birth—and their partners—don't realise that they have the right to refuse any intervention if they don't want to have it. This right is well-recognised in the UK: if neither you nor your baby are in danger, you can refuse any routine interventions which are suggested to you. Sometimes, when you refuse an intervention, you'll be asked to sign a refusal of treatment form (or something similar), which refers to the intervention. Nevertheless, if you're convinced of your decision, if all is going well and if you have supportive people around you, why shouldn't you refuse interventions? Let's not forget that many practices in obstetrics and midwifery came into general use without any research to confirm they were helpful or even safe. Although there is a strong emphasis on evidence-based care now, maternity units have a lot of adjustments to make before care can become completely evidence-based and in cases where research isn't 100% clear in its results, there is cause for differences of opinion and consequently differences in approach. Insurance companies also often push hospitals towards a more, rather than a less interventionist approach because of the ever-present fear of litigation and the need for documentary 'proof' in these cases.

The Coalition for Improving Maternity Services (CIMS) emphases in one of its reviews that a planned vaginal birth is not a 'treatment' as such since it's the inevitable consequence of a pregnancy. In other words, this physiological event usually begins spontaneously at the end of pregnancy... as one hospital in Louisiana confirmed at the time of Hurricane Katrina (2005). When the staff sent home all the women who were due to be induced, and cancelled all the appointments of others who were due to come in for induction, they were astonished to find afterwards that almost all the women had given birth one or two days later—without their help at all! This made several members of staff change their approach to maternity care.

Photo © Erin Brown

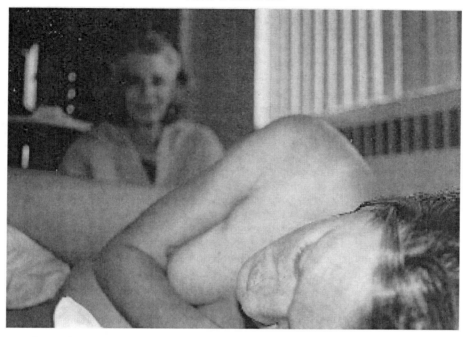

Be confident that your body knows what it's doing and is capable of giving birth. Even though this midwife doesn't look like she's doing anything, her presence is a crucial part of care. She's monitoring and providing support.

You even have the right to refuse another caesarean

On the subject of refusing interventions, you also need to note that you even have the right to refuse to have another caesarean. If your caregiver wants to carry out a caesarean simply because you've already had one (or more than one) beforehand, nobody can force it on you if you don't give your consent. If—against a woman's will—a caesarean is performed—the woman can later sue the consultant for assault. Since this is the case, if a hospital where you're in labour is refusing to help you in your desire to avoid intervention and wants to send you off somewhere else for care, you can contact the media. Tell them this is what you intend to do, because this is probably not what the hospital would want. The only time a hospital can force a woman to have a caesarean is if they take her to court and obtain a court order. Unfortunately, this was done in the USA in the 1980s and 1990s. In Canada and the UK this has happened less often, but it has happened. In the UK there were cases of women who were forced to have a caesarean and who later sued the hospital, successfully. Later, an Appeal Court ruled against compulsory caesareans.[45]

A court order is needed to force a woman to have a caesarean

SHOULD I TRY AND AVOID HAVING AN EPIDURAL IF I CAN?

In one report (written in 1997), WHO questioned whether a labour could be called normal when an epidural had been used by a low risk woman.[46] Perhaps this is why, here in the UK, births involving epidurals are evaluated separately from normal births, in the same way as separate statistics are kept for inductions, instrumental deliveries or ones involving an episiotomy. This is outlined in a document which attempts to offer a standard definition of normal birth and how to promote it.[47] UK bodies, like WHO, treat epidurals as 'non-normal'.

The fact that epidurals are routinely offered to low risk women while they're in labour is a strange development in obstetrics. Because it's considered important to honour a woman's right to control her own body and make a personal choice, some people feel that having an epidural is a woman's basic right and that every woman who wants one should have access to one. Well, yes... we certainly are talking about personal choice here. I did make this choice during my first labour—I had an epidural—and I decided not to in my second labour. Perhaps it's also helpful to know that having an epidural involves the administration of drugs which can have negative effects...

It is indeed often forgotten that the administration of up to three types of drugs is what an epidural involves... These are local anaesthetics, epinephrine and narcotics, such as morphine and its derivatives.[48] As you may know, narcotics—particularly those which can be found in pain-relieving drugs such as Nubain, involve secondary effects. Several studies have shown the negative effects of narcotics on breastfeeding. Narcotics can block the release of endorphins and since they remain in the baby's body for a long time, can also have a negative effect on breastfeeding. If an epidural is administered too near the baby's birth, the narcotics may make it difficult for the baby to breathe. Even the local anaesthetic (xylocaine) can be found in the newborn baby's urine up to 48 hours after his or her birth.[49]

Regional anaesthesia such as an epidural—other forms are spinals and cervical blocks, for example—may also cause maternal hypotension (i.e. low blood pressure), they will increase the need for other obstetric interventions, they make it more difficult for the baby's head to rotate as it should as it's moving down the vaginal passageway, they cause unpleasant itching, and they also slow down labour. They can also cause maternal fever and headaches postnatally, sometimes for several weeks after the birth. Having an epidural also multiplies the risk of having a labour which ends up as a ventouse or forceps delivery (which usually means the need for an episiotomy and consequent perineal injury). It seems that most anaesthetic agents cause uterine relaxation, which consequently could increase the number of caesareans which need to be performed afterwards, as well as increasing the numbers of forceps deliveries and the number of cases of postnatal atonia—which is where the uterus fails to regain its muscle tone after the birth, which is the cause of one serious complication of childbirth: postpartum haemorrhage.[50]

At the moment in the UK, many women have an epidural, although fewer than in North America. According to a recent article in *The Times*,[51] in some hospitals the proportion of first-time mothers now having an epidural is as high as 60%. And the journalist adds: "A British review in 2005 of 21 studies into epidurals involving 6,664 women found the procedure prolonged labour and increased the chance of further medical intervention by 40%." (According to the most recent NHS statistics available—for 2008-9—nationwide the average number of women giving birth with an epidural was 36.5%, which is up from the rate in 2004-5, which was around 20%.)[52] There are indeed times when epidurals may be helpful—for example when labour stops progressing completely, when a woman has been in labour for a very long time (when all other attempts to hurry things along have failed) and in cases where the woman is a survivor of sexual abuse, when the pain of contractions is too reminiscent of the pain the same person felt while being abused. However, as we've already noted, epidural anaesthesia is far from innocuous as far as secondary effects are concerned. From your point of view, perhaps the most important of these is that an epidural often leads to a caesarean (because it necessitates more interventions, which lead to others), particularly when the epidural is administered too early on in labour. You may also want to take into account that epidurals are associated with rectal tears.[53]

Some medical experts are particularly concerned about the use of epidurals. After considering the Cochrane studies on this subject, doctor and researcher Michael Klein concluded that epidurals administered before the active phase of labour more than double the risk of the labour ending with a caesarean.[54] Dr Andrew Kotaska and his colleagues also note that an epidural administered alongside a low dose of synthetic oxytocin (syntocinon) so as to augment labour (when it's slowed down), increases the probability of the labour ending with a caesarean.[55] In addition, an epidural generally forces the woman to remain lying down—often even in cases where the so-called 'mobile' epidural has been administered. As we've already noted, this can affect the progress of labour and cause fetal distress because the vena cava is compressed, so the fetus gets less oxygen. Some caregivers are also worried that an epidural will mask unusual pain which indicates that uterine rupture is occurring (even though no studies have confirmed this), so they're less keen to organise an epidural for a woman attempting a VBAC. Research has certainly shown that babies have more difficulty breastfeeding after an epidural[56] because of a weakened suck,[57] they cry more and they have a higher body temperature.[58] The *duration* of breastfeeding can also be affected if the mother had an epidural during labour.[59] The fact that epidural babies also have more fevers leads to more mother-baby separation (because these babies need to be kept under observation) and more antibiotics end up being administered to these babies so as to prevent infection. In half of the research conducted, effects on babies are clear until they are one month old. Epidural babies are less alert, they have more difficulty getting used to life outside the womb and their motor functions are less well coordinated.[60]

It's best to avoid an epidural if you can

For all these reasons, it's best to avoid having an epidural if you possibly can. The midwife and researcher Denis Walsh argues that the rising demand for epidurals during labour stems from "inadequate service provision and an impoverished approach to labour pain".[61] If you have good support during your labour, access to a bath or birthing pool and access to pain relief which doesn't involve any drugs, you should be able to cope with the pain of contractions.

Photos © Regroupement Les Sages-Femmes du Québec, Canada

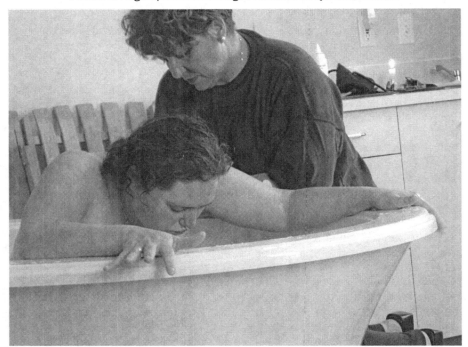

Women usually find they manage to cope with labour when they're able to move round as they wish and use water for pain relief

IS EPISIOTOMY A NECESSARY PROCEDURE?

Brigitte Denis, a woman I spoke to from Montreal, commented that she'd been cut (with a big pair of scissors) from one side to the other, from her vagina to her anus. In her view, she'd had a vaginal caesarean. Fortunately, episiotomy is one intervention which is less and less widespread. For a long time, it was almost (or always) a routine procedure, performed on the pretext that it was beneficial—but the benefits were never confirmed scientifically. Research has since shown that this type of surgery caused more pain than a natural tear, it weakened pelvic muscles, left more scar tissue (than tears) after they've healed up and inhibited sexual activity after the birth.[62] It's possible that lying down or being in a half-sitting position often meant that caregivers needed this procedure so as to get women's babies out. However, even a side-lying position could have helped prevent tears and would have given the baby enough time to gently put pressure on the perineum to allow it to extend—although of course an upright position is even better from this point of view, particularly since the coccyx moves back when a woman is upright, enlarging the exit for the baby considerably. In any case, a woman who has done daily Kegel exercises (see the Glossary) and also had perineal massage towards the end of the pregnancy is far less likely to need an episiotomy. In addition, she is likely to have less perineal pain postnatally. Also, if her perineum is supported (by a caregiver) while she's pushing, and if oil is applied to her perineum, or hot compresses, and if the woman pushes her baby out gently, the vaginal opening will gradually stretch out effectively to allow the baby through. In short, an episiotomy cannot be justified except in an emergency (e.g. in the case of a breech baby whose body has been born, but not his head), or when it's clear (to caregivers) that the woman's perineum is about to tear badly.

IS A POSTNATAL UTERINE EXAMINATION NECESSARY?

This is another procedure that some caregivers carry out after a VBAC has taken place—i.e. after the birth itself. In other words, they take advantage of the fact that the cervix is open at this time and insert their hand into the woman's womb so as to check it out, looking particularly at the state of the scar from the previous caesarean. This procedure isn't absolutely necessary if everything has gone well during the labour and birth and it's certainly an uncomfortable procedure, which can be painful. It can also involve risks, particularly the risk of uterine infection. In addition, since the procedure needs to be carried out quickly, it often involves rapidly pulling out the placenta, after having cut the umbilical cord quickly too. The rhythm of the birth and what comes afterwards therefore becomes rushed as a result of this procedure, and the woman isn't able to follow her own and her baby's natural rhythms. It also gives some women a very nasty surprise after a beautiful vaginal birth, involving no intervention at all, when suddenly an over-zealous consultant makes the woman jump to the ceiling—going ahead with this examination without any warning or anaesthesia. Having said all that, if a separation of the uterine scar is suspected, if the new mother has lost a lot of blood or if she is still experiencing suspicious pain, the situation is obviously very different and this intervention would be entirely appropriate.

Overall, when deciding whether or not to accept an intervention, you need to take all factors into account, remembering too that childbirth is not a performance. Even though it's important for many women to succeed in having a vaginal birth after one or more caesareans—an act which only a woman can perform—it's even more important to like and accept yourself, however you give birth. According to Rahima Baldwin and Terra Palmarini Richardson, the authors of *Pregnant Feelings: Developing Trust in Birth* (Celestial Arts, 1995), even women who try and have a VBAC and succeed in doing so are often hard on themselves. Perhaps they didn't manage to meet all the demands they imposed on themselves. You need to accept that attempting a VBAC in our society is a courageous move. Even if you don't succeed, it's important to know how to congratulate yourself for having tried and to forgive yourself for not managing to 'reach the grade'. You might feel resentful towards your consultant, if your wishes weren't respected during your labour and birth, but often—and usually unconsciously—women bear a grudge against themselves for not having been capable of living up to what they wanted. If this proves to be the case (or if it was the case the last time you went into labour) you mustn't forget that right in the middle of labour a woman is not always in a state of mind where she can defend her rights. The task which is occupying her is very intense and she is in a very vulnerable state. For all these reasons, let's be a little less hard on ourselves and, above all, let's be well prepared so we're able to articulate and express our real wishes clearly and effectively. Let's get these wishes put on record and let's make sure we have people around us in labour to support us, so we can have the birth we really want to have. Then, if not everything goes as we want it to, let's try not to feel guilty. We'll have plenty of time to feel guilty when we bring up our children! After all, childbirth is not an examination which we either pass or fail. It's about the birth of a baby.

To summarise...

Things to avoid if you want to optimise your chances of a VBAC

- Avoid anything which is intended to soften the cervix before induction of labour.
- Avoid any induction of labour before 41 complete weeks of gestation are over, unless there is a clear medical reason for induction.
- Low risk mothers should avoid continuous electronic fetal monitoring and simply have intermittent monitoring, using a Sonicaid or a fetoscope (Pinard)
- Avoid having a third trimester scan to assess fetal growth and evaluate the probability of a vaginal birth occurring because scans can be an unreliable way of estimating fetal weight for the purpose of 'allowing' a VBAC (or not).
- Avoid having your waters broken routinely (amniotomy).
- Avoid having a routine drip set up (an IV).
- Avoid having an epidural, particularly when you're less than 4cm dilated or before the baby's head is engaged in the pelvis.
- Don't let anyone challenge your right to freedom of movement while you're in labour.
- Avoid lying down.
- Avoid pushing while you're lying down and avoid pushing with your legs in lithotomy stirrups.
- Avoid going into hospital before you're in active labour unless your situation presents special risk factors of uterine rupture. (See Chapter 3 for more information on this, especially pages 84-95.)

Things to do to facilitate a vaginal birth

- Make sure you receive the emotional and physical support you need.
- If you're low risk, make sure you have midwifery care and consider giving birth in a birth centre or midwifery-led-unit rather than in a large hospital.
- Keep mobile while you're in labour. (Walk around. Frequently change position. Use a birthing ball.)
- Keep your energy reserves up and keep yourself hydrated by eating and drinking whenever you want to.
- Use hot water (when you're more than 5cm dilated).
- Express yourself on an emotional level, particularly if something is not as you would like it to be.
- Rest whenever you need to.
- Use a position which *isn't* lying down on your back when you give birth.

Note: In fact the above points apply to *all* vaginal births, not just VBACs.

Answers to frequently asked questions about labour and birth

- Be ready to challenge normal hospital protocols in preparation for your labour.
- A consultant may not need to be present while you're in labour, especially if your VBAC is low risk. However, it's helpful if your midwife can easily make contact with him or her, if necessary.
- You can refuse any intervention because any intervention might disturb your labour. This even means you have the right to refuse EFM. Medical opinion is divided on whether or not EFM is useful for monitoring labour in potentially high risk situations. It also means you can refuse other interventions—even if they're offered for reasons of safety—but you have a right to full information at all times, so always feel free to ask questions.
- An epidural can have negative effects on labour, i.e. it can increase its length, cause the baby to become malpositioned and it can result in more instrumental deliveries. It can have negative effects on you too, i.e. it can result in a whole series of other interventions, it can cause a fever, and it can cause low blood pressure (hypotension) as well as postnatal headaches, etc. An epidural can also have negative effects on the baby. Sometimes it can cause a worrying, but temporary depression of the fetal heartbeat. It can also cause problems with breastfeeding.
- There is usually no need for an episiotomy during a vaginal birth.
- It is not necessary to have a uterine examination after your baby's born.

In the next chapter...

- Current trends and the quest to reclaim birth
- Birth as a reflection of values...
- Why should you want to give birth yourself?
- But how on earth do you do it?
- Whatever happens, keep a sense of perspective

Birthframe 18

Encountering complete lack of support in hospital

Estelle phoned when she was 10 weeks' pregnant. Her first caesarean had been performed under general anaesthetic after her labour failed to progress. She felt as if she'd been tossed aside. Then she had a repeat caesarean, because her baby was presenting breech. Later, she had pelvimetry and sought the opinion of three consultants. According to one of them, her first caesarean had been justified because of a short umbilical cord, which wasn't even five inches long. However, he felt the pelvimetry indicated she would be capable of birthing 10lb (4.54kg) babies. One of the consultants she asked about the possibility of having a VBAC wasn't encouraging. He stipulated various conditions—she would have to give birth at 36 or 37 weeks, etc. Then her own consultant frightened her husband: "You're putting your wife in the hands of her creator. When I open up a woman after two caesareans I see the baby lying across the uterus." The third consultant she consulted contradicted the opinions of the first two and confirmed the results of the pelvimetry. She certainly did not have—as she had been told was the case—a 'small, flat pelvis'. He said: "At the other hospital the doctors are young and they just freak out, and the old doctors just aren't up-to-date." In his opinion, she had an 80% chance of having a successful VBAC and he said she could have a doula if she wanted to. He was happy to let her go beyond her due date without inducing her (up to 42 weeks) and he said if her baby presented breech, he would still be happy for her to try for a VBAC. However, two months later, the consultant who frightened her partner (whose work regularly brought him into contact with consultants) made him afraid once again. The husband came home looking worried, not at all sure that he wanted to take the risk. But he knew that Estelle was determined.

In the end, Estelle went into labour and had a long latent phase lasting more than two days. She then had a long active labour in the hospital, where her midwife kept her company. During the night, the anaesthetist came to see them. He offered to set up an epidural before he left, emphasising that he was now going home. He said he knew that the contractions would get worse and he didn't want to be 'disturbed' in the middle of the night. Estelle didn't want to have an epidural, because she had the impression this was the first step towards having a caesarean. The consultant on duty declared that if, in a few hours' time—it was then the middle of the night—things hadn't progressed, he would 'open her up'. Estelle said to her partner: "Pack my case. We're going to give birth in the car park." Her partner managed to convince the consultant to give her a bit more time, because he knew his wife wouldn't change her mind. Even though her labour was slow, the baby's heartbeat was fine. Then, when the waters broke, it really sped things up. Estelle went from 5cm to 10cm very quickly and in three pushes her son was born, with an Apgar score of 9, 10 and 10 (at birth, one minute and five minutes). Her labour and birth had been entirely normal, even though she did have an episiotomy. Baby William weighed 9lb 2oz (4.14kg).

When I spoke to Estelle a few years later, she was extremely happy to have given birth in that way and happy to have fought against having another caesarean. She told me she'd had postnatal depression after the birth, which she felt had been caused by having had to fight so hard for the VBAC. For her, it was vital to bring her third baby into the world herself. She said she had come out of the experience feeling stronger.

Make wise decisions during labour 213

Birthframe 19
A twin VBAC with wise care during labour

We had our first baby by caesarean. In the eighth month of my pregnancy I lost a friend and the shock of her death made the baby turn—I felt a huge movement in my belly. At my next antenatal appointment, the consultant told me the baby was breech. "Come in next Monday and we'll give you a caesarean." In a state of shock, we basically agreed without saying a word. The caesarean was carried out with an epidural, but my husband wasn't present.

Two and a half years later, I was pregnant again. This time, we wanted to have a normal birth. A friend who was a midwife wanted to attend our birth at the hospital. Unfortunately, though, I went in far too early when I went into labour. I was in labour for 21 hours, strapped up to the electronic fetal monitor, unable to walk around. Even though I'd taken Lamaze antenatal classes, I was terrified by the whole experience. The consultant suggested an epidural. In the end he pulled the baby out with forceps, after giving me an episiotomy which meant I had to have 25 stitches afterwards.

> The consultant suggested an epidural. He pulled the baby out with forceps, after an episiotomy which meant 25 stitches. That experience made me realise birth shouldn't be like that.

That experience made me realise that birth shouldn't be like that. I started to read a lot. Then, when I got pregnant for the third time, we decided to have a home birth. Loads of people were against the idea. And I had a long labour, which stopped and started over three long days. I had a lot of support, though, and it was a magnificent experience.

Soon after that, I found I was pregnant again. A scan confirmed that there were two babies. We decided to register with a hospital in a nearby town, and we had no trouble finding a consultant there, who agreed to let me give birth vaginally—even though he was rather apprehensive about the idea.

I went into labour three weeks before my due date and we went round a friend's house, accompanied by a midwife. When I was 7cm, despite me begging them not to take me anywhere else—"Please! I want to give birth here!"—I was taken into the hospital. The consultant was worried because he couldn't hear one of the babies' heartbeats very well. He threatened my husband and told me that if I hadn't given birth within the next half hour, I'd be given a caesarean. The midwife who was with me suggested I walk around. Then, suddenly, I grabbed hold of the bed and squatted down. The hair of one baby's head was showing and he was born with me pushing from a squatting position. It was a boy... I felt so relaxed and happy! I stayed in that position and after half an hour the other baby was born—it was a girl. Both babies weighed 5lb 12oz (2.60kg). They were two perfect births.

At the end of the day, I had more or less what I wanted at the hospital and my consultant was there too.

Birthframe 20
An important glimmer of positivity amongst all the negativity

Nicole: I knew it was possible to give birth vaginally after a caesarean, even before I had the caesarean for our first one, because I knew women who'd done it. So when my doctor told me during his postnatal visit that I would always have to have caesareans because of the narrowness of my pelvis, it didn't make much of an impression on me. "VBAC is dangerous," he said. "Your uterus could explode and you could lose the baby." Since I wasn't pregnant any more, I wasn't very vulnerable. And in the three years between the two pregnancies we kept on wanting to have a VBAC the next time round.

Our first baby had been poorly positioned and he hadn't managed to rotate his head as he came down. So he stopped at the bottom of my spine, the narrowest part of the pelvis. I should say at this point that I hadn't been moving around much during my labour, especially when I'd been pushing. What's more, when the pushing stage began, without any form of explanation I was told I was in danger of needing a caesarean. Then they put a limit on the amount of time I was allowed to push… And after pushing for three hours I was exhausted.

Raymond: I think the mere fact of speaking to her like that stopped her labour!

Nicole: The caesarean itself wasn't really traumatic and afterwards I was very disappointed. It was several months before I bonded with my baby. Fortunately, I breastfed for a long time. Then, three years later—in my second pregnancy I wondered why it had all happened like that.

Raymond: To prepare for the VBAC we read *Silent Knife* (Bergin & Garvey, 1983).

Nicole: We went to a meeting about caesareans, which a consultant at the hospital had told us about. Besides, one of our friends had also given us the name of a midwife who did manual pelvic exams. We went to see her and she really restored my confidence. In her opinion, my pelvis was quite big. She said I'd just need to be careful not to give birth in a half-sitting position because of a slight problem at the base of my spine. After that, we went to see another consultant and we agreed on the kind of birth we wanted. We also went to antenatal classes run by midwives and they were a great help. A local birthing group also helped us a lot. The only thing which depressed me, which I took a while to get over, was a comment a midwife made when we went for an appointment with our consultant. She said, "You know, it doesn't work out very often." But I hadn't decided to have a VBAC without giving it a lot of thought. The first time, I pushed for three hours to no avail. I was a bit frightened the same thing would happen again. But this fear didn't stop me.

Raymond: In the end another consultant happened to be on duty.

Nicole: We'd met him two weeks before and he'd been very encouraging. We went into the hospital with a doula when I was completely dilated. (We waited that long so as to avoid having interventions I didn't want.) During the second stage, the consultant was relaxed and non-interventionist. After one and a half hours pushing, Francois was born. I had absolutely no intervention at all, except for intermittent monitoring. I gave birth in the position I wanted to, but the bed was so narrow I was afraid of falling off! Apart from that, I wasn't afraid of anything throughout the whole labour and birth.

Raymond: She gave birth squatting on the bed, holding on to a special kind of bar, that they have at that hospital. She turned her back on the consultant. He'd never had that happen before but he let her get on with it... but then the other staff insisted she change position. In the end, the consultant excused himself for a couple of minutes and our doula, who was also a midwife, was obliged to catch the baby. When Nicole had finally gone to sleep after the birth, they woke her up to suggest she take a sleeping tablet! We came out of hospital that same evening because it was impossible for Nicole to get any rest there. It took us two hours of hassle to get discharged against hospital instructions. We even had to sign a refusal of treatment form, but doing that did at least keep them quiet, as long as we agreed to have our midwife come and see us the next day to check that everything was OK.

Nicole: Psychologically, going home had an enormous effect on us. And on the second or third day, I suddenly felt enormously proud. I felt very happy with my body! It had done its job. I'd got back to normal so much faster than the first time... and this time I fell in love with my baby only 24 hours after giving birth.

Raymond: Personally, I also felt incredibly proud of having won, despite everyone's negativity, apart from that one consultant. People were negative all around us, everywhere we looked.

Photo © Regroupement Les Sages-Femmes du Québec, Canada

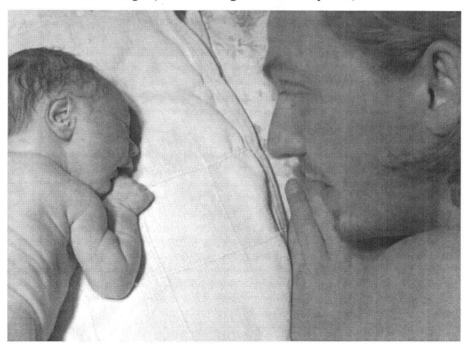

A new father contemplates his newborn baby

Birthframe 21

Learning how to do it normally: a VBAC after two caesareans

When I got pregnant for the first time, I'd been wanting to get pregnant for five years. We were living in the countryside then. I had animals, I went walking every day and I worked hard. I decided to have a home birth at a nearby town, with a midwife I knew in attendance.

I got my dates mixed up and I was waiting for this happy event at a friend's house. I waited and waited... There I was in exile, and nothing was happening. Under family pressure and under pressure from the friend I was staying with, I started doubting when I was due. In the end, we decided I was due later and we reckoned the birth would take place around 10 February. The baby was still not engaged, my cervix was still long and firmly closed. We couldn't believe this baby would ever come out! Nevertheless, I was ready.

At the end of February, at the last possible moment, I gratefully agreed to be induced with an acupuncture treatment. After three treatments I woke up one morning, realising that my waters had broken and that I was having contractions. I went back to sleep for a few hours and then contractions started up again. I was hot, I was cold. It went on for a long time... I was in pain. My husband was somewhere else— he was meditating! I felt alone, even though midwives were with me. With my consent they broke my waters—they hadn't gone completely before—and everything was going well. But the baby was so small and he was in a posterior position (i.e. his back was against mine). At that point I was 7cm dilated.

We decided to go into the hospital. My consultant had some family business to attend to, so he couldn't be there. I dealt with his replacement, which I only met four hours later, through a pethidine haze. He told me my baby would probably manage to be born vaginally, but he suggested I have a caesarean because I was so tired. (I'd been in labour for three days.) I agreed. I would have agreed to have hara-kiri at that moment and I would have said 'thank you'.

I was given a general anaesthetic for the caesarean so I didn't see my baby, Gabriel, until four hours after his birth. He was a stranger to me. He could have been another woman's baby. The next day I had no memory of him. I was only aware of the post-caesarean pain. I felt guilty... What had gone wrong with my labour? I just wasn't up to it. When I saw the midwives who'd offered me so much support I felt disappointed and embarrassed. And the feelings which stayed with me were incompetence and distress.

One and a half years later I was pregnant again. Fortunately, I was more determined than ever to start over and really give birth this time round. At the same time, I was training to be a midwife. My pregnancy was taking place while other women around me were giving birth. In my eyes, it was amazing that all these women could give birth vaginally. I still felt the agony of my first birth, though. I got support, but I have to say I still couldn't accept myself.

I still felt the agony of my first birth...

Once again, I went into town to give birth, but this time I didn't stay still. I worked alongside the midwife I was attached to (as a student). I felt good having this new responsibility. Then one week before my due date I decided to leave my partner. Suddenly, I tried to recover from my inertia, my passivity. And once again, during my labour, I had the feeling I just wasn't up to it... that I was being carried along, instead of standing on my own two feet. Everything stopped for four hours. (I was 6cm dilated and had done 24 hours of labour at that point.) So I had another caesarean under general anaesthetic because they didn't offer regional anaesthesia at the weekends. Before they put me out I spoke to my baby and told him what was going to happen. I told him I wouldn't see him straight away, but that I'd be with him. And while I'd been in labour I had somehow managed to cope with the pain in such a way that although it hurt, it never became unbearable, like it had the first time.

After the caesarean, since I was running a bit of a fever and they were worried I would 'contaminate' my daughter, I didn't see her until two days later, but then I felt as if my heart would burst with love. My immense joy of having a daughter made me suppress my sadness at having had another caesarean. Still, I did promise myself I'd have another go and would not stop trying, even if it meant having 10 children!

Six years later, I got pregnant again. I was happy but worried at the same time, and also calm. I now lived in town and by that time I'd become a fully-qualified midwife. All the births I saw taking place among ordinary women seemed extraordinary to me. I'd worked out how to love myself, despite my desire to be perfect. I'd accepted my faults and my limitations. Isn't that what life is for... getting to know ourselves and accepting who we are? And Hélène lent me this book, while it was still just a manuscript.

It did work out the third time round. My last child, Diego-Ely, was finally born in October, vaginally, after six and a half hours of active labour. I was in the countryside and my labour started spontaneously one Saturday afternoon. That night I tried to get to sleep between contractions. The next day after lunch, I decided to go back into town. After dinner my contractions were coming five minutes apart. I took a bath and things really started moving. I was so comfortable in the bath! But two hours later, I no longer felt relaxed, either in the bath or anywhere else. I phoned my birth attendants. When they examined me for the first time at 9.30pm it turned out I was only 1cm dilated. I was really disappointed. It was hurting and the contractions were coming every three minutes! I walked back and forth from the toilet to the rocking chair, then up to my bed, etc. Anyway, by about midnight I was 5cm to 6cm dilated. I felt like pushing but my cervix was swelling up... I was gasping for breath. In the end, at about 2.30 in the morning they let me push. Oh the pleasure at last! I'd been waiting two hours for this moment to arrive... Actually, I'd been waiting for eight years! How I love pushing! I felt the baby's head with my fingers. Then I saw his hair. Then I felt a burning sensation! Then Diego-Ely was born, making me into an ordinary woman. I'd at last had a normal birth. Three months later, I remember two things. First, I remember that burning sensation on my perineum. Before, when a woman in labour used to tell me 'it's burning', I'd say: "That's normal. You're just stretching." I won't say that any more. Instead I'll say: "Yes, I know. It's burning." Now I know the strange pleasure, which is so intimately linked with pain and happiness... the pleasure of bringing life into the world.

CHAPTER 7:

Remember the reasons for birthing vaginally

I hesitated for a long time before writing this final chapter. It may be difficult for some women who've had one or more caesareans to read about birth and to understand what giving birth can mean to women.

> It may be difficult for some women who've had one
> or more caesareans to read about birth and to understand
> what giving birth can mean to women

Nevertheless, I decided to talk about this, given the incredible rise in caesarean rates around the world—to as high as 95% in some urban centres in China and 90% in some private hospitals in Brazil (as we've seen), and to well above the rates recommended by the World Health Organization (10-15%) in Britain (24% in 2006/2007)[1] and the USA (32.3% in 2008)[2]. Given the craze among certain women for this kind of surgery and given its new 'ordinary' status in the minds of modern citizens, it seems to me it's important to consider why giving birth vaginally can be so important in a woman's life and even essential for some women. Finally, given the power of vaginal birth to deeply affect women, we must also take into account the positive effect it might have on society. I hope this chapter will not only help you to think through the value of vaginal birth... I'm hoping it will also help to motivate you to do it yourself and understand better how it happens, because I've also included some additional tips.

Actually, in a way, talking about the advantages of vaginal birth is similar to talking about the advantages of breastfeeding. For a long time, there was no talk of the benefits of breastfeeding, or people spent little energy focusing on them—simply because they didn't want to make women using formula feel bad. However, for quite a few years now, WHO and many other official organisations have been freely promoting breastfeeding. And it's easy to understand why... Even though babies who are brought up on formula develop normally, there do seem to be many advantages for babies if they're breastfed, and it also seems to be better for the mother's long term health. (Research has shown that breastfeeding helps to reduce the risk of the mother getting certain illnesses like Type 2 diabetes, breast cancer and depression, etc[3].) We're looking at the same kinds of differences when we talk about vaginal birth. Yes, it's true that babies who are born abdominally develop normally, but being born vaginally seems to prepare babies better for life outside the womb. And giving birth to their own babies (rather than having them 'extracted' or 'delivered') can bring women and society as a whole important benefits, which people have only recently started understanding.

Remember the reasons for birthing vaginally

Photo © Yeshi Neumann

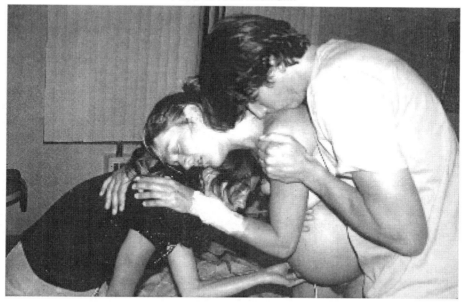

Above and below: *Pregnancy and birth represent journeys to be shared.*

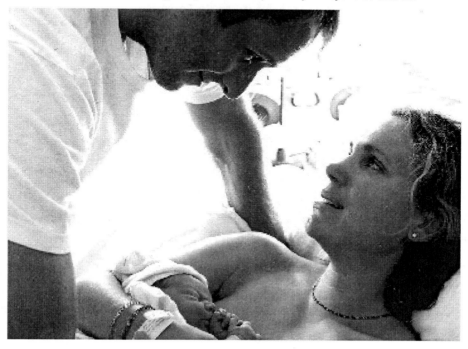

Photo © Elayne Klein

Current trends and the quest to reclaim birth

So why have people only recently started thinking about the value of vaginal birth? Perhaps it's because of the ongoing trend towards intervention and abdominal birth... After all, in our society, giving birth is now viewed as a medical event. With the rise in the caesarean rate, it's even also beginning to be viewed as a surgical event. Women who give birth now are no longer put to sleep (as they were around 40 years ago), but there certainly is more intervention and surgery than there was in the past.

In reaction to this, a movement which is trying to demedicalise childbirth sprang up in the 1970s in North America and Britain (with people like Suzanne Arms in the States and Sheila Kitzinger in the UK) and this movement soon started migrating around the world. This reconception of birth has now also been taken up by other groups—both grassroots and official—including AIMS (the Association for Improvements in Maternity Services), MIDIRS (the research organisation which was originally an off-shoot of the ARM—the Association of Radical Midwives) and the NCT (National Childbirth Trust) in Britain—not to mention the RCM (the Royal College of Midwives) with its 'Campaign for Normal Birth', Childbirth Connection and CIMS (the Coalition for Improving Maternity Services) in the USA and the research-based World Health Organization internationally. All of these organisations have consistently advocated an emphasis on normality for the sake of safety. In other, non-English-speaking areas of the world, similar organisations are promoting vaginal birth in the same way. In France there is AFAR (l'Alliance Francaise pour l'Accouchement Respecté) and CIANE (le Collectif Interassociatif autour de la Naissance); in Italy there is the Associazione Nazionale Culturale Ostetriche Parto a Domicilio e Casa Maternita; in Latin America there is RELACAHUPAN (Red Latinoamericano y el Caribe por la Humanizacion del Parto y Del Nacimiento; in Brazil specifically there is REHUNA (le Rede Pela Humanizaçao do Parto e Nascimento); and in Quebec (Canada), where I live, there is the Regroupement Naissance-Renaissance—to mention just a few organisations. See the Useful contacts section at the back of this book for contact details for UK organisations—the ones mentioned and others—and find others via Google.

Like the organisations which are trying to promote a new vision of childbirth, certain individuals have also been very active over the last 40 years or so. The antenatal teacher and anthropologist Sheila Kitzinger, the consultant-turned-midwife Michel Odent, the Brazilian consultant Ricardo Herbert-Jones, and many others, have worked to bring people's attention back to the physiology of birth and the needs of women and babies while this event is taking place.

Sheila Kitzinger, for example, has pointed out how, during the second half of the twentieth century, a woman giving birth became stripped of her own essential being in the name of hygiene from the moment she set foot in a hospital. In Kitzinger's view, at the point when that happened giving birth in a hospital came to signify—and, unfortunately, it still does in some establishments—a primitive rite of passage comprising the following elements:

- **Separation** The woman is isolated from her 'significant others', including her other children. Often, she can't have a friend or even her own mother beside her.
- **Depersonalisation** She is given an ID bracelet, her jewellery is whisked away, she is given a hospital gown and she finds herself in unfamiliar surroundings.
- **Purification** The woman is 'prepared' ('prepped'). In certain institutions this means she has her pubic hair shaved off, she is given an enema, and other 'rites' are performed.
- **Fear** An atmosphere of fear is created from the fact of being in hospital, because of all the medical hardware on display, the noises and cries from other women in labour, and also because the woman doesn't know who's going to provide care or when this person has to go off duty, etc.
- **Evaluation** This is the evaluation of the birth itself, carried out by the hospital (through its record-keeping) and the wider social circle (family, friends, etc).
- **Celebration** "Thank God it's over! I thought I was going to die, but somehow I got through it OK." This element is about the relief and celebrations which usually follow a birth, however informal and improvised.

As far as Sheila Kitzinger is concerned, the way in which a birth takes place in hospital forces women to participate in a ritual and in procedures which benefit the institution, to the detriment of the individual. In order to re-establish birth as the specifically feminine event which it is, she says it's first of all necessary to change our own way of conceiving birth and realise that giving birth helps to increase our self-esteem and our power as women.[4] She says the type of environment which facilitates birth is the same as that which facilitates lovemaking.[5]

To improve outcomes we could decrease the quantity of drugs prescribed, reduce the number of interventions and make sure fewer babies are separated from their mothers

Michel Odent has also always put a lot of emphasis on the importance of creating an environment which facilitates the smooth-running of physiology—in both his writing and his medical practice. In his view, in typical modern hospitals, even if we tried we could hardly do more to decrease the perinatal mortality rate. What we could do, though—and this may improve outcomes, in my opinion—is decrease the quantity of drugs prescribed to women in labour, reduce the number of interventions and make sure that fewer babies get separated from their mothers. He feels that this alone would improve our knowledge of birth and help us to recognise the importance of the environment in which it takes place. Ever since a certain Dr Mauriceau introduced 'labour wards' early on in the twentieth century and made women lie on their backs, consultants have wanted to take control of birth, without asking if controlling it might not also mean *disturbing* it.

Michel Odent was inspired by the findings of the researcher Niles Newton, who was working in Chicago. Back in the 1960s, she discovered that if mice were made to labour in an unfamiliar place, if they were placed in a well-lit glass cage where they felt observed, instead of in a cage with dim lighting and opaque walls, their labours would become longer, more difficult and riskier.[6] Odent tested out her observations on women in his own practice and consequently made the Pithiviers Maternity Hospital (which he was in charge of) a place where good birth was practised. There, as the resident consultant, he worked in harmony with six midwives. Odent soon noticed that the more a woman is undisturbed during labour, the more quickly she will give birth. He concluded that in order for her to give birth herself, with her own hormones, the woman needs to cut herself off from the world. With this in mind, Odent says it's pointless repeatedly carrying out vaginal examinations so as to find out how dilated the woman is. In the right environment, if the woman feels free to act as she wants to, simply observing the noises she makes will tell a caregiver that in a few contractions' time the baby will be born. For example, when the woman is in transition, he says the woman is likely to show a sudden desire to grab hold of something or she is likely to be seized by a sudden, fear-filled panic. For Odent, in contrast to the usual view, women who are the most likely to experience difficulties and the ones who are considered highest risk are the ones who are most in need of the favourable conditions for labour, i.e. discrete support with minimal disturbance, dim lighting and comfortable surroundings.

According to Jean Saint-Arnaud, a Canadian GP who was one of the first doctors in Quebec to collaborate with midwives, in the field of childbirth the expert is the woman giving birth. Why, he asks, should specific interventions which may be needed for high-risk situations be applied to all births? Saint-Arnaud says that people tend to confuse high and medium risk births. Also, he says that when there are actually *no* particular risks associated with a woman's labour she is categorised as being 'low risk', not zero risk. He adds that what women experience during labour is demanding and often difficult—painful, in fact. Sometimes there is also fear. And when it's expressed it can change the whole course of a labour. He says that if a couple's emotional experience of labour is overlooked, the most essential part is disregarded. After all, blockages are often located in the emotions. Caregivers, he says, can at least check out what's going on (in terms of the woman's emotions). Saint-Arnaud feels it's important for a woman to express her emotions when she's giving birth since the hypothalamus is the seat of the emotions—and the secretion of endorphins has some connection with the hypothalamus. In addition, the hypothalamus controls the posterior pituitary gland, which releases the hormone oxytocin, which in turn facilitates the work of the uterus. The more emotional expression is encouraged, the more the level of endorphins will rise, he says. Labouring rooms which allow a woman's nearest and dearest to be present not only facilitate the physiological processes, they also support the emotional and social realities of birth. The more that a context is created, which allows women to forget everything they know during labour, the more women will get back in touch with their instinctual knowledge, their bodies and their emotions—all of which will facilitate the production of oxytocin and endorphins. During birth a woman has to let herself go completely, let go of what she's 'learnt'. And one of the ways of doing this is to focus on the baby who's on its way.

The Brazilian consultant, Ricardo Herbert-Jones, says it was the birth of his eldest son which 'opened his eyes'. (These are the very words he used when I interviewed him in Mexico in July 2005[7].) For the first time, he explained, he observed the power of a woman giving birth herself, with her own resources, when he was a medical student. This consultant then radically changed his practice, teaming up with his partner, a midwife, and a doula, so as to help women bring their babies into the world in the place they preferred—whether this was at hospital or at home. More often than before, he did nothing during women's labours and just sat in a corner, reading a journal or taking photos, and later making beautiful slide shows to give to the women who'd given birth.

Dr Odent, Dr Saint-Arnaud and Dr Herbert-Jones have a different view of birth to many of their colleagues. In this respect, they're swimming against the tide in terms of our modern view of birth...

Birth as a reflection of values...

Clearly, the way in which society sees birth is not separate from the values which it promotes. In a society where everything goes fast, where the slightest problem makes us resort to technology, birth is not allowed to take its time. We have to 'help' it along using medical interventions, instead of offering emotional support or questioning why things are happening in a particular way. In a report issued by the British Colombia Perinatal Health Program (in 2008), it was noted that both caregivers and users (labouring women) now seem much more relaxed about technology and more wary of taking any risks.[8]

Our reactions towards the pain of labour are also often coloured by the values which society promotes. Advertising—amongst other things—conditions us to prefer to avoid the slightest headache and it encourages us to rush to the latest form of analgesia (i.e. drug-based pain relief), instead of taking a walk in the fresh air, getting a massage from someone we love, or talking about whatever it is that's bothering us. Taking this into account, it's hardly surprising that antenatal classes usually focus on ways of avoiding pain, suppressing fears and acquiring techniques which might allow women to control the whole process of birth. Therapist, Claudia Panuthos, wonders whether these techniques actually increase fear and sensitivity to pain. In her view, adequately preparing for pain—let's dare to talk about it!—as well as understanding and recognising our fears, would facilitate birth much more effectively than what people typically do now.[9]

Our reactions towards the pain of labour are also often coloured by the values which society promotes

People seem to forget that when women experience pain during labour it doesn't mean that something is going wrong or that they're in danger.[10] Labour pain is normal! Facing it also doesn't mean accepting suffering in a masochistic way. It's possible to grow as a result of a difficult experience of a limited duration. During painful contractions maintaining eye contact with someone and taking his or her hand can be really helpful, so the pain of birth prompts us to ask for support from people around us. Labour also triggers the release of endorphins and these help us to experience sensations as being less painful. The hormones which course through our body when the baby is finally in our arms also make us feel euphoric. At that point the pain we felt is no longer important—even if we do remember it for the rest of our lives.

Actually, the way in which childbirth is viewed really is different in different places around the world. For example, in some countries birth is seen as a natural process. People have confidence in women's bodies and they assume a woman 'knows' how to give birth. This is the case in Holland, where my mother-in-law was told by her doctor "Hop on your bike and come on over" when she phoned him in labour! In Sweden, birth is considered an intense event, which is an opportunity for self-realisation. In the USA, it's essentially seen as a medical event. How do you think it's viewed in the UK? Has this been changing over the last few decades?

Unsurprisingly, different perceptions of birth colour maternity practices in different places. For example, the presence of other children when a baby is born is regarded warily in the States, because people are afraid of germs going where they shouldn't. The situation is very different in Europe, where children are welcomed, because their presence is considered important for family interaction. The presence of children at births in Mexico is actually taken for granted, simply because women tend to give birth at home in that part of the world.[11] Other aspects of birth are also affected by different viewpoints. For example, pain is regarded differently in different places—depending on whether birth is seen as a medical event, a family event or even just a natural event. And one of the dimensions which we often forget (which, as I've already noted, is not forgotten in all cultures around the world) is the psychological dimension of childbirth and this is perhaps a shame because it helps us to understand why it's valuable to give birth yourself, vaginally, without the help of surgery.

Why should you want to give birth yourself?

At a time in history when some women are beginning to ask their consultants to carry out caesareans for no medical reason, without necessarily having experienced birth beforehand, we must consider why other women yearn to bring their babies out into the world on their own. In my view, it's because giving birth is not just a biomedical event (far from it), as is usually the view in Britain and America. Giving birth to another human being is actually an event which takes places on several levels, all of which are important. As we shall see, many people believe that how a woman brings her babies into the world really can have an enormous impact on her.

BIRTH IS AN EMOTIONAL EXPERIENCE SO IT NEEDS TO BE TAKEN SERIOUSLY

In *Rediscovering Birth* (Little Brown, 2000) Sheila Kitzinger points out that all our physiological functions are affected by our state of mind and she says that labour is profoundly affected by our emotions, our beliefs and our interpersonal relationships. Stress has long been known to slow down or stop labour, she says, and it can cause contractions which are ineffective and extremely painful.

Even by the end of the 1980s the sociologist Maria De Koninck was stressing that the affective (emotional) dimension of birth is often neglected.[12] The antenatal teacher Penny Simkin[13] also noted how well a woman will remember her birth, even many years afterwards. She came to this conclusion after asking women about their births 20 years after the event for a research project. She was impressed by how clearly women remember their caregivers' attitudes towards them and she concluded that these attitudes seemed to have a long-lasting effect on the women. Simkin notes that bad memories don't fade with time... quite the opposite happens, in fact. In a similar way, other authors have noted that caregivers' attitudes towards labouring women can lead to either feelings of *empowerment* or to extreme discouragement—depending on what the caregivers' attitudes were.[14]

Pregnancy and birth can make us feel vulnerable as women

Pregnancy and birth can make us feel vulnerable as women—a fact that several traditional societies have clearly understood very well because they make efforts to protect pregnant women from harm. Research carried out in the 1990s confirmed the possible impact of birth on women's minds. As we saw before, some women experience post-traumatic stress disorder after giving birth.[15] And this isn't only true for women who've had a caesarean because, as we also noted before, a traumatic vaginal birth can also cause post-traumatic stress disorder. Whatever the cause, post-traumatic stress disorder can make a woman experience difficulties in normal daily life, it can make her avoid sex and it can result in difficulties with parenthood.[16] One study even notes that most women who are diagnosed with post-traumatic stress disorder have had a vaginal birth which the medical community would consider 'normal'.[17]

There certainly seem to be links between the way in which a woman is treated by caregivers during her labour and the way in which she sees herself afterwards.[18] The researcher and therapist, Gayle Peterson,[19] emphasises the effects of the way in which women are criticised when they're in labour on their self-esteem and their family relationships. The sociologist, Ann Oakley,[20] also sees a connection between the emotional well-being of mothers and the extent to which technology was used during their labours and births. It's not surprising that birth affects so many women, because it's a major rite of passage, which profoundly influences all aspects of a woman's life, her body image, and her sense of self.[21] One study concluded that women have important expectations of human relations while they're in labour and giving birth... they expect them to be central, while in fact they're often considered unimportant.[22]

In *Of Woman Born: Motherhood as Experience and Institution* (Virago, 1977), Adrienne Rich claims that changing women's experience of childbirth involves changing their relationship with fear and impotence, changing their relationship with their bodies and their children. She says that birth has important implications on a psychological level and even on a political level.

In her thesis,[23] the researcher Lucy H Johnson, responds to the question which some people might ask: "If the outcomes [of a birth] are good, what's lost?" (If both mother and baby are in good health, surely nothing's missing?) She says that when birth is medicalised, something which is crucial for the development of the family is indeed irrevocably lost. This is what she argued throughout her whole thesis. For her, technology infantilises the woman and prevents her from being in control of the experience which involves projecting her inner world on to the outside world—according to psycho-analytical theory. By contrast, a pregnancy and birth which are experienced naturally (particularly the birth)—and not masked and changed by drugs and interventions—can have the effect of enabling the woman to mature. Considering these events to be as important as those occurring during puberty, Johnson emphasises that giving birth gives women the opportunity to confront their primitive fears and go beyond them—a process which she describes as involving an act of creation, which is an important accomplishment. Women emerge from the experience with new psychological strength and their internal psychological world will also have been profoundly changed, just as it was during adolescence. This experience of growth is a phenomenon which continues and unfolds, ultimately integrating and changing the woman in new ways all through her life.

But—even if you agree that birth is an *emotional* event—why is actually giving birth so important? One French consultant, Serge Bizieau, helps us to understand why. He reports excellent results, basing the care he provides on a respect for the physiology of childbirth. He emphasises the benefits of this approach for mothers, their babies and even for the health professionals which are at the woman's side during labour and birth. The first principle he observes is to respect the integrity of the labouring woman. He makes sure the woman is kept in an intimate atmosphere (perhaps with her partner there too). And afterwards she feels happy to have gone through this challenge. She achieves a new level of confidence in herself and in her baby, and the connections she's made with her baby during the labour and birth are very strong. There is less mother-baby separation or father-baby separation. The mother is more capable of caring for her baby and she spends more time with him or her. She breastfeeds for longer. She is less likely to become depressed postnatally. She moves around more freely postnatally too—because she is less likely to have had an episiotomy, forceps or a caesarean. This doctor confirms that babies born naturally have better Apgar scores than those born in medicalised births. He also sees babies perform better in neurological terms in the first month of their lives. The mothers seem to be in a state of serenity and seem more confident around their babies—who also cry less. He emphasises the quality of human engagement he feels when he attends physiological births. He says he feels happy to have attended these women, to have helped them feel more confident.[24]

GIVING BIRTH CAN BE SATISFYING AND TRANSFORMATIONAL

It may seem an obvious thing to say, but pregnancy and birth transform a woman into a mother, particularly when they occur for the first time. All over the world pregnancy and birth are seen as a period of transition, of transformation[25]. Nowadays, it seems to be becoming increasingly important to ask if birth can be an opportunity for psychological growth.[26] As modern people in a post-modern society, we don't have any ceremonies or rites to mark this transformation, which nevertheless takes place, even though the world keeps spinning round. The psychological dimension of pregnancy and birth means that a woman's identity is affected by the way in which she gives birth. What's more, her sense of fulfilment and her development as a mother also obviously affect her relationship with her baby. In fact, when a woman has a negative view of how she gave birth this can affect how competent she feels as a mother, how well she bonds with her child and her development as a parent.[27]

We rarely talk about how pregnancy and birth might allow women to develop. We rarely consider the personal growth or even transformation which might come as a result. When I did a literature review in 2004 I discovered some studies on these issues, but not many.[28] Towards the end of the 1990s one study into the humanisation of birth carried out in Brazil showed the importance of this aspect of birth.[29] Transformation was shown to be a characteristic of 'humanised' births in general, but was found to be particularly characteristic of home births, when women are able to be themselves and go deep inside themselves to find the inner resources to bring their babies out into the world. It seems clear to me that wherever we give birth—whether at home, in a hospital or at a birth centre—bringing a child into the world really can mean a process of profound transformation, which can affect every aspect of our lives.

Fulfilment is particularly important for human beings—something I would like to call having a 'feeling of accomplishment'.[30] The experience of giving birth can give us this feeling...[31] Some research which was carried out in hospital environments has actually confirmed the capacity of birth to bring a sense of accomplishment and self-transformation. For example, in Finland,[32] research has shown that people there see pregnancy and birth as experiences of growth and well-being, which take place on various dimensions. What makes the experience work for Finnish women is a strong feeling of confidence in their ability to give birth—they feel "I can do it!"—a confidence which influences their perception and the way they deal with labour. They feel ready to experience and survive any pain, seeing birth as one of life's challenges, and afterwards they have a particularly strong feeling of accomplishment. Similar results were found in nearby Sweden—another Scandinavian country.[33] (It's noteworthy that Scandinavia is a region where women usually give birth with midwives in attendance, as long as there are no complications.) The experience of accomplishment and self-transformation, which was observed through the research, corresponds with what numerous women feel after they've had a VBAC—as the accounts in this book show.

One woman who wrote to me—a woman called Caroline—said: "My baby was finally with us and she came out the right way—to the delight of her parents! I'm happy I succeeded and I'm sure it's affected all kinds of things in my life. If I'd had another caesarean, I wouldn't have breastfed, I wouldn't have been that close to my baby and I would have stopped having children. Now, I feel as if everything's possible. I know I'm capable of giving birth and I'm really happy about that! This second pregnancy and birth made me learn a lot about myself. I discovered within myself a determination to face anything whatsoever and a new confidence in myself. I now have a new way of seeing challenges which life throws at me and I've discovered an inner strength I didn't know existed. I discovered a capacity to go beyond what I'd done before, which amazed me. All this helped me come to terms with the past in various respects, especially my previous caesareans, but also very difficult periods I've gone through in my life." This woman would certainly lead us to conclude that in certain circumstances giving birth can give women a real feeling of accomplishment and a profound experience of transformation.

GIVING BIRTH PROVIDES AN OPPORTUNITY FOR A UNIQUELY FEMININE EXPERIENCE

In her study of home birth,[34] the midwife Céline Lemay, concluded that birth is an essentially feminine act, that it represents an opening which is not only physical, but also an opening up to the unknown, to oneself and even to life itself. She also concluded that it is a force we can work with and not just be controlled by. In her view, birth is an act which takes place deep inside oneself right up to the birth of the baby. She concluded that it stimulates instinctual behaviour and that it's an opportunity to discover what one really is, to evolve and experience a link with all women, since women have brought their children into the world for millennia. Her research also made her conclude that birth is an event which can change for ever a woman's personal and social identity.

For the anthropologist and antenatal teacher, Sheila Kitzinger, childbirth is also linked to women's power—to the power of the feminine. The contact women have with their own power can give them a feeling of unity, a feeling of union with birth and the rest of creation—with nature, in fact. This feeling of non-separation is particularly characteristic of Eastern cultures. Traditionally, women from different cultures have invoked the powers of goddesses and the energy of all women, from all time, during labour and during the birth of their babies. In several cultures, such as Namibia, women give birth alone and they consider birth to be a rite of transformation. They feel they're guided by a spiritual energy. These women believe that their only enemy is fear. Their labour is seen as an important process of maturation, which signifies their entry into life as a responsible adult, who is productive and who possesses power.

For some women, having a good experience of a normal birth can be an opportunity to get in touch with their instincts again and their intuition. Often, women who choose to give birth at home have previously given birth in a hospital and had a difficult or medicalised birth. In the study carried out by the researcher Klassen (who found that women give birth alone),[35] there was an extreme case (a woman called Nina—not the one mentioned elsewhere in this book) who, after three homebirths, decided to follow her instincts and give birth unassisted. During her labour she reached a meditative state, which helped her to birth her baby alone. She said, "I was my own midwife." She also said this last experience of birth led her to a level of spiritual and physical maturity in other areas of her life. Another person who took part in this study (Miriam) emphasised that her last home birth was an incredible experience. While it was going on she was overwhelmed by a very strong feeling of love for the whole universe—and this led her afterwards to continue a spiritual journey which honours the feminine principle in life and honours the power of women to bring their children into the world.

So why is it that so many women deny themselves the opportunity to have this uniquely feminine experience? At a time in history when extreme sports are valued, when so many people seek out dramatic experiences which either allow them to go beyond pain or transcend it, why do women seem to forget that bringing a child into the world constitutes a unique opportunity in their lives? Why do they forget that it's their chance to experience something intense, which has the power to make them transcend their normal day-to-day perceptions, which could affect them for the rest of their lives?

But how on earth do you do it?

One Finnish woman, who was interviewed by the researcher Kirsi Viisainen, said she gave birth believing in all her strength. She said we women have so much power in us, as long as we know how to use it and dare to follow the path which inspires us, even if it isn't the approach valued by the society in which we live. In her view, we need to dare to do what we see as right.[36]

In *Pregnant Feelings* (Celestial Arts, 1986) author Rahima Baldwin explains that childbirth is a process which we need to abandon ourselves to, not resist— just as we do when we have sex... During sex we 'abandon' ourselves so we can have an orgasm. This author says the energy is the same, and he argues that there's really something to be gained from letting go, allowing ourselves to be invaded by something which is more powerful than we are ourselves. Our bodies know how to give birth and we need to have faith in its inner knowledge. After all, childbirth has been going on since the world began and it's not something people have ever 'learnt'—just as we have never learnt how to sneeze or have an orgasm. Nevertheless, this author explains that just as we can stop ourselves from sneezing or having an orgasm, it's also possible for us to disturb the process of birth.[37] This is why—as I've explained before—we need to be so wary of unnecessary interventions and their possible consequences. It's also why we need to make an effort to ensure conditions are as good as they possibly can be, when we go into labour.

But then what? It's like running a marathon. It's hard, it hurts... At a certain point you might reach your limits, but then you go beyond them. You get through the experience and emerge feeling stronger and—most importantly—having the baby who you've been waiting for over nine long months. And if—during labour—you have the feeling that you're never going to get through it, that you were stupid to want a VBAC, that it just hurts too much and you want to ask for another caesarean, let's hope someone reminds you at this moment how much you wanted to have a normal birth and let's hope that he or she helps you to get through transition, when dilation is almost complete, when the baby's almost ready to come out.

At a certain point you might reach your limits, then you go beyond them...

On this subject, one consultant, a certain Dr Porreco, told me about an agreement that was reached at the hospital where he worked with any woman who requested a VBAC. He said the consultants agreed they would support the woman during her labour for as long as everything indicated that both she and her baby were doing well and that her labour was progressing normally. The doctors agreed that it would be normal for her to regret her decision (to have a VBAC) during labour and that this wouldn't indicate that things were going badly. He said: "No woman should be obliged to keep quiet while she's in labour but we told the women clearly that we wouldn't finish their labour off with another caesarean just because they'd changed their minds during labour. We agreed that just 'changing your mind' was not a valid reason to have a caesarean. Instead we encouraged the women to prepare themselves by attending antenatal classes designed for women in the same kind of situation."

To succeed in giving birth, we really do ourselves a favour if we let ourselves go, if we say 'yes' to the whole process, if we accept what's going to happen (even if it's painful), if we stay in touch with the baby who is also doing its part within us. But we can't do any of this with our head—we have to do it with our whole body and with our heart. It isn't easy but it is something we can gradually manage to do, because labour lasts long enough to allow us to get accustomed to it! What really helps is letting go. A woman shouldn't feel embarrassed about expressing herself, making sounds or crying out if necessary; she shouldn't feel bad about groaning or singing... all that can really help! After all, why not *really* experience the event without worrying about keeping up appearances, without worrying about spoiling your well-cultivated image of being a sophisticated person? After all, these days we women give birth so rarely in our lives.

Whatever happens, keep a sense of perspective

We often forget in our society, that childbirth means *giving* birth... bringing a child into the world. A few decades ago, the consultant Frederick Leboyer poetically made us reconsider what childbirth was really about in his book *Birth Without Violence* (Wildwood, 1975). While he was highlighting the inhumanity of practices in obstetrics at that time, his reminder is useful in other respects, since many people focus too much on the *processes* of giving birth. Really, our main focus needs to be on the baby because birth is really about the baby. Personally, I admit that even if during my pregnancies my babies *in utero* were very real to me, when I was actually having my first labour and then a VBAC I didn't think about my baby too much—I found labour and pushing so incredibly intense. I was hardly aware that my baby was trying to make its way through my body, so as to come out. It's easy to fall into this trap during a VBAC, especially if you've had to go to quite a lot of trouble to find a hospital or a caregiver who will agree to support you. Let's not forget this, even though having a vaginal birth is *so* important in our lives...

In any case, if a woman brings her baby into the world herself, everything then looks different. But after that, she will have to let her baby go as it grows up to the point where it will eventually fly the nest.[38] Our adventures will really begin after our baby is born and they will be far more demanding than those few hours of contractions, which sometimes make us feel so very frightened...

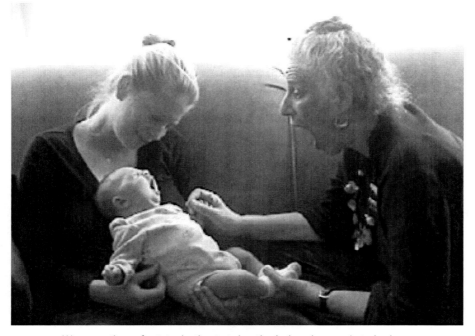

We sometimes forget what's at stake: the baby who needs to be born
Photo © Bliss Dake

To summarise...

Current trends and the quest to reclaim vaginal birth

- Our view of birth has changed radically and it is now often considered a surgical event which involves many risks.
- For quite a few decades various organisations and individuals have been working to reinstate birth as a normal process.

Birth as a reflection of values...

- Our reactions to birth are often coloured by the values of our culture or by the society in which we live.
- The pain of labour doesn't signify that something is going wrong. Instead of using interventions when things appear to be blocked, it may be wise to consider what's happening to the labouring woman emotionally.

Why should you want to give birth yourself?

- Birth is then also experienced as a cultural and social event.
- The bio-medical approach to birth reflects the values of our society. However, our bodies know how to give birth. Giving birth involves using energy, opening up and abandoning oneself to the process—and it can be more fulfilling when it's approached in this way.
- Birth can be a transforming experience.
- The psychological dimension of birth is important.
- Birth is a major rite of passage, in which affective factors are often ignored.
- The feeling of having achieved something is empowering.
- This opportunity for psychological growth can have an impact on the rest of our lives.
- Birth constitutes an exclusively feminine act in an era when people are exploring strong experiences, such as extreme sports.

But how on earth do you do it?

- Abandon yourself to the process—don't resist it.
- Just keep on going, however bad it feels and seek support from your birth attendant(s) while you're in labour and giving birth.
- Discuss with your caregiver what he or she should do if you become discouraged during labour.
- Forget about 'performing' and really become involved in the experience—moving around as you feel you need to, groaning or making other sounds when necessary, and asking for whatever you need as you go along.
- Let yourself go and say 'yes' to the whole process.

Whatever happens, keep a sense of perspective

- Really the most important thing is to get your baby born and then focus on the other adventures you and your partner will no doubt have together with this new human being, after he or she is born.
- As we've seen, birth really can be an empowering and transformative experience but be kind to yourself, whatever your experience, and focus on your baby afterwards!

Birthframe 22

A VBAC after four caesareans and better postnatal recovery

I had four caesarean babies. The first one was carried out because I didn't dilate at all, even though I'd been having contractions—it was a case of false labour over two days. Since my waters had broken, I was given a caesarean. The other caesareans were a repetition of the first scenario. During my fourth pregnancy, my local hospital suggested I might have a VBAC, but they didn't press the point and they didn't offer me the support I would have needed to make a VBAC possible.

Then, a few years later, at the age of 32, when I was pregnant with my fifth daughter, I was fortunate enough to meet a different midwife. When she examined me she said that with my long menstrual cycles—they were regular, but long—it'd be better to calculate my due date from the moment of ovulation and not from the day my last period started (i.e. my LMP). That gave me two more weeks than any other method of calculation! The midwife also made me realise I really could think about having a vaginal birth and she helped me to find a hospital who would take me on.

Once we'd found a hospital—which wasn't easy to do!—I continued seeing the same midwife. She helped me to prepare for my VBAC, getting me to do visualisation exercises and also sending me off to see a chiropractor, who was also an acupuncturist. He did something which he said would ensure my cervix opened up.

On my due date—the one my midwife had established was correct—my contractions started... and I started dilating at 2 o'clock in the afternoon. In the middle of the night, my waters broke and I called the midwife as I wanted her to go into hospital with me. Early in the morning (it was a Friday) we arrived at the hospital and we were welcomed with open arms. Everyone was encouraging me. They were discrete—they respected what it was I had to do—but they were listening to us. I hardly lay down at all for the whole of my labour because I felt uncomfortable lying down. During the afternoon, my labour slowed down but they still let me get on with it. I took a hot bath and around midnight I agreed they should augment contractions a bit using synthetic oxytocin (syntocinon). My baby was born at 3.30am in the presence of her eldest sisters, who were then 10 and 8 years old. The baby stayed with us the whole time. It was a beautiful birth. I felt positive while I was in labour and I felt well prepared. The next morning, we went home. I found the difference in my postnatal recovery—comparing this time with my previous caesareans—quite, quite incredible!

Birthframe 23

Preparing for a VBAC, but deciding to have a section after all

I'm a nurse and I'm married to a doctor. I had both my babies after I was 35, quite close together, but they both ended up being caesareans. I did prepare for a VBAC, though, the second time I gave birth...

My first pregnancy was going very well, but I was three weeks overdue. Towards the end, I was having non-stress tests every two days. The baby wasn't moving about as much, and there was less amniotic fluid, so they decided to induce me. However, it didn't work and my cervix remained firmly closed. There were also decelerations in the baby's heartbeat—once they went as low as 60—and they didn't go up again. So it was an emergency caesarean. By chance, the theatre staff were ready. It turned out the baby was postmature and he had no more room to grow inside me. It's funny, but I thought it would happen that way. Three days before I was induced, I dreamt that I was having a caesarean. Luckily, my baby was in perfect health and he had a three-minute Apgar score of 9 out of 10. I was relieved.

Afterwards, I didn't question that the caesarean had been necessary, but I did ask my consultant many other questions. She came up with various hypotheses, but there were still numerous contradictions.

When I got pregnant again, I decided to go and seek out other answers. I went to a personal development centre and had three rebirthing sessions. (This is a therapy which uses the breath—and it sometimes allows people to relive the experience of their own birth.) Even then, I wasn't satisfied with what was being suggested to me. One idea was that my mother must have had difficulty giving birth... but in fact she had easily given birth to large babies at home. (Having said that, I must say she'd had trouble giving birth to *me*, though!) Anyway, by that time, I'd already had therapy and I was doing all the exercises which had been suggested to me—affirmations, amongst other things—and I really believed in what I was doing. Then, one week before I went into labour, I practised all the exercises again. I meditated, and I spoke to my baby... I sensed that I was with my baby and that everything was going to be fine, no matter how it happened. So I decided to give myself up to the universe and I thought that if it was my path to give birth naturally, that would actually happen. The most important thing for me was for us both to stay healthy.

At the end of the ninth month, there was no sign of my labour starting anytime soon. My consultant suggested that we wait another 15 days, while doing tests. At 41 weeks, still nothing was happening. At the end of the 41st week, my consultant said: "It's the same pattern as before. We've been letting nature do its thing, but nothing's happening. Still, some women do need 42 weeks of pregnancy. It's up to you to choose."

I didn't want to risk having any fetal distress occurring again so I opted to have a caesarean with an epidural. It went very well. I had the feeling I was living out my destiny. I was accepting the limits of my body. I'd prepared to give birth vaginally, I was ready for everything and open—at least, consciously I was. Perhaps I didn't do enough preparation? I don't really want to know whether I did or not. I accept what happened and I feel serene. I no longer feel like I'm not a real woman just because I haven't given birth vaginally. Accidents like that occur in nature so as to make us think. Why does one birth work out but not another one? We'll never know why.

Remember the reasons for birthing vaginally 235

Birthframe 24
A VBAC which didn't work out, but she was pleased she'd tried

At the beginning of my third pregnancy, after two previous caesareans I was very afraid I'd have to have another caesarean, but I'd resigned myself to it. Deep down, I still felt doubtful and angry because I'd been given a second caesarean after a trial of labour. During my third pregnancy I took some VBAC antenatal classes. All my doubts and inner conflicts about routine caesarean came to the surface again. I discussed all the reasons doctors had given me for not allowing me to have a vaginal birth. The teacher who organised the classes encouraged me to look into it more thoroughly and suggested I go and see a consultant who was considered a VBAC pioneer. Although he wasn't very positive about my chances of success, he nevertheless took me on as a client, even though other consultants had refused me. I also carried on seeing my own consultant.

My own consultant's hesitations about VBAC scared me and it wasn't until the seventh month of my pregnancy that I made up my mind... At that moment I started putting all my energy into preparing for the upcoming event. On the one hand, I was relieved to find I wasn't going to have an elective caesarean. On the other, I experienced a whole series of fears, doubts and conflicts. Could I do it? Was it all worth it? Would I be able to stand the disappointment of another caesarean if that's how it turned out? I always came up with the same answer: if I didn't try, I was 100% certain to have a third caesarean. That's why I contacted a doula to support me in my third labour.

On my due date a vaginal examination showed that my cervix was completely closed, and the baby also wasn't engaged. I read and re-read *Silent Knife* (Bergin & Garvey, 1983) and I cried. Then I phoned a local organisation and asked to see a midwife. She gave me a manual pelvic examination and reassured me, telling me that it really would be possible for me to give birth vaginally. 10 days after my due date, at 11.30 on a Friday night, my contractions began... then they stopped on the Saturday morning. They stopped and started like that for three days and all through that time my doula came to my house to massage me and encourage me. My consultant had said he would trust us to judge the moment to go into hospital. On Monday afternoon my labour started up again, but by Tuesday afternoon my contractions were still coming only once every 10 minutes, although at least they were now stronger and longer. At 8.30pm my doula gave me a vaginal examination. I was only 3cm dilated. I just couldn't believe it— after all that time! At that moment my husband wanted us to go into the hospital.

We got there at 9.30pm. The staff were a bit worried because of my two previous caesareans. My consultant was there and he said I was 5cm dilated. He broke my waters and told me he would come back again later. The midwives put me on the electronic fetal monitor, but I refused to stay still like I'd done the first time. I detached myself so I could walk around. By 4 o'clock in the morning I was 7cm. I stayed like that for two hours. My contractions were strong and about five minutes apart. My husband breathed through each one with me and I hung on to my doula. They both told me I was doing very well. I was progressing slowly and I felt I just couldn't keep going right through to the end... But five hours later I was completely dilated and the baby was engaged. I couldn't believe it!

My consultant told me to start pushing, even though I felt no urge to push. Everyone explained to me how to push. My consultant told me he would come back an hour later and I kept on pushing. Then my doula suggested I have a rest. I was very tired and nobody had told me that pushing during contractions would hurt. In the end, I pushed for almost four hours—while everyone watched the monitor and kept on encouraging me. At 12.30 that Wednesday lunchtime, the consultant came back and told me the baby's head was too big. I think he was truly sorry to have to carry out a caesarean. In his opinion, since I was so tired and since he'd waited until the last possible moment, it was preferable for me to have a general anaesthetic. I agreed, but asked not to be given too much anaesthetic and not to have any syntocinon in the drip after the caesarean. On 25 January, at 2 o'clock in the afternoon, I gave birth by caesarean to a boy who was 8lb 11oz (3.94kg). He had a big head, like his father.

Some people might think I must have been disappointed. Quite the opposite... For me, this experience was a big success. First of all, the baby was born when he was ready. Next, he was engaged when I'd been told that not even a 5lb baby could become engaged and I'd completely dilated, when I'd been told I wouldn't be able to dilate to 10cm. All these things were big successes. Also, now I know what it feels like to give birth. I'm proud of having tried and I have no doubts about the reasons why the caesarean was carried out. I know I did my very best and that I was given the best possible chance of success. I feel really grateful that my consultant let me have the kind of birth I'd wanted. He didn't write off any possibility and he let me try and push the baby out for a long time. My doula has a special place in my heart and I feel deeply grateful to the people who encouraged me all through my pregnancy. Without their help, I wouldn't have been able to do it.

My consultant told me afterwards that my uterus was perfect and completely intact. Thinking how determined I'd been, he said that if my next baby were a bit smaller, we could perhaps talk about the possibility of having a VBAC next time...

Birthframe 25

Taking risks or doing the safest thing? Not disturbing labour...

We're Canadian, but Anaïs was born when we were working in Holland. As is usual there, we decided to have a home birth with our GP in attendance. Unfortunately, as we soon found out, he didn't have much experience in obstetrics. He told me to push too early, which made my cervix swell up and become very painful. After 28 hours of labour and after pushing for about an hour and a half, I went to the hospital with Bruce, my husband. When we got there they wanted to knock me out for a few hours, to give me a chance to recover. It didn't work... They then put me on a syntocinon drip, but that didn't work either. Three hours later, after even higher doses of syntocinon, still nothing was happening. Then they scared us by saying: "Look at the monitor! This baby's going to die!" Rather angrily, the consultant broke my waters and then—in the end—they told me it'd be a caesarean, without any more syntocinon. I detached myself from the drip. I was furious! Then I was put to sleep for the caesarean.

I finally woke up and stayed in hospital for a week. I had a reaction to the anaesthetic. They'd given me a vertical (classical) incision and they hadn't done a good job of it. We were constantly fighting with the hospital staff. They didn't want me to breastfeed. ("Look, there's no milk in your breasts!") They wanted to give my baby sugared water. They constantly wanted to weigh her... After two days, we signed a refusal of treatment form for the baby. We finally had her all to ourselves and I was able to breastfeed in peace. They wouldn't let me eat for five days. I felt upset and the baby was also upset. She cried every night for weeks on end. We ended up going home and when we got there, we immediately started thinking about our next baby, which we wanted to have vaginally. We went to see the GP... He was really sorry about how it had all gone and he was aware of his mistake. He told me I would be able to give vaginally next time.

When we flew home three years later, I was pregnant again. Since it was out of the question for me to give birth in hospital, we phoned some midwives. They didn't want to attend me at home. We were refused everywhere. So we called Pithiviers hospital in France. [This was when Michel Odent was in charge there, which was between 1962 and 1985.] No problem: "Come when you want to." It was only going to cost 200 French francs—about 20 Euros (which was worth a lot more in those days, of course). One month before my due date, we moved to France, renting a house for $50 a week, not far from Pithiviers. During my pregnancy, I'd read books by Michel Odent as well as *Spiritual Midwifery* (Book Publishing Company, 2002) by Ina May Gaskin and a little book about VBAC. I was convinced it was all going to work out fine.

My second labour started at 3 o'clock in the morning. I had a shower. Then at 7 o'clock we went into the maternity unit. My contractions were coming every three minutes. We were given a good welcome and nobody seemed stressed out. I was put on an electronic fetal monitor for just 10 minutes. Then we were left on our own—me and Bruce—in the 'salle sauvage' (the 'wild room'). About once an hour the midwife and Michel Odent came in to check on me. At around 11 o'clock in the morning, I felt like pushing. I was advised to wait a bit so, to stop myself, I sang some Mozart operatic arias with Bruce. That made me understand the value of breathing exercises! It was becoming a whole concert, though... In the end, standing up, I gave birth to our first son. He was blue. We left the cord intact and the staff gently stimulated him by rubbing his back. He turned his head, gave a little cough and looked all around. He didn't need to cry. We were both left alone for about half an hour. Then our new son was given a little bath, I cut the cord and my husband and daughter came back into the room. The placenta had come out and I was stitched up, because I'd torn. The atmosphere was like a celebration. Two hours later, we went home with a baby who turned out to be a 'dream baby'—he hardly ever cried.

Two years later I was pregnant again. Still not finding anyone who would support our wish for a home birth, we decided to go and see Michel Odent, who happened to be in in our town. He agreed to attend us in London, where he lived if we could get there. So in February the next year, we flew to London. We rented a house near where he lived and went to see him again. Not long after that my contractions started.

Although Michel Odent had agreed to support a home birth, I'd also been to register at a hospital before I went into labour—because that was the law in England at the time. While I was there they kept me waiting for two hours because a consultant took my blood pressure and found it a bit high. He told me I was risking my own life and also that of our baby, but he didn't get angry. In any case, after these 'encouraging' words, my blood pressure rose even higher!

My third labour was different from the first two. For two hours I had irregular contractions and I was able to rest between them. We called Michel Odent and he arrived soon afterwards, armed with his fetoscope, etc... as well as his pyjamas! He went to bed. At around midnight, my contractions changed. Then, at 3 o'clock in the morning, Michel came in to see me. He had trouble finding the baby's heartbeat, but he did find it in the end. He also apparently confirmed (but didn't say anything till later) that the baby was a face presentation and that I hadn't started dilating. At around 6 o'clock, Bruce went in to see him. Michel suggested leaving me on my own for a while. I was furious, but I tried to keep going. Between contractions I was 'floating' with the birds, who were singing the dawn chorus outside. Half an hour later, I saw Bruce and Michel come in. This time, Michel was dressed. I asked him if I could push—because the first time that's what had seemed to be the problem, that made them to decide on a caesarean. He didn't reply. At 7.30am Jacob was born, with me standing up again. He cried a little and also looked all around him. Michel went out of the room and Bruce stood back. I was with my baby. At 8 o'clock our other children woke up and were very happy to see the new arrival. Life went on. This baby didn't cry much either.

After the birth I tried to go and see the consultant I'd seen at the hospital in London. After really insisting that I see him and after telling the secretary that I wanted to talk about my birthing experience on Swedish television before flying back to Canada (which I did actually do, several days later) I managed to get him on the phone. I told him what had happened and asked him what he would have done with this baby—given that it was a face presentation and there was no sign of any dilation after several hours of intense contractions. He told me he would have broken my waters, put me on a drip, and also attached an internal fetal monitor—a scalp electrode, attached to the baby's head. When I told him what had happened, he told me I'd been very lucky it had all gone so well. Nevertheless, without any intervention, the baby had turned all on his own and within the space of three and a half hours, I'd gone from 0cm to 10cm dilation with a consultant who'd been very discrete and relaxed. Michel encouraged women to give birth a bit like animals do because he thinks this makes labours shorter. Perhaps it had been a bit too animalistic for me? Anyway, it had worked out fine.

Michel Odent came to see us twice a day for five days after Jacob was born, then once a day for the next five days. On the 10th day, we remembered we owed him his fee, which turned out to be $1,600. We'd forgotten to ask him how much he charged! In the end, this birth, which had been as beautiful as the one before, cost us quite a bit more, since the cost of living in London was much higher. But nowadays, we give birth so rarely in our lifetime and it's something so important... why not make it as good as it possibly can be? Yes, it hurts—it hurts a lot. But between contractions there are sometimes some very special moments. It was as important for me as it was for my husband.

Now, if we were to have a fourth child, we would want it to be another home birth, but in Canada this time!

Birthframe 26
Seeing the benefits of antenatal rather than postnatal pain

André: For our first child we wanted to have a normal birth. However, at the hospital right at the beginning of labour the consultant noticed that our baby was breech. For this reason he got Christine to have a pelvic examination and then he announced that her pelvis wasn't big enough. He told us there was a chance the baby would die. Hearing this, we accepted a change of plan and Christine was given a general anaesthetic.

Christine: Afterwards, I put on a brave face and convinced myself not to get beaten up about what had happened thanks to this 'change of plan'. Two years later, when I found I was pregnant again, I asked my consultant if I could give birth vaginally. "Never in your whole life!" he answered, churning out horror stories, which to this day give me the heebie-jeebies. Basically, he was saying: "If the uterus ruptures, the baby almost always dies and sometimes the mother does too." So the consultant picked out a date for my caesarean. I was anxious to see my baby. But the day before the operation was due to take place, I burst into tears. I was terrified. I felt as if I was preparing for the gallows.

André: Since Christine wanted to give birth near where we lived, and since the nearest hospital didn't allow caesareans to take place with an epidural, she was given another general anaesthetic. The year after the caesarean was very difficult. Christine suffered from hypoglycaemia—that's low blood sugar—and was very depressed. It tore her apart. I was just starting a new business and I didn't realise the seriousness of what she was experiencing. But we got through it in the end.

Christine: It was when the consultant told me that hypoglycaemia couldn't be cured that I reacted strongly—for the very first time. I decided to take charge of my own health. My body would somehow recover. It took months and months, but managing it confirmed to me that the human body has hidden resources.

André: In August that year, Christine was pregnant again. This time, the consultant told us that if we'd only had one caesarean a VBAC might have been possible—but after two, it was out of the question. And when a scan revealed that the baby had a kidney problem we were transferred to another hospital. There, we again asked if we could have a vaginal birth. After lots of hesitation, the medical team finally told us it was impossible after two previous caesareans.

Christine: So we kept on asking our consultant questions. "No, the baby's kidney isn't a contraindication for a VBAC, but nevertheless..." In the end we found out the real reason for their refusal: they were afraid of legal consequences if anything should go wrong. It's true, there was a big chance of me having problems. After all, I'd had two caesareans already and I was extremely 'old' at 35!

André: But this time, we didn't let a refusal stop us. During the other pregnancies without realising what I was doing, I realise now I'd left Christine to deal with her fears and her anxieties—and with the refusals—all on her own. Not this time. After attending a conference on VBAC when Christine was seven months pregnant, we felt surer than ever. Christine and I are both on the same wavelength in terms of attitude...

we're both ready to run the extra mile. She talked to me about finding a doula to support us. I was relieved to hear this idea. And when someone recommended a doula, we found we immediately liked her. A friend also told us about a hospital where she'd had a VBAC after two caesareans. We made an appointment to see a consultant there and he seemed receptive to what we were saying. He listened to us and he agreed to take us on. Leaving his office, I said to Christine: "This time I feel sure you're going to have a vaginal birth."

We really got into preparing for this birth and the nearer we got to the due date, the more our confidence increased. The doula helped us to explore what we wanted for this birth—as well as our fears and doubts. And she gave us lots of information. She also helped us deal with the fears people around us had expressed at one time or another. We also talked a lot, Christine and I. Every evening, she'd read me bits from articles on birth, pain and VBAC.

Christine: In the end my labour began with a latent phase which lasted three days. I had regular contractions, every five or 10 minutes, and sometimes they stopped altogether. I dozed throughout the night. The doula came to visit me twice. Then, on the evening of the third day, by which time I'd dilated to 4cm, we went into the hospital. Our consultant wasn't on duty... but that wasn't a problem for me. I took each contraction as it came, one after the other, aware that each one was opening up my cervix a little more. I drank apple juice and that gave me energy. André, the doula and I made a good team. Between contractions, we talked, had a laugh about little things that happened, which were all part of labouring in a hospital. I was very aware and extremely lucid, even though it was hurting. I walked around a lot. On several occasions I refused interventions that were suggested to me. No one pushed the point.

Between 3 o'clock and 8 o'clock in the morning, I 'stagnated' at 8cm. It was only during that morning that I had a single moment of real discouragement in the whole of my labour. It was when the consultant announced that he'd have to speed things up because the anaesthetist was going off duty at 1 o'clock in the afternoon. (Let him go, I thought. What's he got to do here?!) Then a hospital midwife came in with a crochet hook in her hand, ready to break my waters. She waited between my legs, waiting for me to consent to this. I hesitated. I looked at my doula. She didn't say a word. I thought that if she agreed, she would signal her agreement to me, so I said 'no'—for fear that the rhythm of my labour would change. So the midwife went off after that.

André: I was bowled over by all Christine's physical and moral force. She spent the rest of her labour sitting on the toilet, which did actually speed things up.

Christine: Then it was time to push. My doula helped me to get into different positions. I felt safe, even though I was tired. When I was on the bed I took hold of the horizontal bar, while I was squatting down. I felt the baby move down. Then, for the very first time I suddenly believed he really was going to come out that way. The consultant respected the note in my birth plan which said 'no episiotomy' and just massaged my perineum. I felt a burning sensation, but I somehow relaxed through it. My perineum was gradually stretching... I must say, before the consultant arrived, I'd surreptitiously smeared a bit of sweet almond oil on myself too!

About an hour later our baby started showing her head. The moment she came out, she looked at me. I still remember the sensation of her little body, which was all hot, soft and gooey. I was intact and so was she. I just couldn't believe it. At last she was here and. despite the prediction of a non-functioning kidney, she was actually in perfect health. André was overjoyed!

André: Mission accomplished. We'd won the bet to have a normal birth after two caesareans—despite all the obstacles which had been put in our path. What a difference it made to me to see Christine in good health, welcoming this baby we'd been waiting for, for so long! She was on cloud nine—really on top form. The whole thing really brought us closer together and it also made us mature a lot.

Christine: I really enjoyed giving birth. Between a caesarean and a VBAC there's so much difference... They really are a world apart. The pain of giving birth is active pain—it's positive pain. And when the baby arrives, the pain disappears. When a woman has a caesarean, it's afterwards that she's in pain—so it makes no sense! And it was much easier for me to submit to the laws of nature than it was to deal with the rules of the medical profession.

Photo © Regroupement Les Sages-Femmes du Québec, Canada

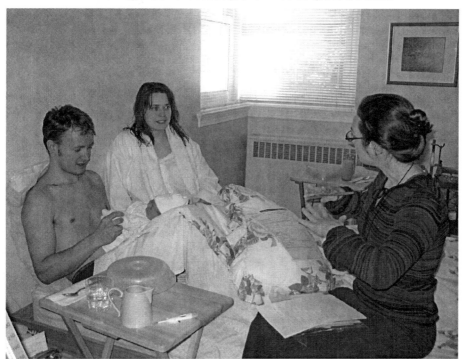

New parents talk to their midwife after a normal birth

Birthframe 27

Consequences of unsupportive and supportive environments

I experienced tremendous joy when I finally gave birth on my own... but that was not the beginning of the story.

When my daughter was born in 2005 I had no idea what a VBAC was. And I had even less idea that 'ordinary' interventions could lead to a caesarean. I'd had a normal pregnancy but since I had gestational diabetes I was told I was at risk of having an unusually big baby. Having gone past my due date, my consultant didn't want to wait much longer. I was therefore induced one an a half weeks after my due date. The induction quickly led to a runaway cascade of interventions (intense and very painful contractions, epidural, drip, amniotomy, etc) which in turn led to fetal distress—. worrying decelerations in the fetal heartbeat. It was this fetal distress which led to the caesarean. Afterwards, although I was disappointed not to have been able to bring my baby into the world myself, I was aware that without the caesarean, my baby's life might have been in danger.

Since I then had trouble breastfeeding, I became a real breastfeeding expert. That meant I ended up attending numerous conferences on the subject. It was at one of these conferences that I heard the word 'VBAC' for the first time. Out of sheer curiosity, I asked a few questions and then I immediately knew that this was what I wanted for my own next birth.

A few months later, I found I was pregnant again and from my first antenatal appointment onwards, I made it clear that I wanted to have a VBAC. My consultant supported me and was 100% in favour of my decision. I found a doula to help me prepare to face 'the unknown'. And, once again, my pregnancy went well, except the baby remained breech for a long time, which put my hopes for a VBAC in jeopardy. An attempt at external cephalic version was successful, but since I'd already had a large baby, I was not allowed to go more than one week overdue. Since, at that stage, the baby still hadn't appeared and since I was booked in for a caesarean the very next day, I then took some castor oil, hoping it would help me go into labour.

My wish was granted when contractions woke me up in the middle of the night. And when we got to the hospital everything was still going well. My contractions were coming regularly and I was slowly but surely dilating. My consultant, who was on duty when we arrived, gave me lots of encouragement and assured me that everything was proceeding normally. At the end of the day, when he finished his shift, I was 7cm dilated, and he assured me there was a good chance my VBAC would take place successfully during the night. The other consultant, who arrived soon after that, immediately started lecturing me about my decision to have a VBAC and about the 'risks' I was taking, etc. Then it was the anaesthetist's turn—someone I hadn't seen before, during the day. He came and explained that he was leaving so if I had to have an emergency caesarean it would be without an epidural, and I would be put to sleep. Both the consultant and the anaesthetist then took turns coming to see me, several times over. Feeling exhausted—for hours I'd hardly had anything to eat or drink and had had very little sleep—my contractions then started to slow down, and they stopped altogether when I was 7½cm dilated. The consultant then insisted I have a caesarean

Remember the reasons for birthing vaginally 243

and since I was so tired I couldn't put up a fight at all—even though there was nothing to indicate a potential uterine rupture... My doula said afterwards that, in her view, a little rest would have got my contractions started up again.

After that caesarean, which took place in June 2007, I found it very difficult to accept the fact that my birth had been 'stolen' from me—to accept that I wasn't capable of looking after my baby myself, not to mention my 2-year-old daughter (who also didn't understand why Mummy couldn't pick her up). I also couldn't come to terms with the fact that my own health had been put at risk by a major operation, which hadn't been necessary. At that point, I almost abandoned my dream of having a large family.

Nevertheless, knowing that I could still try for a VBAC next time round, I got pregnant two years later and immediately started preparing for a second attempt at a VBAC, with the help of my doula. During the nine months of my pregnancy, I worked very hard on myself. I went to see a psychologist, who helped me deal with my grief over my two previous births. I also did a lot of visualisation and worked on being positive. I worked hard on reducing my stress levels and learnt how to let go, so as to be able to accept that I couldn't control everything. I also transferred to another caregiver, choosing this time to see a GP who had a more positive view of birth and who was very supportive of VBAC.

My pregnancy went extremely well. In fact, it was the best pregnancy of all three. It was the one where I had the least nausea and the most energy... I went for walks and did all kinds of activities with my older two children. It was only another diagnosis of gestational diabetes which spoilt my pleasure to some extent, but with a few dietary changes, my diabetes was very much under control all through the pregnancy.

One day, two days after my due date, I got up in a very bad mood. I was annoyed about being pregnant and all the physical constraints made me feel really grumpy. Then, that same afternoon, my mucous plug went and during the night I started having contractions. It wasn't anything serious enough to wake up my partner, but nevertheless, pretty strong contractions were coming every 20 minutes. The next day, we decided that my partner would not go to work, just in case, but during the morning, my contractions became weaker and more and more spaced out. As a result, we decided to start walking around and then go shopping—in the hope that it would start me off again. But I had nothing more than a few small contractions over the next few hours. After lunch, my partner suggested we go for another walk and go and have an ice cream. (Since I was about to give birth, I could spoil myself a bit, despite my gestational diabetes.) When we got back, I went to lie down, so as to have a nice nap. Later on, feeling well rested and in a much better mood, we had dinner and it was then that the contractions started up again, coming along every 20 minutes. Over the course of the evening, they started coming closer together and became somewhat more intense. I then phoned my doula so as to let her know what was happening. She suggested I rest, in case it all happened during the night, especially as she knew I tended to have slow labours (judging by my first attempt at VBAC). So I took a bath and while I was there, my contractions quickly became more painful and they were coming closer together too. Then, quite suddenly they started coming every two or three minutes. That's when my partner decided we'd better go into the hospital.

He phoned my mother to ask her to come over and look after our other two children and, when she arrived, she helped me to deal with each contraction, while my partner quickly had a shower. Just before we left home, my waters broke. I remember the car journey as extremely unpleasant and painful.

When we got to the hospital, I was examined—they checked both my own and my baby's vital signs. My doula arrived while they were doing that. Then the midwife wanted to give me an internal, so as to check how far along I was. What a surprise! I was completely dilated and the baby's head was already visible! At that point, the rhythm of the whole thing changed... The midwife rushed out to arrange for a room to be made ready, and she came back in with a wheelchair.

I was vaguely aware that she was running when she wheeled me to my room. Then, as soon as she got me onto the bed, the baby pushed himself out all by himself, even though the consultant who was on duty was with another woman at that point, who was also giving birth. We then briefly wondered if we should go and call the other consultant on duty, but the GP who was on evening duty turned up, just in time to see me give birth. I only pushed for 20 minutes before having my warm son on my chest. His Apgar score was far better than those of my caesarean babies' and I finally found I was able to look after my baby myself—right from the first moment onwards.

It all happened very quickly—even too quickly. Of course, it wasn't how I imagined it would be. In my birth plan I'd said I wanted to give birth in a calm atmosphere, in dim lighting, with soft music playing in the background. I wanted to be free to choose a position of my choice for pushing, etc. Nevertheless, I had the main thing: the joy of bringing my baby out into the world all by myself. It's true, I do have three children... but I've only experienced one birth and I am very proud that I was able to experience that fully, without any anaesthesia.

So it's with great pride that I did what I did that day... I'm still amazed by it. And I realise now that I was right to insist on experiencing this wonderful moment. I realise it really was the best thing for my baby as well as me (both physically and psychologically). I was up on my feet much sooner afterwards. You just couldn't compare that time to what I experienced postnatally after my caesareans!

Baby Felix, who was born on 22 May 2009, is a very calm child, who doesn't cry much. He seems much more serene and much less stressed out than my other two babies. That also affected the breastfeeding and it had an effect on his well-being, as well as on my own. I would encourage any woman who's previously had a caesarean to try and have a VBAC next time, and not just accept that a caesaeran is inevitable. It really is possible to give birth normally. I'm living proof!

I feel enormously grateful towards my partner and my doula, who helped me prepare for this second VBAC, but I would also like to thank everyone else who believed in me and who encouraged me to keep persevering with this wonderful idea... which resulted in the birth of my baby.

It wasn't how I imagined it would be....
It wasn't what I put in my birth plan. But I had the main thing:
the joy of bringing my baby out into the world, all by myself.

Remember the reasons for birthing vaginally

Photo © Regroupement Les Sages-Femmes du Québec, Canada

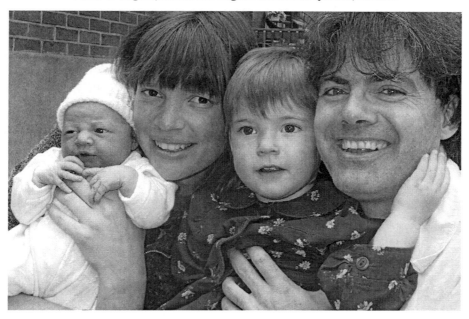

Above and below: *Happy families! The woman in the photo below is Judith, whose account appears in Birthframe 4*

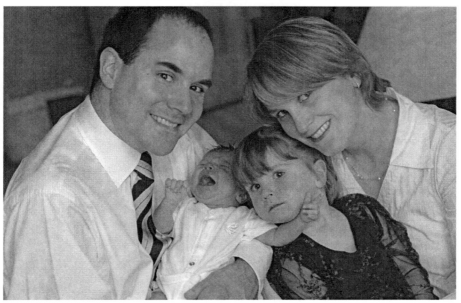

Useful contacts

AIMS (Assoc. for Improvements in the Maternity Services) – www.aims.org.uk
Tel: 0870 765 1433.
Support and information about parents' rights and choices. Provides information on complaints procedures.

Active Birth Centre – www.activebirthcentre.com
Tel: 020 7281 6760.
Classes for mothers interested in active, physiological birth. Can put you in touch with local groups and supply birth pools.

Association of Radical Midwives (ARM) – www.radmid.demon.co.uk
Tel: 01243 671673.
Support for midwives. Helpline for pregnant women.

Birth Choice UK – www.birthchoiceuk.com
No phone number
Information to help you make choices about caregivers and places of birth.

Doula UK – www.doula.org.uk
Tel: 0871 433 3103.
Information about birth and postnatal doulas working in your area.

Independent Midwives Association – www.independentmidwives.org.uk
Tel: 0845 4600 105 (leave message on answering machine).
Association for independent midwives. Can provide list of independent midwives in your area, experienced in homebirth.

International Cesarean Awareness Netwework (ICAN) – www.ican-online.org
Information and support for women who wish to avoid a repeat caesarean.

Meet-a-Mum Association (MAMA) – www.mama.co.uk
Tel: 0845 120 6162. Helpline: 0845 120 3746 Mon-Fri, 7pm-10pm.
Support for mothers who feel lonely, isolated or depressed. Can put you in touch with other mothers in a similar situation.

Useful contacts

The National Childbirth Trust (NCT) – www.nct.org.uk

Tel: 0300 330 0770 (enquiries), 0300 330 0772 (pregnancy and birth), 0300 330 0774 (shared experiences) or 0300 330 0773 (postnatal)

Maternity sales: 0141 636 0600. Pregnancy and birth line: 0870 444 8708.

Information and support for all aspects of pregnancy and birth. Antenatal classes and network of informal postnatal groups.

The Nursing & Midwifery Council (NMC) – www.nmc-uk.org

Information on the code of conduct by which midwives work.

Parentalk – www.parentalk.co.uk

Tel: 020 7921 4234.

Support for parents in the workplace, as well as for employers and professionals who support parents.

Patients' Association – www.patients-association.org.uk

Tel: 020 8423 9111. Helpline: 0845 608 4455.

Forum for NHS users to raise or share concerns about health care.

Primal Health Research Centre – www.birthworks.org/primalhealth

Information on various aspects of primal health. Publishes a quarterly newsletter (available by subscription).

Twins and Multiples Births Association (TAMBA) – www.tamba.org.uk

Tel: 01483 304 442. Helpline: 0800 138 0509.

Encouragement and support for parents of twins or more.

VBAC Information and Support – no website – but see instead: www.vbac.org.uk

Tel: 01243 868440.

Information about VBAC offered by volunteers.

What Doctors Don't Tell You – www.wddty.com

Tel: 0870 444 9886.

Information on medicine and health. Publishes newsletter and booklets.

Bibliography

A Good Birth, A Safe Birth. Korte D and Scae R. 1992. Harvard Common Press. ISBN: 9780553340686.

A Guide to Effective Care in Pregnancy and Childbirth. Enkin M, Keirse M, Neilson J, Crowther C, Duley L, Hodnett, E, Hofmeyr J. 2000. Oxford University Press. ISBN: 9780192631732.

A Woman in Residence. Harrison M. 1993. Fawcett. ISBN: 9780449222386.

Birth: Countdown to Optimal. Donna S. 2011. Fresh Heart Publishing. ISBN: 9781906619190.

Birth Without Violence. Leboyer F. 1975. Wildwood. ISBN: 9780704501713.

Impact of Birthing Practices on Breastfeeding—Protecting the Mother-Baby Continuum. Kroeger and Smith. 2004. Jones & Bartlett. ISBN: 9780763763749 (for 2nd edition, 2009).

Impact of Cesarean Childbirth. Affonso D. 1981. Davis. ISBN: 978083600348.

Living Through Personal Crisis. Kaiser Stearns A. 1992. Random House. ISBN: 9780883471661.

Of Woman Born: Motherhood as Experience and Institution. Rich A. 1977. Virago. ISBN: 9780860680314.

Pregnancy as Healing. Mehl L and Peterson G. 1984. Mindbody Press. ISBN: 9780939508044.

Pregnant Feelings. Baldwin R. 1986. Celestial Arts. ISBN: 9780890874233.

Pregnant Feelings: Developing Trust in Birth. Baldwin R and Palmarini Richardson T. 1996. Celestial Arts. ISBN: 9780890874233.

Silent Knife. Cohen N and Estner L. 1983. Bergin & Garvey. ISBN: 9780897890274.

Spiritual Midwifery. Gaskin IM. 2002. Book Publishing Company. ISBN: 9781570671044.

The Vaginal Birth After Cesarean Experience—Birth Stories by Parents and Professionals. Baptisti Richards L. 1987. Greenwood Press. ISBN: 9780897891202.

The VBAC Experience. Baptisti Richards L. 1987. Bergin & Garvey. ISBN: 9780897891202.

Transformation Through Birth. Panuthos C. 1984. Greenwood Press. ISBN: 9780897890380.

Understanding the Dangers of Cesarean Birth: Making Informed Decisions. Jukelevics N. 2008. Praeger. ISBN: 9780275999063.

Vivre sa Grossesse et son Accouchement—Une Naissance Heureuse. Brabant I. 2003. Chronique Social. ISBN: 9782850085109.

Vaginal Birth After Caesarean: The VBAC Handbook. Churchill H, Savage W. 2008. Middlesex University Press. ISBN: 9781904750215.

Further reading

Books relating to caesareans and VBAC

- *Understanding the Dangers of Cesarean Birth: Making Informed Decisions* by Nicette Jukelevics. Praeger, 2008. ISBN: 9780275999063.
- MIDIRS Leaflet No.17: *Caesarean birth and VBAC*. Midwives Information and Resource Service. Available by post from MIDIRS, Freepost 9, Elmdale Road, Clifton, Bristol BS8 1ZZ or by emailing via their website at www.infochoice.org
- NCT Information Sheet: *Vaginal birth after caesarean*. National Childbirth Trust. Available from the NCT (see 'Useful contacts').
- *Vaginal Birth After Caesarean* by Helen Churchill and Wendy Savage. Middlesex University Press, 2008. ISBN: 9781904750215.
- *The Caesarean* by Michel Odent. Free Association Books 2004. ISBN: 9781853437182.

Classics:

- *Silent Knife: Caesarean Prevention and Vaginal Birth After Caesarean* by Nancy Cohen and Lois Estner. Bergin & Garvey, 1983. ISBN: 9780897890274.
- *Open Season: A survival guide for natural childbirth and VBAC in the 1990s* by Nancy Wainer Cohen. Greenwood Press 1991. ISBN: 9780897892728.

Books relating to problems in modern maternity care

- *Impact of Birthing Practices on Breastfeeding—Protecting the Mother-Baby Continuum* by Linda Smith. Jones & Bartlett, 2010. ISBN: 9780763763749.
- *Pushed: The Painful Truth about Childbirth and Modern Maternity Care* by Jennifer Block. Da Capo Press 2008. ISBN: 9780738211664.
- *Born in the USA: How a broken maternity system must be fixed to put women and children first* by Marsden Wagner. University of California Press 2006. ISBN: 9780520245969.
- *The Farmer and the Obstetrician* by Michel Odent. Free Association Books 2002. ISBN: 9781853435652.
- *The Scientification of Love* by Michel Odent. Free Association Books 1999. ISBN: 9781853434761.
- *Birth Crisis* by Sheila Kitzinger. Routledge 2006. ISBN: 9780415372664.

Classics:

- *Immaculate Deception II* by Suzanne Arms. Celestial Arts 1994. ISBN: 9780890876336.
- *Birth Traditions and Modern Pregnancy Care* by Michel Odent and Jacqueline Vincent-Priya. Element Books 1992. ISBN: 9781852303211.

Books about birth generally, which will help you prepare

- *Birth: Countdown to Optimal* by Sylvie Donna. Fresh Heart Publishing, 2011. ISBN: 9781906619190.
- *A Guide to Effective Care in Pregnancy and Childbirth* by Murray Enkin, *et al.* Oxford University Press, 2000. ISBN: 9780192631732.
- *Home Birth: A Practical Guide* by Nicky Wesson. Pinter & Martin, 2006.
- *Gentle Birth, Gentle Mothering: A Doctor's Guide to Natural Childbirth and Gentle Early Parenting Choices* by Sarah J Buckley. Celestial Arts, 2009. ISBN: 9781587613227.
- *Surprising, Inspiring Birth* by Sylvie Donna. Fresh Heart Publishing, 2010. ISBN: 9781906619121.
- *Birth and Breastfeeding* by Michel Odent. Clairview Books, 2003 [first published in 1992]. ISBN: 9781902636481.
- *Is There Sex After Childbirth?* by Juliet Rix. HarperCollins 1995. ISBN: 9780722529570.
- *Easy Exercises for Pregnancy* by Janet Balaskas and Anthea Sieveking. Frances Lincoln Publishers, 1997. ISBN: 9780711210486.

For caregivers:

- *Promoting Normal Birth: Research, Reflections & Guidelines,* an international collaboration, Sylvie Donna (ed). Fresh Heart Publishing 2010. ISBN: 9781906619060.
- *Normal Childbirth: Evidence and Debate* by Soo Downe (ed.). Churchill Livingstone, 2008. ISBN: 9780443069437.
- *Informed Choice in Maternity Care* by Mavis Kirkham. Palgrave Macmillan, 2004. ISBN: 9780333998434.
- *Birth Models That Work* edited by Robbie Davis-Floyd, Lesley Barclay, Betty-Anne Daviss and Jan Tritten, 2009. University of California Press. ISBN: 9780520258914.
- *The Mother-Midwife Relationship* by Mavis Kirkham. Palgrave Macmillan, 2000. ISBN: 9780333760536.
- *Birth Pain: Explaining Sensations, Exploring Possibilities* by Verena Schmid. Fresh Heart Publishing, 2011. ISBN: 9781906619145.

Books to support you in motherhood—read them in advance!

- *Breast is Best* by Penny Stanway. Pan Books, 2005. ISBN: 9780330436304.
- *The Womanly Art of Breastfeeding* by Judy Torgus (ed.). Plume Books, 2004. ISBN: 9780452285804.
- *Diaper Free! The Gentle Wisdom of Natural Infant Hygiene* by Ingrid Bauer. Natural Wisdom Press, 2001. ISBN: 9780452287778.
- *Mother and Baby* by Miranda Castro. Pan Books, 1996. ISBN: 9780330349253.
- *Sleeping with Your Baby: A Parent's Guide to Cosleeping* by James McKenna. Platypus Media, 2007. ISBN: 9781930775343.

Notes and references

Chapter 1—The current situation

1. Bertrán AP, Merialdi M, Lauer JA *et al*, 2007. Rates of cesarean section: analysis of global, regional and national estimates. *Paediatrics and Perinatal Epidemiology*, 21: 98-113.

2. Canadian Institute for Health Information, 2007. *Giving Birth in Canada: Regional Trends from 2001-2002 to 2005-2006*. Ottawa.

3. • Lumbiganon P, Laopaiboon M, Gülmezoglu AM *et al*, 2010. Method of delivery and pregnancy outcomes in Asia: the WHO global survey on maternal and perinatal health 2007-2008. *Lancet*, 375(9713): 490-499
   • Festin MR, Laopaiboon M, Pattanittum P *et al*, 2009. Caesarean section in four East Asian countries—Reasons for, rates, associated care practices and health outcomes. *BMC Pregnancy Childbirth*, 9: 17. doi: 10.1186/1471-2393-9-17
   • http://www.ncbi.nlm.nih.gov/pmc/articles/PMC2695422/
   • http://www.medicalnewstoday.com/articles/176128.php

4. • Villar J, Valladares E, Wojdyla D *et al*, 2006. Caesarean delivery rates and pregnancy outcomes: The 2005 WHO global survey on maternal and perinatal health in Latin America. *Lancet*, 367(9525) : 1819-1829 - www.thelancet.com, DOI: 10.1016/50140-6736(06)68704-7
   • http://www.ans.gov.br/portal/site/_hotsite_parto_2/publicacoes/ Villar_et_al_Lancet_2006_AC.pdf

5. Bertrán AP, Merialdi M, Lauer JA *et al*, 2007. Rates of cesarean section: analysis of global, regional and national estimates. *Paediatrics and Perinatal Epidemiology*, 21: 98-113.

6. See http://www.cdc.gov/mmwr/preview/mmwrhtml/mm5737a7.htm

7. Young D, 2003. The push against vaginal birth. *Birth*, 30(3): p 151.

8. Schulman H, 1984. Quoted by Norwood C in *How to Avoid a Cesarean Section*. New York: Simon and Schuster, p 11.

9. Brabant I, 2003. *Vivre sa Grossesse et son Accouchement: Une Naissance Heureuse*. Lyon, France: Chronique Sociale.

10. Bouchez C, 2006. Caesarean on rise despite risks to baby, mom. www. FoxNews.com

11. St-Amant S, 2006. La construction medico-médiatique du concept de 'césarienne sur demande'. *Mamanzine*, 10(1): 27-30.

12. • Declercq E, Sakala C, Corry M *et al*, 2006. *Listening to Mothers II: The Second National US Survey of Women's Childbearing Experiences*. New York: Childbirth Connection. Available at www.childbirthconnection.org/listeningtomothers/
    • McCourt C, Weaver J, Statham H *et al*, 2007. Cesarean section and decision-making: a critical review of the literature. *Birth*, 34(1): 65-79
    • Weaver JJ, Statham HH, Richards M, 2007. Are there 'unnecessary' cesarean sections? Perceptions of women and obstetricians about cesarean sections for nonclinical indications. *Birth*, 34(1): 32-41
    • Turner CE, Young JM, Solomon.J *et al*, 2008. Vaginal delivery compared with elective caesarean section: the views of pregnant women and clinicians. *BJOG*, DOI: 10.1111/ j.1471-0528.2008.01892.x.

13. Declercq ER, Sakala C, Corry MP, *et al*, 2006. *Listening to Mothers II: The Second National US Survey of Women's Childbearing Experiences*. New York: Childbirth Connection. Available at www.childbirthconnection.org/listeningtomothers/

14. *La césarienne sur demande*. Enjeux [a radio programme]. Radio-Canada, October 2005.

15 • Fédération Internationale de Gynécologie et d'Obstétrique (FIGO) Committee for the Ethical Aspects of Reproduction and Women's Health. *Recommendations on Ethical Issues in Obstetrics and Gynecology*. London, 2003
   • Société des obstétriciens et gynécologues du Canada (SOGC), 2004. *La position de la SOGC au Sujet des Césariennes de Convenance* – Avis de la SOGC, Ottawa, March 10.

16 ACOG, 2003. New ACOG opinion addresses elective cesarean controversy. *ACOG New Release*, October 31, 2003, www.acog.org

17 • ACOG, 2006. Cesarean delivery associated with increased risk of maternal death from blood clots, infection, anesthesia. *ACOG News Release,* August 31
   • ACOG, 2000, *Evaluation of Cesarean Delivery*, Washington, DC.

18 ACOG, 2006. News release: *Patient-requested cesarean update*. Washington, DC.

19 According to the Canadian researcher, Nils Chaillet, RCT QUARISMA, 2006, quoting:
   • Morrison J, MacKenzie IZ, 2003. Cesarean section on demand. *Semin Perinatol*, 27(1): 20-33
   • Devendra K, Arulkumaran S. Should doctors perform an elective caesarean section on request? *Ann Acad Med Singapore*, 32(5): 577-581
   • Gamble JA, Creedy DK, 2000. Women's request for caesarean section: a critique of the literature. *Birth*, 27(4): 256-263.

20 • Saisto T, Salmela-Aro K, Nurmi JE, *et al*, 2001. A randomized controlled trial of intervention in fear of childbirth. *Obstet Gynecol* 98(5): 820-826
   • Nerum H, Halvorsen L, Sorlie T, *et al*, 2006. Maternal request for cesarean section due to fear of birth: can it be changed through crisis-oriented counseling? *Birth*, 33(3): 221-228

21 Ponte W, 2007. Cesarean: birth in a culture of fear. *Mothering*, 144. Interview with Robbie Davis-Floyd.

22 Rioux-Soucy LM, 2007. Femmes enceintes, femmes négligées. *Le Devoir*, December 8-9, p A-1, A-6, A-7.

23 Diane Francoeur, President of the Association des Obstétriciens et Gynécologues du Québec in the report: *Pregnant Women, Neglected Women. Le Devoir,* December 8-9, 2007, p A-7.

24 Klein M, 1988. Do family physicians 'prevent' caesarean sections? A Canadian exploration. *Fam Med*, 20(6): 431-436.

25 Klein M, Lloyd I, Redman C, *et al*, 1983. A comparison of low-risk pregnant women booked for delivery in two systems of care: shared-care (consultant) and integrated general practice unit. I. Obstetrical procedures and neonatal outcome. 1983, *Brit J. Obst & Gyn* 90(2): 118-122.

26 • According to OECD, quoted in News, 2007, *Birth*, 34(1): 92
   • Roan S, Girion L, 2010. Rising maternal mortality rate causes alarm, calls for action. *Los Angeles Times*, May 22

27 Affonso D. *Impact of Cesarean Childbirth*. Philadelphia: FA Davis, p 6.

28 Baptisti-Richards L, 1987. *The VBAC Experience*. Westport, CT, USA: Bergin & Garvey.

29 Declercq E, 2010. VBAC 2010: *Establishing the link between research, evidence and practice*. Normal Labour & Birth Research Conference: The Benefits & Challenges of Preserving Physiologic Birth, Vancouver, 2010.

30 Korte D, 1998. Infant mortality, cesarean and VBAC rates. *Mothering*, No 89, July-August 1998.

31 Canadian Institute for Health Information, 2007. *Giving Birth in Canada: Regional Trends from 2001-2002 to 2005-2006*. Ottawa.

32 Ministry of Health and Social Services, Quebec, Canada, 2008.

33 Centers for Disease Control and Prevention – National Center for Health Statistics, 2004.

Notes and references 253

34 • Thomas J and Paranjothy S, 2001. *National Sentinel Caesarean Audit Report.* Royal College of Obstetricians and Gynaecologists Clinical Effectiveness Support Unit. London: RCOG Press
   • Warwick C, 2010. The impact of national professional associations on normal birth. Normal Labour & Birth Research Conference: The Benefits & Challenges of Preserving Physiologic Birth, Vancouver, 2010.

35 • Keutchman M, King VJ, *et al*, 2007. Changing policies on vaginal birth after cesarean: impact on access. *Birth*, 34(4): 316-322
   • Declercq ER, Sakala C, Corry M.P, *et al*, 2006. *Listening to Mothers II – The Second National U.S. Survey of Women's Childbearing Experience.* New York: Childbirth Connection. Available at: www.childbirthconnection.org/listeningtomothers/

36 • Canadian Institute for Health Information, 2004. *Giving Birth in Canada: Providers of Maternity and Infant Care,* Ottawa
   • Lalonde A, 2008. La pénurie de ressources humaines en obstétrique au Canada est à nos portes. *Communiqué SOGC*, April 2008, p 3.

37 Hueston WJ, Lewis-Stevenson S, 2001. Providers distribution and variations in state wide cesarean section rates. *Journal of Community Health*, 26(1): 1-10.

38 • Lacoursière A, 2008. Les sages-femmes auront du renfort. *La Presse*, May 1 2008
   • Rioux-Soucy LM, 2007. Femmes enceintes, femmes négligées. *Le Devoir*, December 8-9, p A-1, A-6, A-7.

39 • Gagnon A & Waghorn K, 1996. Supportive care by maternity nurses: a work sampling study in an intrapartum unit. *Birth,* 23(1): 1-6
   • McNiven PE, Hodnett E, O'Brien-Pallas LL, 1992. Supporting women in labor: a work sampling study of the activities of labor and delivery nurses. *Birth*, 19(1): 3-8.

40 Jimenez V. 2004. Naissances: les intervenantes ont-elles vraiment le choix? Annual conference of the Association pour la Santé Publique du Québec, November 23-24. Montreal, Canada.

41 • Hofberg K Ward M, 2003. Fear of pregnancy and childbirth. *Postgraduate Medical Journal* 79:505-510
   • Wijma K, 2003. Why focus on 'fear of childbirth'? *Journal of Psychosomatic Obstetrics and Gynecology*, 24(3): 141-143

42 Veloso CM, 2006. Medication use of childbirth and unplanned cesarean sections: associations with stress and coping. State University of New York at Stony Brook.

43 • Weaver JJ, Statham H, Richards M, 2007. Are there 'unnecessary' cesarean sections? Perceptions of women and obstetricians about cesarean sections for nonclinical indications. *Birth*, 34(1): 32-41
   • McCourt C, Weaver J, Statham H, *et al.* Elective cesarean section and decision making: a critical review of the literature. *Birth*, 34(1):65-79

44 Green JM, Baston HA, 2007. Have women become more willing to accept obstetric interventions and does this relate to mode of birth? Data from a prospective study. *Birth*, 34 (1): 6-13.

45 • Vadeboncoeur H, 2004. La naissance en 2004: qu'est-ce que l'humanisation? Association pour la Santé Publique du Québec, Montréal
   • Vadeboncoeur H, 2004. La naissance au Québec à l'aube du troisième millénaire: de quelle humanisation parle-t-on? Doctoral thesis. Sciences humaines appliquées. Université de Montréal
   • Hivon M, Jimenez V, 2006. Perception d'une naissance et naissance d'une perception: où en sont les femmes? Centre de Recherche et de Formation, CSSS de la Montagne, Montréal
   • Hunter N, 2008. Mums having procedures without consent. www.irishealth.com/ index.html ?level=4etid=13216

46   Kroeger M, Smith LJ, 2004. *Impact of Birthing Practices on Breastfeeding– Protecting the Mother and Baby Continuum.* Sudbury, MA, USA: Johns & Bartlett. See revised 2010 edition.

47   Coalition for Improving Maternity Services, 2007. *Evidence basis for the ten steps of mother-friendly care. Journal of Perinatal Education,* 16(1): Supplement. Available at http://www.motherfriendly.org/products.php

48   • Lajoie F, 2007. Femmes libres tenues dans l'ignorance. Dossier périnatal. *L'Actualité médicale,* 28(10)
      • March 21, 2007, interview with the midwife Céline Lemay

49   Fédération des Médecins Omnipraticiens du Québec. Survey SOM, 2006, in Lajoie F, 2007. Femmes libres tenues dans l'ignorance. Dossier périnatal. *L'Actualité Médicale,* 28(10).

50   Vadeboncoeur H, 2004. La naissance au Québec à l'aube du troisième millénaire: de quelle humanisation parle-t-on? Doctoral thesis. Sciences humaines appliquées. Université de Montréal.

51   Martin JA, Hamilton BE, Sutton PD *et al,* 2009. *Births: Final Data for 2006. Natl Vital Stat Rep* 57(7). Centers for Disease Control and Prevention National Center for Health Statistics, 2004.

52   Canadian Institute for Health Information, 2007. *Giving Birth in Canada: Regional Trends from 2001-2002 to 2005-2006.* Ottawa.

53   Maternity Care Working Party, 2008, *Making Normal Birth a Reality,* Consensus Statement, Royal College of Midwives and Royal College of Obstetricians & Gynaecologists, UK.

54   www.sogc.org

55   https://www.cpass2.umontreal.ca/quarisma/

56   Hartmann KE, 2006. *Development of the Global Mother-Friendly Childbirth Initiative.* Survey by the Center for Women's Health Research, University of North Carolina. Presented in June 2006, Geneva.

57   World Health Organization, 1985. Appropriate technology for birth. *Lancet,* August 24.

58   SOGC, 1986. Sommaire de la déclaration définitive du panel de la Conférence nationale d'unanimité sur les aspects de l'accouchement par césarienne. *Bulletin de la SOGC,* March-April 1986, p 8-9.

59   *Vaginal Birth After Cesarean.* ACOG Practice Bulletin, No 5, 1999.

60   • Guise JM, McDonagh M, Hashima J. *et al,* 2003. Agency for Healthcare Research and Quality. *Vaginal Birth after Cesarean Summary Evidence Report.* Technology Assessment No 71.
      • Dr Michael Klein's study on Canadian maternity care providers reveals that the changes are generational and not necessarily gender-based. See Klein M, Kaczorowski J, Tomkinson J *et al,* 2010. Survey of Canadian family physicians who provide intrapartum care and those that do not. Do they view childbirth differently and does it matter? Normal Labour and Birth Research Conference, Vancouver, 2010

61   Guise JM, McDonagh M, Hashima J, *et al,* 2003. Agency for Healthcare Research and Quality. *Vaginal Birth After Cesarean (VBAC).* Evidence Report/Technology Assessment No 71, March 2, Chapter 3: Question 1, Likelihood of Vaginal Delivery. Referring to the following study: McMahon M J, Luther E R, Bowes W A. *et al.* Comparison of a trial of labor with an elective second cesarean section. *N Engl J Med.* 1996; 335(10): 689–95

62   Chang JJ, Stamilio DF, Macones GA, 2008. Effect of hospital volume on maternal outcomes in women with prior cesarean delivery undergoing trial of labor. *American Journal of Epidemiology Advanced Access,* 167(6):711-718.

63   American College of Obstetricians and Gynecologists, 2010. Vaginal birth after previous cesarean delivery. Practice Bulletin 115.

64   Declercq ER, Sakala C, Corry MP, *et al,* 2006. *Listening to Mothers II – The Second National US Survey of Women's Childbearing Experience.* New York: Childbirth Connection. Available at www.childbirthconnection.org/listeningtomothers/

Notes and references 255

65 British Columbia Perinatal Health Program, 2008. *Caesarean Birth Task Force Report.* Vancouver. February.

66 Cesarean section – Why does the national US cesarean section rate keep going up? December 2007. Available at http://www.childbirthconnection.org/pdf.asp? PDFDownload=cesarean bookletsummary

67 • ACOG News Release, May 6, 2006. Patient-requested cesarean update. www.acog.org
 • Ponte W, 2007. Cesareans – why so many? *Mothering,* September-October 2007, available at http://www.childbirthconnection.org/pdf.asp?PDFDownload=cesarean-birth-mothering-ponte

68 • McCourt C, Weaver J, Statham H, *et al,* 2007. Elective cesarean section and decision making: a critical review of the literature. *Birth* 34(1): 65-79
 • Faundes A, de Padua KS, Duarte Osis MF, *et al.* 2004. Opinião de mulheres e médicos brasileiros sobre a preferência pela via de parto. *Rev Saúde Pública* 38(4): 488-494
 • Weaver JJ, Statham H, Richards M, 2007. Are there 'unnecessary' cesarean sections? Perceptions of women and obstetricians about cesarean sections for nonclinical indications. *Birth* 34(1): 32-41

69 Declercq ER, Sakala C, Corry MP, *et al,* 2006. *Listening to Mothers II: The Second National US Survey of Women's Childbearing Experiences.* New York: Childbirth Connection. Available at www.childbirthconnection.org/listeningtomothers/

70 Gagnon AJ, Meier KM, Waghorn K. 2007. Continuity of nursing care and its link to cesarean birth rate. *Birth,* 34(10): 26-31.

71 Declercq ER, *et al.* 2006. *Listening to Mothers II: The Second National US Survey of Women's Childbearing Experiences.* New York, Childbirth Connection. Available at www.childbirthconnection.org/listeningtomothers

72 Potter JE, Hopkins K, Faúndes A, *et al,* 2008. Women's autonomy and scheduled cesarean sections in Brazil: a cautionary tale. *Birth,* 35(1): 33-40.

73 Gamble J, Creedy D, McCourt C, *et al,* 2007. A critique of the literature on women's request for cesarean section. *Birth,* 34(4): 331-340.

74 Bertrán AP, Meridaldi M, Lauer JA, *et al,* 2007. Rates of caesarean section: analysis of global, regional and national estimates. *Paediatric and Perinatal Epidemiology,* 21:98-113.

75 Codes 6903 and 6912 of the Rules for Health Insurance in Quebec, Canada.

76 NIH Consensus Development Conference: Vaginal Birth After Cesarean: New Insights, Bethesda, Maryland, March 8-10, 2010.

Chapter 2—The risk element, whatever your decision

1 Quéniart A. 1988. Le corps paradoxal: regards de femmes sur la maternité. Montreal: Éditions Saint-Martin.

2 Klein M. Personal communication with Dr. Vania Jimenez. Quoted by her in 2004 in her presentation: Naissances: les intervenantes ont-elles vraiment le choix? Annual conference of the Association pour la Santé Publique du Québec, Canada, November 23-30, 2004: Obstétrique et santé publique: élargir les perspectives sur la réalité de la naissance.

3 National Institute of Health Consensus Development Conference Statement on Cesarean, September 22-24, 1980. *Cesarean Childbirth,* 3(6) 1-30.

4 World Health Organization, 1985, Appropriate Technology for Birth, *Lancet,* Aug 24.

5 See the following:
 • NICE caesarean section clinical guidelines at http://guidance.nice.org.uk/CG13 - National Collaborating Center for Women's and Children's Health, Cesarean – Clinical Guidelines, commissioned by the National Institute for Clinical Excellence, RCOG Press, p 95

6 Beckett VA, Regan L, 2001. Vaginal birth after caesarean: the European experience. *Clinical Obstetrics and Gynecology*, 44: 594-603.

7 Bujold E, *et al*. 2005. Single versus double layer closure and the risk of uterine rupture. *Am J Obstet Gynecol*, 193: S20.

8 Beckett VA, Regan L, 2001. Vaginal birth after caesarean: the European experience. *Clinical Obstetrics and Gynecology*, 44: 594-603.

9 Flamm B, 2001. Vaginal birth after caeserean and the New England Journal of Medicine: a strange controversy. *Birth*, 2 8(4): 276.

10 Beckett VA, Regan L, 2001. Vaginal birth after caesarean: the European experience. *Clinical Obstetrics and Gynecology*, 44: 594-603.

11 Royal College of Obstetricians and Gynaecologists, 2007. *Birth after previous caesarean birth*. Green-Top Guideline No 45.

12 Lieberman E, 2001. Risk factors for uterine rupture during a trial of labor after a cesarean section. *Clin Obstet & Gynecol*, 44: 609-621.

13 Baskett TF, Kieser KE, 2001. A 10-year, population-based study of uterine rupture. *Obstet Gynecol*, 97(4) Suppl 1:S69.

14 Lieberman E, Ernst EK, Rooks JP, *et al*, 2004. Results of a national study of vaginal birth after cesarean in birth centers. *Obstet Gynecol*, 104 (5 Part 1): 933-:942.

15 Landon MB, Hauth JC, Leveno KG, *et al*, 2004. Maternal and perinatal outcomes associated with a trial of labor after prior caesarean delivery. *NEJM*, 351(25): 2581-2589.

16 Coalition for Improving Maternity Services (CIMS), 2007. Evidence basis for the ten steps of mother-friendly care. *Journal of Perinatal Education*, 16(1): Supplement. Winter 2007. Available at http://www.motherfriendly.org/products.php

17 Hugues WM, 2005. *Out-of-hospital VBAC: assessing the risks for midwives*. Seattle Midwifery School.

18 Chauhan SP, Martin JN, Henrichs CE, *et al*. 2003. Maternal and perinatal complications with uterine rupture in 142,075 patients who attempted vaginal birth after cesarean delivery: a review of the literature. *Am J Obstet Gynecol*, 189(2): 408-417.

19 NIH Consensus Development Conference. Vaginal Birth After Cesarean: New Insights, Bethesda, Maryland, March 8-10, 2010. Final statement, Bethesda, Maryland, USA. See: http://consensus.nih.gov/2010/images/vbac/vbac_statement.pdf

20 Guise JM, McDonagh MS, Osterweil P, *et al*, 2004. Systematic review of the incidence and consequences of uterine rupture in women with previuous caesarean section. *BMJ*, 329 (7456): 1-7.

21 Seeds JW. 2004. Diagnostic mid trimester amniocentesis: how sage? Am J Obstet Gynecol 191(2): 607-615.

22 Guise JM, McDonagh M, Hashima J, *et al*, 2003. Vaginal birth after cesarean (VBAC). Evidence Report/Technology Assessment No. 71. Agency for Healthcare Research and Quality, March 2.

23 • Guise JM, McDonagh MS, Osterweil P, *et al*, 2004. Systematic review of the incidence and consequences of uterine rupture in women with previuous caesarean section. *BMJ*, 329 (7456): 1-7
    • Landon, MB, Hauth, JC, Leveno, KG, *et al*, 2004. Maternal and perinatal outcomes associated with a trial of labor after prior caesarean delivery. *NEJM*, 351(25): 2581-2589

24 NIH Consensus Development Conference: Vaginal Birth After Cesarean: New Insights, Bethesda, Maryland, March 8-10, 2010.

25 Lydon-Rochelle M, Holt VL, Easterling TR *et al*, 2001. Risk of uterine rupture during labor among women with a prior cesarean delivery. *NEJM* 345(1): 3-8.

26 • Flamm B, 2001. Vaginal birth after cesarean and the New England Journal of Medicine: a strange controversy. *Birth*, 28(4):276

Notes and references 257

- Anonymous, 2000. Use of hospital discharge data to monitor uterine rupture. Massachusetts Dept of Public Health. *MMWR Morb Mortal Wkly Rep*, 49(12): 245-248

27   Bujold E, 2006. L'accouchement vaginal après césarienne. Congrès annuel de la CAM: L'effet cascade pour le normal: reconquérir la confiance dans la naissance. Ottawa, October 18-20, 2006

28   Landon MB, Hauth JC, Leveno KG, *et al*, 2004. Maternal and perinatal outcomes associated with a trial of labor after prior caesarean delivery. *NEJM*, 351(25): 2581-2589.

29   Goer H, 2004. When research is flawed: is planned VBAC safe? Lamaze Institute for Normal Birth. See www.lamaze.org/institute/flawed/vbac1.asp .

30   See http://nctwatch.wordpress.com/2009/05/07/new-nhs-maternity-statistics-released/

31
- Lerchl A, 2005. Where are the Sunday babies? Observations on a marked decline in weekend births in Germany. *Naturwissenschaften* 92: 592-594. DOI 10.1007/s00114-005-0049-y
- Lerch A, Reinhard SC, 2008. Where are the Sunday babies? II. Declining weekend birth rates in Switzerland. *Naturwissenschaften* 95: 161-164
- Lerch A, Reinhard SC, 2008. Where are the Sunday babies ? III. Cesarean sections, decreased weekend births, and midwife involvement in Germany. *Naturwissenschaften* 95: 165-170

32   Lydon-Rochelle M, Holt VL, Easterling TR, *et al*. 2001. Risk of uterine rupture during labor among women with a prior cesarean delivery. *NEJM* 345(1): 3-8.

33   Kaczmarczyk M, Sparén P, Terry P, *et al.*, 2007. Risk factors for uterine rupture and neonatal consequences for uterine rupture: a population-based study of successive pregnancies in Sweden. *BJOG*, 114(10): 1208-1214.

34   Lydon-Rochelle M, Holt VL, Easterling TR, *et al*, 2001. Risk of uterine rupture during labor among women with a prior cesarean delivery. *NEJM* 345(1): 3-8.

35   Buhimschi CS, Buhimschi IA, Patel S, *et al*, 2005. Rupture of the uterine scar during term labour: contractility or biochemistry? *BJOG*, 112(1): 38-42.

36   Bujold E, 2006. L'accouchement vaginal après césarienne. Congrès annuel de la CAM: L'effet cascade pour le normal: reconquérir la confiance dans la naissance. Ottawa, October 18-20, 2006

37   Kwee A, Bots ML, Visser GHA, *et al*, 2007. Obstetric management and outcome of pregnancy in women with a history of caesarean section in the Netherlands. *European Journal of Obstetrics et Gynecology and Reproductive Biology*, 132(2): 171-176.

38   Kolderup L, McLean L, Grullon K, *et al*, 1999. Misoprostol is more efficacious for labor induction than prostaglandin E2, but is it associated with more risk? *Am J Obstet Gynecol* 180(6): 1543-1550.

39
- Plaut MM, Schwartz ML, Lubarsky SL, 1999. Uterine rupture associated with the use of misoprostol in the gravid patient with a previous cesarean section. *Am J Obstet Gynecol*, 180(6): 1535-1542;
- May Gaskin I, 2000. Cytotec: dangerous experiment or panacea? See http://archive.salon.com/health/feature/2000/07/11/cytotec/print.html

40   SOGC, 2001. Induction of labour at term. Clinical Practice Guideline No 107. See http://www.sogc.org/guidelines/public/107E-CPG-August2001.pdf

41   See NICE caesarean section clinical guidelines at http://guidance.nice.org.uk/CG13

42   Lieberman E 2001. Risk factors for uterine rupture during a trial of labor after a cesarean section. *Clin Obstet & Gynecol*, 44: 609-621.

43
- Blanchette H, Blanchette M, McCabe J, *et al*, 2001. Is vaginal birth after cesarean safe? Experience in a community hospital. *Am J Obstet Gynecol*, 184(7): 1478-1484
- Zelop CM, Shipp TD, Repke JT, *et al*, 1999. Uterine rupture during induced or augmented labor in gravid women with one prior cesarean delivery. *Am J Obstet Gynecol*, 181(4): 882-886

44   Declercq ER, Sakala C, Corry MP, *et al*, 2007. Listening to Mothers II: Report of the Second National U.S. Survey of Women's Childbearing Experience. *Journal of Perinatal Education*, 16 (4): 9-14.

45   Flamm B, 2001. Vaginal birth after cesarean (VBAC). *Best Pract Res Clin Obstet Gynaecol*, 15(1):81-92.

46   Bujold E, 2006. Prise en charge de scénarios d'AVAC. Congrès des omnipraticiens en obstétrique, SOGC, Montreal, Canada, November 17.

47   Royal College of Obstetricians and Gynaecologists, 2007. Birth after previous caesarean birth. Green-Top Guideline No 45.

48   • Leung A, Leung E, Paul R, 1993. Uterine rupture after previous caesarean delivery: maternal and fetal consequences. *Am J Obstet Gynecol*, 169:945-950
      • Grubb DK, Jjos SL, Paul RH, 1996. Latent labor with an unknown uterine scar. *Obstet Gynecol*, 88: 351-355

49   Macones GA, Peipert J, Nelson DB, *et al*, 2005. Maternal complications with vaginal birth after cesaean delivery: a multicenter study. *Am J Obstet Gynecol*, 193(5): 1656-1662.

50   Goyet M, Bujold E, 2006. Conference of the Society for Maternal-Fetal Medicine. Jan 30-Feb 4, 2006, Miami Beach, Florida, USA. Quoted in: *Medscape OB/GYn & Women's Health*, 11 (1), 2006.

51   Heffner LJ, Elkin E, Fretts RC, 2003. Impact of labor induction, gestational age, and maternal age on caesarean delivery rates. *Obstetrics and Gynecology*, 102(2): 287-293.

52   Coalition for Improving Maternity Services (CIMS), 2007. Evidence basis for the ten steps of mother-friendly care. Journal of Perinatal Education, 16(1): Supplement. Winter 2007. Available at http://www.motherfriendly.org/products.php

53   • Flamm B, 2001. Vaginal birth after cesarean (VBAC). *Best Pract Res Clin Obstet Gynaecol*, 15(1): 81-92
      • Lieberman E, 2001. Risk factors for uterine rupture during a trial of labor after a cesarean section. Clin Obstet et Gynecol, 44: 609-621

54   • Shipp TD, Zelop CM, Repke JT, et al, 1999. Intrapartum uterine rupture and dehiscence in patients with a prior lower uterine segment vertical and transverse incision. *Obstet Gynecol*, 94(5 Pt 1):735-740
      • Naef RW 3rd, Ray MA, Chauhan SP, *et al*, 1995. Trial of labor after caesarean delivery with a lower-segment, vertical uterine incision: is it safe? *Am J Obstet Gynecol*, 172 (6):1666-1673

55   This information was posted at www.vbac.com. These types of incision are between 4% and 9% at risk of uterine rupture.

56   • American College of Obstetricians and Gynecologists, 2010. *Vaginal birth after previous cesarean delivery*. Practice Bulletin No 115, August 2010
      • Rosen MG, Dickinson JC, Westhoff CL, 1991. Vaginal birth after caesarean section: a meta-analysis of morbidity and mortality. *Obstet Gynecol*, 77: 465-470
      • Flamm B, 2001. Vaginal birth after caesarean and the New England Journal of Medicine: a strange controversy. *Birth*, 28 (4): 276

57   Durnwald D, Mercer B, 2003. Uterine rupture, perioperative and perinatal morbidity after single-layer and double-layer closure at caesarean delivery. *Am J Obstet Gynecol*, 189 (4):925-929.

58   Koppel E, Struzyk B, Zbieszczyk J, 1983. Cesarean section using singlelayer tansisthmic uterine sutures. *Zentralbl Gynakol*, 105(23): 1522-1525.

59   Durnwald D, Mercer B, 2003. Uterine rupture, perioperative and perinatal morbidity after single-layer and double-layer closure at caesarean delivery. *Am J Obstet Gynecol*, 189 (4):925-929.

60   Bujold E, Goyet M, Marcoux S, *et al*, 2010. The role of uterine closure in the risk of uterine rupture. *Obstetrics & Gynecology*, 116(1): 43-50.

Notes and references

61 National Perinatal Epidemiology Unit, United Kingdom, 2006. Caesarean section surgical techniques. See www.npeu.ox.ac.uk/caesar

62 Coalition for Improving Maternity Services (CIMS), 2007. Evidence basis for the ten steps of mother-friendly care. *Journal of Perinatal Education*, 16(1): Supplement. Winter 2007. Available at http://www.motherfriendly.org/products.php

63 The consensus on the definition of normal birth comes from the *Joint Policy Statement on Normal Birth*, Joint Policy Statement No 22, December 2008, and is a summary of policies in the following associations:
  - Society of Obstetricians and Gynecologists
  - Association of Women's Health
  - Obstetric and Neonatal Nurses of Canada (AWHONN Canada)
  - Canadian Association of Midwives (CAM)
  - College of Family Physicians of Canada (CFPC)
  - Society of Rural Physicians of Canada (SRPC)

64 American College of Obstetricians and Gynecologists, 2010. Vaginal birth after previous cesarean delivery. Practice Bulletin No 115, August 2010.

65 SOGC, 2005. Guidelines for Vaginal Birth After Previous Caesarean Birth. Clinical Practice Guideline No 155. See www.sogc.org/guidelines/public/155E-CPG-February2005.pdf

66 Wagner M, 2001. What every midwife should know about ACOG and VBAC: Critique of ACOG, Practice Bulletin No 5. July 1999. See www.midwiferytoday.com/articles/acog.asp .

67 - Foureur M, Ryan CL, Nicholl M, *et al*, 2010. Inconsistent evidence: analysis of six national guidelines for vaginal birth after cesarean section. *Birth* 37(1): 3-10
  - See http://dx.doi.org/10.1111/j.1523-536X.2009.00372.x

68 SOGC, 2005. Guidelines for Vaginal Birth After Previous Caesarean Birth. Clinical Practice Guideline No 155. See www.sogc.org/guidelines/public/155E-CPG-February2005.pdf

69 Leung A, Leung E, Paul R, 1993. Uterine rupture after previous caesarean delivery: maternal and fetal consequences. *Am J Obstet Gynecol*, 169:945-950.

70 Quoted in Vadeboncoeur H, 1989. *Une autre césarienne?* Montréal: Éditions Québec-Amérique.

71 NIH Consensus Development Conference: Vaginal Birth After Cesarean: New Insights, Bethesda, Maryland, March 8-10, 2010. Final statement. See: http://consensus.nih.gov/2010/images/vbac/vbac_statement.pdf

72 Schneider ME, 2005. Insurers set criteria for VBAC coverage. *OB/GYN News*, Feb 1 2005.

73 Thompson S. 2003. VBAC litigation paranoia. *The Female Patient*. See www.femalepatient.com

74 Hugues WM, 2005. *Out-of-Hospital VBAC: Assessing the Risks for Midwives*. Seattle Midwifery School, USA.

75 This is what I also talk about in the chapter of the book *Evidence-Based Midwifery*, Munro J, Spiby H (forthcoming). Is there a link between the VBAC decline since the 2nd half of the 90s and scientific studies on the risks of VBAC? Oxford: Blackwell Publishing.

76 Zinberg S, 2000 Recommendation on VBAC based on risk of uterine rupture. Washington, DC, *ACOG Today*, April 2000: 2.

77 Perreault M, 2007. Le monitoring foetal pas facile à remplacer. *La Presse*, Feb 11 2007.

78 Wagner M. 2001. What every midwife should know about ACOG and VBAC. Critique of ACOG Practice Bulletin, No 5, July 1999. See www.midwiferytoday.com/articles/acog.asp

79 Discussion group of North American family practitioners (GPs) online, 2008.

80 American Academy of Family Physicians, 2005. Trial of labour after caesarean (TOLAC). Formerly: Trial of labor versus elective repeat caesarean section for the woman with a previous caesarean section: a review of the evidence and recommendations. American Academy of Family Physicians. Available at http://www.aaafp.org/online/etc/medialib/aafp_org/documents/clinical/clin_recs/tolacpolicy.Par.0001.File.dat/clinicalrec_tolac.pdf

81   • Janssen PA, Ryan EM, Etches DJ, *et al*, 2007. Outcomes of planned hospital birth
      attended by midwives compared with physicians in British Columbia. *Birth*, 34(2): 140-
      147
      • Blais R, Joubert P, Collin J, *et al*, 1998. Que nous apprend l'évaluation des projets-pilotes
      de la pratique des sages-femmes. *Interface* 19(3):26-37
      • Johnson KC, Daviss BA, 2005. Outcomes of planned home births with certified
      professionnel midwives: large prospective study in North America, *British Medical Journal*,
      330(7505): 1416-1427

82   Albers LL, 2005. Safety of VBACs in birth centers: choices and risks. *Birth*, 32(3): 229-231.

83   Wagner M, 2001. What every midwife should know about ACOG and VBAC: critique of ACOG,
      Practice Bulletin No 5. July 1999. See www.midwiferytoday.com/articles/acog.asp .

84   Avery MD, Carr CA, Burkhardt P, 2004. Vaginal birth after caesarean section: a pilot study of
      outcomes in women receiving midwifery care. *Journal of Midwifery and Women's Health*, 49
      (2): 113-117.

85   Amelink-Vergurg MP, Verloove-Vanhorick SP, Hakkenberg RMA, *et al*, 2007. Evaluation of
      280,000 cases in Dutch midwifery practices: a descriptive study. *BJOG*, 2008 115: 570-
      578.

86   Turner LA, Cyr M, Kinch RAH, *et al*, 2002. Underreporting of maternal mortality in Canada: a
      question of definition. *Chronic Diseases in Canada*, 23(1).

87   • Hogan MC, Forman KJ, Naghavi M, *et al*, 2010. Maternal mortality for 181 countries,
      1980-2008: a systematic analysis of progress towards Millennium Development Goal 5.
      Lancet, 375(9726): 1609-1623
      • National Health Services, 2009.
      • See http://www.ic/nhs.uk/default.asp?
      sID=1172577414129&sPublicationID=1237192136859&sDocID=4969
      • American College of Obstetricians and Gynecologists, 31 August 2006. *ACOG News
      Release*

88   Wen SW, Rusen ID, Walker M, *et al*, 2004. Comparison of maternal mortality and morbidity
      between trial of labor and elective caesarean section among women with previous
      caesarean delivery. *American Journal of Obstetrics and Gynecology*, 191(4): 1263-1269.

89   Health Canada, 2004. *Special Report on Maternal Mortality and SevereMorbidity in Canada*,
      Maternal Health Study Group of the Canadian Perinatal Surveillance System.

90   Minino AM, Heron MP, Murphy SL, *et al*, 2007. Deaths: Final Data for 2004. *National Vital
      Statistics Reports*, 55(19), Aug 21.

91   • Merialdi M, 2005. As novas pesquisas da OMS sobre cesariana. II Conferência
      International sobre Humanização do Parto et Nascimento. Rio de Janeiro, Brazil
      • Villar J, Valladeres E, Wojdyla D, *et al*, 2006. Caesarean delivery rates and pregnancy
      outcomes: the 2005 WHO global survey on maternal and perinatal health in Latin
      America. *Lancet* 367(9525):1819-1829.

92   Hall MH, Bewley S, 1999. Maternal mortality and mode of delivery. *Lancet*, 354:776.

93   Ramos GJL, *et al*, 2003. Morte maternal em hospital terciario do Rio Grande do Sul – Brasil:
      um estudo de 20 anos. *Re Bras Ginecol Obstet* 25(6):431-436. Quoted by Diniz SG, Duarte
      AC, 2004. *Parto normal o casarea? O que toda mulher deve saber (e todo homem também.*
      São Paulo, Editora UNESP.

94   Government of Ontario, Office of the Chief Coroner, 2006. *Second Annual Report – Maternal
      and Perinatal Death Review Committee.* Toronto, Ontario, Canada.

95   NIH Consensus Development Conference: Vaginal Birth After Cesarean: New Insights,
      Bethesda, Maryland, March 8-10, 2010.

96   Villar J, Valladeres E, Wojdyla D, *et al*, 2006. Caesarean delivery rates and pregnancy
      outcomes: the 2005 WHO global survey on maternal and perinatal health in Latin America.
      Lancet, 367(9525):1819-1829.

97   Liu S, Liston RM, Joseph KS, *et al*, 2007. Maternal mortality and severe morbidity associated with low-risk planned caesarean delivery versus planned vaginal delivery at term. *Canadian Medical Association Journal*, 176(4): 455-476.

98   Public Health Agency of Canada. See http://www.phac-aspc.gc.ca/rhs-ssg/srmm-rsmm/page2-eng.php

99   Kramer MS, Rouleau J, Baskett TF, *et al*, 2006. Amniotic-fluid embolism and medical induction of labour: a retrospective, population based cohort study. *Lancet*, 368(9545): 1444-1448.

100   Coalition for Improving Maternity Services (CIMS), 2007. Evidence basis for the ten steps of mother-friendly care. *Journal of Perinatal Education*, 16(1): Supplement. Winter 2007. Available at http://www.motherfriendly.org/products.php

101   • Van Hoover C, 2004. Impact of birthing practices on breastfeeding: protecting the mother and baby continuum. *Journal of Midwifery and Women's Health*, 49(4): 370-371
      • Leung GM, Lai-Ming H, Tai-Hing L. 2002. Breast-feeding and its relation to smoking and mode of delivery. *Obstet & Gynecol* 99(5 Pt 1), p 785-794
      • Forster DA, McLachlan HL. Breastfeeding initiation and birth setting practices: a review of the literature. *J Midwifery Women's Health*, 2007; 52(3): 273-280

102   • Torvaldson S, Roberts CL, Simpson JM, Thompson JF, Ellwood DA, 2006. Intrapartum epidural analgesia and breastfeeding: a prospective cohort study. *Int Breastfeeding J*, 1:1-24
      • Jordan S, Emery S, Bradshaw C, Watkins A, Friswell W, 2005. The impact of intrapartum analgesia on infant feeding. *BJOG*, 112: 927-934

103   • Otamiri G, Berg G, Leden T, *et al*, 1991. Delayed neurological adaptation in infants delivered by elective caesarean section and the relation to catecholamine levels. *Early Human Dev* 26:51-60
      • Nissen E, Uvnas-Moberg K, Svensson K, *et al*, 1996. Different patterns of oxytocin prolactin but not cortisol release during breastfeeding of women delivered by caesarean section or by the vaginal route. *Early Hum Dev* 45:103-118
      • Rowe-Murray H, Fisher J, 2001. Operative intervention in delivery is associated with compromised early mother-infant interaction. *Br J Obstet gynecol*, 108:1068-1075
      • Note: The above studies were quoted in Kroeger M, Smith L, 2004. *Impact of Birthing Practices on Breastfeeding – Protecting the Mother and Baby Continuum*. Sudbury, MA, USA: Jones & Bartlett.

104   • Pare E, Quinones JN, Macones GA, 2006. Vaginal birth after caesarean section versus elective repeat caesarean section: assessment of maternal downstream health outcomes. *BJOG*, 113(1): 75-85
      • Cohain JS, 2006. Vaginal birth after caesarean section: seeing the bigger picture. *British Journal of Midwifery*, 14(7): 424-426

105   Morales KJ, Gordon MC, Bates GW Jr, 2007. Postcesarean delivery adhesions associated with delayed delivery of infant. *Am J Obstet Gynecol*, 196(5): 461-466.

106   Declercq E, Cunningham DK, Johnson C, *et al*, 2008. Mothers' reports of postpartum pain associated with vaginal and cesarean deliveries: results of a national survey. *Birth*, 35(1): 16-24.

107   • NIH Consensus Development Conference on VBAC, 2010. Final statement, Bethesda, Maryland, March 8-10. See: http://consensus.nih.gov/2010/images/vbac/vbac_statement.pdf
      • Childbirth Connection. Comparing risks of cesarean and vaginal birth to mothers, babies, and future reproductive capacity: a systematic review. New York: Childbirth Connection, April 2004. See http://www.childbirthconnection.org/article.asp?ck=10166&ClickedLink=274&area+27#future_birth

108   • Ananth CV, Smulian JC, Vintzileos AM, 1997. The association of placenta previa with history of cesarean delivery and abortion: a metaanalysis. *Am J Obstet Gynecol*, 177(5): 1071-1078

- Grobman WA, Gersnoviez R, Landon MB, 2007. Pregnancy outcomes for women with placenta previa in relation to the number of prior cesarean deliveries. *Obstetrics & Gynecology*, 110(6): 1249-1255

109 Kirn TF, 2001. Cesarean rate portends rise in placenta accrete. *Ob Gyn News*. March 1, 36 (5): 23.

110 MacDorman MF, Declercq E, Menacker F, *et al*, 2008. Neonatal mortality for primary cesarean and vaginal births to low-risk women: application of an 'intention-to-treat' model. *Birth* 35 (1): 3-8.

111 Zweifler J, Garza,A, Hugues S, *et al*, 2006. Vaginal birth after caesarean in California – before and after a change in guidelines. *Annals of Family Medicine*, 4:228-234.

112 Levine EM, Ghai V, Barton JJ, *et al*, 2001. Mode of delivery and risk of respiratory diseases in newborns. *Obstetrics and Gynecology*, 97(3): 439-442.

113 Villar J, Valladeres E, Wojdyla D, *et al*, 2006. Caesarean delivery rates and pregnancy outcomes: the 2005 WHO global survey on maternal and perinatal health in Latin America. *Lancet,* 367(9525): 1819-1829.

114 Hansen AK, Wisborg K, Uldbjerg N, *et al*, 2007. Risk of respiratory morbidity in term infants delivered by elective caesarean section: cohort study. *British Medical Journal*, Dec 11, 2007.

115 Hansen AK, Wisborg K, Uldbjerg N, *et al*, 2007. Risk of respiratory morbidity in term infants delivered by elective caesarean section: cohort study. *British Medical Journal*, Dec 11 2007.

116 • Madar J, Richmond S, Hey E, 1999. Surfactant-deficient respiratory distress after elective delivery at "term. *Acta Paediatr* 88: 1244-1248
- DeNoon D.J., 2007. C-section before 39th week ups baby breathing problems. *WebMD Medical News*, from the following Danish study, in university hospital of Aarhus: Hansen AK, Wisborg K, Uldbjerg N, *et al*, 2007. Risk of respiratory morbidity in term infants delivered by elective caesarean section: cohort study. *British Medical Journal*, Dec 11, 2007

117 • Levine EM, Ghai V, Barton JJ, *et al*, 2001. Mode of delivery and risk of respiratory diseases in newborns. *Obstet Gynecol*, 97: 439-442
- Morrison JJ, Rennie JM, Milton PJ. 1995. Neonatal respiratory morbidity and mode of delivery at term: influence of timing of elective caesarean section. *Br. J. Obstet Gynaeocol*. 102: 101-106; Richardson BS, Czilck MJ, daSilva O. et al. 2005. The impact of labor at term on measures of neonatal outcome. *Am J Obstet Gynecol* 192: 219-226

118 Silva AA, Lamy-Filho F, Alves, MT, 1998. Trends in low birth weight: a comparison of two birth cohorts separated by a 15-year interval in Ribeirão Preto, Brazil. *Bull World Health Organ* 76 (1): 73-84. Quoted by Diniz SG, Duarte AC, 2004. Parto normal ou cesarea ? O que toda mulher deve saber (e todo homem também). São Paulo, Editora UNESP.

119 • Kapla M. Caesarian sections may increase asthma risk. *Nature* (online, October 29, 2007)
- Sullivan MG, 2003. Asthma associated with planned caesarean - large retrospective study. *Ob/Gyn News*, May 15, 2003.

120 Coalition for Improving Maternity Services (CIMS), 2007. Evidence basis for the ten steps of mother-friendly care. *Journal of Perinatal Education*, 16(1): Supplement. Winter 2007. Available at http:/www.motherfriendly.org/products.php

121 Smith GCS, Pelle JP, Dobbie R, 2003. Caesarean section and risk of unexplained stillbirth in subsequent pregnancy. *Lancet,* 362(29): 1779-1784.

122 Smith GCS, Pell JP, Dobbie R, 2003. Caesarean section and risk of unexplained stillbirth in subsequent pregnancy. *Lancet,* 362(29): 1779-1784.

123 Tollanes MC, Melve KK, Irgens LM, *et al*, 2007. Reduced fertility after cesarean delivery: a maternal choice. *Obstetrics & Gynecology*, 110(6): 1256-1263.

124 SOGC, 2007. Mid-trimester amniocentesis fetal loss rate. Committee Opinion, *Journal of Obstetrics and Gynecology Canada*, No 194, p 586-590. Note: the following study shows

Notes and references   263

that the risk of miscarriage after an amniocentesis is 0.06%: Eddleman KA, Malone FD, Sullivan L, *et al*. Pregnancy loss rates after midtrimester amniocentesis. *Obstet Gynecol*, 108:1067-1072. However, previous studies all show a higher risk, similar in degree to the risk of uterine rupture during a VBAC.

125 • Source of the Paling scale: Stalling SP, Paling JP, 2001. New tool for presenting risk in obstetrics and gynecology. *Obstet Gynecol* 98(2):345-349.
   • Source of the data for the risk of amniocentesis: 0.6% according to Seeds JW, 2004. Diagnostic mid trimester amniocentesis: how safe? *Am J Obstet Gynecol*, 191(2):607-615.
   • Source on accidents in the home and on the stairs: Putting risks into perspective. November 1997; 45-5. See www.medicine.ox.ac.uk/bandolier/band45/b45-5.html
   • Source for the data on pedestrian accidents: SAAQ for the year 2000 .
   • Source of data on the risk of VBAC: Chauhan SP, Martin JN, Henrichs CE, *et al*, 2003. Maternal and perinatal complications with uterine rupture in 142,075 patients who attempted vaginal birth after caesarean delivery: a review of the literature. *Am J Obstet Gynecol*, 189(2):408-417

126 Enkin M, Keirse MJNC, Neilson J, *et al*, 2000. *A Guide to Effective Care in Pregnancy and Childbirth*, 3rd ed. Oxford: Oxford University Press, 2000. The chapter on VBAC is available at http://www.childbirthconnection.org/article.asp?ClickedLink=194&ck=10218&area=2

127 Dauphin F, 2003. Les mythes de l'accouchement. *Les Dossiers de l'Obstétrique*, No 317, pp 21 -22.

128 The chapter on VBAC (Enkin M, *et al*, 2000) is available at http://www.childbirthconnection.org/article.asp?ClickedLink=194&ck=10218&area=2

129 See http://www.childbirthconnection.org/article.asp?ClickedLink=274&ck=10168&area=27#learn

130 • Gerten KA, Coonrod DV, Bay RC, *et al*, 2005. Cesarean delivery and respiratory distress syndrome: does labor make a difference? *Am J Obstet Gynecol*, 193(3), Part 2: 1061-1064; 163
   • Richardson BS, Czikk MJ, daSylva O, *et al*, 2005. The impact of labor at term on measures of neonatal outcomes. *Am J Obst Gynecol*. 192(1):219-226

131 Choquet, J, 2007. Primum non nocere, impact des interventions obstétricales sur l'allaitement. Journée Programme Périnatalité Petite Enfance, CSSS de la Pommeraie, Cowansville. Note: This was a presentation at a conference.

132 Li W, Weiyuan Z, Yanhui Z, 1999. The study of maternal and fetal plasma catecholamines levels during pregnancy and delivery. *Journal of Perinatal Medicine*, 27(3): 195-198.

133 Lagercrantz H, Slotkin TA, 1986. The stress of being born. *Scientific American*, 254(4): 100-107.

134 • Heritage CK, Cunningham MD, 1985. Association of elective repeat cesarean delivery and persistent pumonary hypertension of the newborn. *Am J Obstet Gynecol*, 152:726-729
   • Leder ME, Hirschfeld S, Faranoff A, 1980. Persistent fetal circulation: an epidemiologic study. *Pediatr Res*, 14:490
   • Reece EA, Moya F, Yazigo R, *et al*, 1987. Persistent pulmonary hypertension: assessment of perinatal risk factors. *Obstet Gynecol*, 70:697-700

135 Phjavuori M, Fyhrquist F, 1980. Hemodynamic significance of vasopression in the newborn infant. *Journal of Pediatrics* 97(3): 462-465

136 Hugues WM, 2005. *Out-of-Hospital VBAC: Assessing the Risks forMidwives*, Seattle Midwifery School, USA.

137 Sulyok L, Csaba LF, 1986. Elective repeat cesarean delivery and persistent pulmonary hypertension of the newborn, *Am. J. Obstet Gynecol*, 155:687-688.

138 Hansen AK, Wisborg K, Uldbjerg, N, *et al*, 2007. Risk of respiratory morbidity in term infants delivered by elective caesarean section: cohort study. *British Medical Journal*, Dec 11, 2007.

139 Choquet, J, 2007. Primum non nocere, impact des interventions obstétricales sur l'allaitement. Journée Programme Périnatalité Petite Enfance, CSSS de la Pommeraie, Cowansville. Note: This was a presentation at a conference.

140 The study published in 1995 was quoted in: Richardson B, Czikk MJ, da Silva O, et al, 2005. The impact of labor at term on measures of netonatal outcomes. Am J Obstet Gynecol, 192:219-226.

141 Morrison JJ, Rennie JM, Milton P, 2005. Neonatal respiratory morbidity and mode of delivery at term: influence of timing of elective caesarean section. BJOG, 102: 101-106.

142 Madar J, Richmond J, Hey K, 1999. Surfactant-deficient respiratory distress after elective delivery at 'term'. Acta Paediatr, 88(11):1244-1248.

143 Szejer M, 2004. Qu'en est-il à moyen et à long terme? Association pour la Santé Publique du Québec, Canada. Obstetrique et santé publique: élargir les perspectives sur les réalités de la naissance, Montréal, Canada.

Chapter 3—Persuasive reasons to have a VBAC

1 Coalition for Improving Maternity Services (CIMS), 2007. Evidence basis for the ten steps of mother-friendly care. Journal of Perinatal Education, 16(1): Supplement. Winter 2007. Available at http:/www.motherfriendly.org/products.php

2 • Leeman LM, Plante LA, 2006. Patient-choice vaginal delivery? Annals of Family Medicine, 4(3): 465-268
 . Jukelevics, N, 2004. Once a cesarean, always a cesarean: the sorry state of birth choices in America. Mothering, No 123: 46-55.

3 Ribeyron T, 1991. La plus belle histoire de peau. Guide-Ressources, p 21-27.

4 • Christensson K, Cabrera T, Christensson E, et al, 1995. Separation distress call in the human neonate in the absence of maternal body contact, Acta Paediatr, 84(5):468-473
 . Michelsson K, Christensson K, Rothganger H, et al, 1996. Crying in separated and non-separated newborns: sound spectrographic analysis. Acta Paediatr, 85(4): 858-865
 . Note: The above were quoted by Le Brenn C, 2007. Les soins administrés à la naissance au nouveau-né présumé bien portant sont-ils tous pertinents? Les Dossiers de l'Obstétrique,364: 21-24

5 Widström AM, et al, 1990. Short term effects of early suckling and touch of the nipple on maternal behaviour. Early Human Development, 21:153-163. Quoted by Le Brenn, 2007 in: Les soins administrés à la naissance au nouveau-né présumé bien portant sont-ils tous pertinents? Les Dossiers de l'Obstétrique,364: 21-24.

6 • Widström AM, et al, 1990. Short term effects of early suckling and touch of the nipple on maternal behaviour. Early Human Development, 21:153-163. Quoted by Le Brenn, 2007 in: Les soins administrés à la naissance au nouveau-né présumé bien portant sont-ils tous pertinents? Les Dossiers de l'Obstétrique,364: 21-24.
 . Nissen EE, Lilia G, Widström A, et al, 1995. Elevation of oxytocin levels early postpartum in women. Acta Obstet Gynecol Scand, 74(7): 530-533
 . Note: The above were quoted by Le Brenn, 2007 in: Les soins administrés à la naissance au nouveau-né présumé bien portant sont-ils tous pertinents? Les Dossiers de l'Obstétrique,364: 21-24

7 Dr Gremmo-Feger, 2004. L'accueil du nouveau-né en salle de naissance: les dogmes revisités, xxixe Journées niçoises de pédiatrie. October 2. Quoted by Le Brenn, 2007 in: Les soins administrés à la naissance au nouveau-né présumé bien portant sont-ils tous pertinents? Les Dossiers de l'Obstétrique,364: 21-24.

8 • Mikami K, Takahashi H, Kimura M, et al, 2009. Influence of maternal bifidobacteria on the establishment of bifidobacteria colonizing the gut in infants. Pediatr Res 65(6): 669-674

- Keski-Nisula L, Katila ML, Remes S, *et al*, 2009. Intrauterine bacterial growth at birth and risk of asthma and allergic sensitization among offspring at the age of 15 to 17 years. *J Allergy Clin Immunol*, 123(6):1305-1311

9
- Finigan V, Davies S, 2004. 'I just wanted to love, hold him forever': women's lived experience of skin-to-skin contact with their baby immediately after birth. *Evidence Based Midwifery*, 2(2): 59-65
- Feldman R, Weller A, Zagoory-Sharon O, *et al*, 2007. Evidence for a neuroendocrinological foundation of human affiliation. *Psychological Science*, 18(11): 965-970

10   Chaparro CM, Lutter C, 2007. Beyond survival: integrated delivery care practices for long-term maternal and infant nutrition, health and development. Pan American Health Organization, WHO, Washington, DC, USA. See www.paho.org

11   Le Brenn C, 2007. Les soins administrés à la naissance au nouveau-né présumé bien portant sont-ils tous pertinents? *Les Dossiers de l'Obstétrique*, 364: 21-24.

12
- Widström AM, Ransio-Arvidson AB, Christensson AB, *et al*, 1987. Gastric suction in healthy newborn infants: effects on circulation and developing feeding behaviour. *Acta Paediatr Scand*, 76(4): 566-572
- Richard L, Alade OM, 1990. Effects of delivery room routines on success of first feed. *Lancet*, 336: 1105-1107
- Janson UM, *et al*, 1995. The effects of medically-oriented labour ward routines on prefeeding behaviour and body temperature in newborn infants. *J Trop Pediatrics*, 41: 360-363. Quoted by Le Brenn, 2007, Les soins administrés à la naissance au nouveau-né présumé bien portant sont-ils tous pertinents ? *Les Dossiers de l'Obstétrique*, 364 : 21-24

13   Kroeger M, Smith L, 2004. *Impact of Birthing Practices on Breastfeeding – Protecting the Mother and Baby Continuum,* Sudbury, MA, USA: Jones & Bartlett. See revised 2010 edition.

14   Erlandsson K, Dsilna A, Fagerberg I, *et al*, 2007. Skin-to-skin care with the father after cesarean birth and its effect on newborn crying and prefeeding behaviour. *Birth* 34(2): 105-113.

15
- Farnworth A, Pearson PH, 2007. Choosing mode of delivery after previous caesarean birth. *British Journal of Midwifery*, 15(4): 188, 190, 192-194
- Eden KB, Hashima JN, Osterweil P, 2004. Childbirth preferences after caesarean birth: a review of the evidence. *Birth* 31(1): 49-60

16   McClain CS, 1985. Why women choose trial of labor or repeat caesarean section. *Journal of Family Practice*, 21(3): 210-216.

17   Moffat MAQ, Bell JS, Porter MA, *et al*, 2007. Decision making about mode of delivery among pregnant women who have previously had a caesarean section: a qualitative study. *BJOG*, 114(1): 86-93.

18   Meddings F, Philipps FM, Haith-Cooper M, *et al*, 2007. Vaginal birth after caesarean section (VBAC): exploring women's perceptions. *Journal of Clinical Nursing*, 16(1): 160-167.

19
- If you want something to help you make a decision, go to: http://www.healthwise.net/cochranedecisionaid/Content/StdDocument.aspx?DOCHWID=aa37799&SECHWID=aa37799-Intro
- For research on this, see Montgomery AA, Emmett CL, Fahey T, *et al*, 2007. Two decision aids for mode of delivery among women with previous caesarean section: randomised controlled trial. *BMJ*, 334: 1305. doi:10.1136/bmj.39217.671019.55

20   Moffat MAQ, Bell JS, Porter MA, *et al*, 2007. Decision making about mode of delivery among pregnant women who have previously had a caesarean section: a qualitative study. *BJOG*, 114(1): 86-93.

21   Koelker K, 1981. *Vaginal Birth After Cesarean.* Norwalk, CT, USA: The Penny Press, p 2.

22   Mehlan G, 1986. Cesarean rate criticized at Chicago Conference. *C/Sec Newsletter*, 12(4):3.

23   Johnson SR, *et al*, 1986. Obstetric decision-making: responses to patients who request a cesarean delivery. *Obstetrics and Gynecology*, 67(6): 850.

24   Lajoie F, 2007. Se faire materner en toute autonomie - Dossier périnatalité. *L'Actualité médicale*, 28(11).

25   Belizan JM, Althabe F, Barros FC, *et al*, 1999. Rates and implications of cesarean sections in Latin America: Ecological study. *British Medical Journal*, 319: 1397-1400.

26   National Institute for Health and Clinical Excellence, 2007. Intrapartum care – care of healthy women and their babies during childbirth. NICE Clinical Guideline 55. See www.nice.org.uk

27   Hannah ME, Hannah WJ, Hewson SA, 2000. Planned caesarean section versus planned vaginal birth for breech presentation at term: a randomized multicentre trial. Term Breech Trial Collaborative Group. *Lancet* 356(9239): 1375-1383.

28   • Glezerman M, 2006. Five years to the term breech trial: the rise and fall on a randomized controlled trial. *Am J Obstet Gynecol*, 194(1):20-25
     • Vendittelli F, Pons JC, Lemery D, *et al*, 2006. The term breech presentation: neonatal results and obstetric practices in France. *European Journal of Obstetrics and Gynecology and Reproductive Biology*, 125(2): 176-184

29   Hannah ME, Whyte H, Hannah AWJ, *et al*, 2004. Maternal outcomes at 2 years after planned caesarean section versus planned vaginal birth for breech presentation at term: the international randomized term breech trial. *Am J Obstet Gynec*, 191: 917-927.

30   Cesario SK, 2004. Reevaluation of Friedman's Labor Curve: a pilot study. *J Obstet Gynecol Neonatal Nurs*, 33(6): 713-722.

31   • Vercoustre L, Roman H, 2006. Essai de travail en cas de césarienne antérieure – revue de la littérature. *J Gynecol Obstet Biol Reprod*, 35: 35-45
     • NIH Consensus Development Conference: Vaginal Birth After Cesarean: New Insights, Bethesda, Maryland, March 8-10, 2010. Final statement. See: http://consensus.nih.gov/2010/images/vbac/vbac_statement.pdf

32   • Lieberman E, Ernst EK, Rooks JP, *et al*, 2004. Results of a national study of vaginal birth after cesarean in birth centers. *Obstet Gynecol*, 104(5 Part 1): 933-942; 215
     • Guise JM, McDonagh M, Hashima J, *et al*, 2003. *Vaginal birth after cesarean (VBAC)*. Evidence Report/Technology Assessment No 71, Agency for Healthcare Research and Quality, March 2
     • Coalition for Improving Maternity Services (CIMS), 2007. Evidence basis for the ten steps of mother-friendly care. *Journal of Perinatal Education*, 16(1): Supplement. Winter 2007. Available at http:/www.motherfriendly.org/products.php

33   Coalition for Improving Maternity Services (CIMS), 2007. Evidence basis for the ten steps of mother-friendly care. *Journal of Perinatal Education*, 16(1): Supplement. Winter 2007. Available at http://www.motherfriendly.org/products.php

34   Mercer BM, Gilbert S, Landon MB, *et al*, 2008. Labor outcomes with increasing number of prior vaginal births after cesarean delivery. *Obstetrics and Gynecology*, 111:285-291

35   Royal College of Obstetricians and Gynaecologists, February 2007. *Birth after previous caesarean birth*. Green-top Guideline No 45. See http://www.rcog.org.uk/womens-health/clinical-guidance/birth-after-previous-caesarean-birth-green-top-45

36   NICE, National Collaborating Centre for Women's and Children's Health, 2004. Caesarean section clinical guideline. See http://www.nice.org.uk/nicemedia/live/10940/29334.pdf

37   Society of Obstetricians and Gynaecologists of Canada, 2005. Guidelines for vaginal birth after previous cesarean birth. SOGC Clinical Practice Guidelines No 155. See http://www.sogc.org/guildelines/public/155E-CPG-February2005.pdf

38   American College of Obstetricians and Gynecologists, August 2010. Vaginal birth after previous cesarean delivery. Practice Bulletin No 115 – Clinical Management Guidelines for Obstetrician-Gynecologists. See http://www.ourbodiesourblog.org/wp-content/uploads/2010/07/ACOG_guidelines_vbac_2010.pdf

39   NIH Consensus Development Conference: Vaginal Birth After Cesarean: New Insights, Bethesda, Maryland, March 8-10, 2010. Final statement. See: http://consensus.nih.gov/2010/images/vbac/vbac_statement.pdf

40   • Rosen MC, Dickinson JC, Westhoff GL, 1991. Vaginal birth after cesarean: a meta-analysis of morbidity and mortality. *Obstet Gynecol*, 77: 465-470
      • Brill Y, Windrim R, 2003. Vaginal birth after caesarean section: review of antenatal predictors of success. *J Obstet Gynaecol Can*, 25(4): 275-286

41   Rosen MC, Dickinson JC, Westhoff GL, 1991. Vaginal birth after cesarean: a metaanalysis of morbidity and mortality. *Obstet Gynecol*, 77: 465-470.

42   • Bujold E, Gauthier RJ, 2001. Should we allow a trial of labor after a previous caesarean for dystocia in the second stage of labor? *Obstet Gynecol* 98(4): 652-655
      • Flamm B, 2001. Vaginal birth after cesarean (VBAC). *Best Pract Res Clin Obstet Gynaecol*, 15(1):81-92
      • Van Bogaert LJ, 2004. Mode of delivery after one cesarean section. *International Journal of Gynecology and Obstetrics*, 87(1): 9-13

43   • Bujold E, Gauthier RJ, 2001. Should we allow a trial of labor after a previous caesarean for dystocia in the second stage of labor? *Obstet Gynecol* 98(4): 652-655
      • Flamm B, 2001, Vaginal birth after cesarean (VBAC). *Best Pract Res Clin Obstet Gynaecol*, 15(1):81-92
      • Van Bogaert LJ, 2004, Mode of delivery after one cesarean section. *International Journal of Gynecology and Obstetrics*, 87(1): 9-13

44   • Durnwald C, Mercer B, 2004. Vaginal birth after caesarean delivery: predicting success, risks of failure. *J Matern Fetal Neonatal Med*, 14:388-393
      • Hoskins IA, Gomez JL. 1997. Correlation between maximum cervical dilatation at caesarean delivery and subsequent vaginal birth after caesarean delivery. *Obstet Gynecol* 89:591-593.

45   • Mercer BM, Gilbert S, Landon MB, et al, 2008. Labor outcomes with increasing number of prior vaginal births after cesarean delivery. Obstetrics and Gynecology, 111:285-291
      • Shimonovitz S, Botosneano A, Hochner-Celnikier D, 2000. Successful first vaginal birth after cesarean section: a predictor of reduced risk for uterine rupture in subsequent deliveries. *Indian Med Assoc J*, 2: 526-528
      • Cahill AG, Stamilio DM, Odibo AO, *et al*, 2006. Is vaginal birth after caesarean (VBAC) or elective repeat caesarean safer in women with a prior vaginal delivery? *American Journal of Obstetrics and Gynecology*, 195(4): 1143-1147
      • Hendler I, Bujold E. 2004. Effect of prior vaginal delivery or prior vaginal birth after cesarean delivery on obstetric outcomes in women undergoing trial of labor, Obstet Gynecol 10492) : 273-277
      • Guise JM, Eden K, Emeis C, *et al*, 2010. Agency for Healthcare Research and Quality – Evidence Report/Technology Assessment Number 191: *Vaginal Birth After Cesarean: New Insights*, Publication No 10-E001
      • Landon MB, Hauth JC, Leveno KJ. *et al*, 2004. National Institute of Child Health and Human Development Maternal-Fetal Medicine Units Network. Maternal and perinatal outcomes associated with a trial of labor after prior caesarean delivery. *NEJM* 351: 2581-2589

46   • Guise JM, Eden K, Emeis C, *et al*, 2010. Agency for Healthcare Research and Quality – Evidence Report/Technology Assessment Number 191, *Vaginal Birth After Cesarean: New Insights*, Publication no 10-E001
      • Hender I, Bujold E, 2004. Effect of prior vaginal delivery of prior vaginal birth after cesarean delivery on obstetric outcomes in women undergoing trial of labor. *Obstetrics & Gynecology*, 104: 273-277
      • Mercer BM, Gilbert S, Landon MB, *et al*, 2008. Labor outcomes with increasing number of prior vaginal births after cesarean delivery. *Obstetrics and Gynecology*, 111:285-291

47   Guise JM, Denman MA, Emeis C, 2010. Evidence-based practice center presentation II: maternal benefits and harms, and relevant factors. NIH Consensus Development Conference: Vaginal Birth After Cesarean: New Insights, Bethesda, Maryland, March 8-10, 2010.

48   Coalition for Improving Maternity Services (CIMS), 2007. Evidence basis for the ten steps of mother-friendly care. *Journal of Perinatal Education*, 16(1): Supplement. Winter 2007. Available at http:/www.motherfriendly.org/products.php

49   • American College of Obstetricians and Gynecologists, 2010. Vaginal birth after previous cesarean delivery. *Practice Bulletin* No 115.
      • Lieberman E, 2001. Risk factors for uterine rupture during a trial of labor after a caesarean section. *Clin Obstet & Gynecol*, 44: 609-621
      • Flamm B, 2001. Vaginal birth after cesarean (VBAC). *Best Pract Res Clin Obstet Gynaecol*, 15(1):81-92
      • Landon MB, Spong CY, Thom E, *et al*, 2006. Risk of uterine rupture with a trial of labor in women with multiple and single prior caesarean delivery. *Obstetrics and Gynecology*, 108 (1): 12-20
      • Brill Y, Windrim R, 2003. Vaginal birth after caesarean section: review of antenatal predictors of success. *J Obstet Gynaecol Can*, 25(4): 275-286

50   Cahill A, Tuuli M, Odibo A, *et al*, 2010. Vaginal birth after caesarean for women with three or more prior caesareans: assessing safety and success. *BJOG* 2010; DOI: 10.1111/j.1471-0528.2010.02498.x.

51   Lieberman E, Ernst EK, Rooks JP, *et al*, 2004. Results of a national study of vaginal birth after cesarean in birth centers. *Obstet Gynecol*, 104 (5 Part 1): 933-942

52   • Landon MB, 2010. Predicting uterine rupture in women undergoing trial of labor after prior cesarean delivery. NIH Consensus Development Conference: Vaginal Birth After Cesarean: New Insights, Bethesda, Maryland, March 8-10, 2010
      • Giamfi C, Juhasz G, Gyamfi P, *et al*, 2006. Single-versus double-layer uterine incision closure and uterine rupture. *Journal of Maternal-Fetal and Neonatal Medicine*, 19(10): 639-643
      • Durnwald D, Mercer B, 2003. Uterine rupture, perioperative and perinatal morbidity after single-layer and double-layer closure at caesarean delivery. *Am J Obstet Gynecol*, 189 (4):925-929
      • Koppel E, Struzyk B, Zbieszczyk J, 1983. Cesarean section using single-layer tansisthmic uterine sutures. *Zentralbl Gynakol*, 105(23): 1522-1525
      • Coalition for Improving Maternity Services (CIMS), 2007. Evidence basis for the ten steps of mother-friendly care. *Journal of Perinatal Education*, 16(1): Supplement. Winter 2007. Available at http:/www.motherfriendly.org/products.php
      • Enkin MW, Wilkinson C, 2000. Single versus two layer suturing for closing the uterine incision at caesarean section. *Cochrane Database Syst Rev*, (2): CD000192 Cochrane Library Issue 2, Oxford, 2001
      • Bujold E, *et al*, 2005. Single versus double layer closure and the risk of uterine rupture. *Am J Obstet Gynecol*, 193: S20
      • National Perinatal Epidemiology Unit, United Kingdom, 2006. Caesarean section surgical techniques. See www.npeu.ox.ac.uk/caesar

53   Bujold E, Goyet M, Marcoux S, *et al*, 2010. The role of uterine closure in the risk of uterine rupture. *Obstet Gynecol* 116(1): 43-50.

54   Sciscione A, Landon MB, Leveno KJ, *et al*, 2008. National Institute of Child Health and Human Development Maternal-Fetal Medicine Units Network. Previous preterm caesarean delivery and risk of subsequent uterine rupture. *Obstet Gynecol*, 111:648-653.

55   • Rochelson B, Pagano M, Conetta L, *et al*., 2005. Previous preterm cesarean delivery: identification of a new risk factor for uterine rupture in VBAC candidates. *Journal of Maternal-Fetal and Neonatal Medicine*, 18(5): 339-342

Notes and references 269

- Sciscione, *et al*, 2006. Drexel University College of Medicine, Philadelphia, Pennsylvania, research results presented at the Conference of Society for Maternal-Fetal Medicine, Jan 30 - Feb 4, 2006, Miami Beach, Florida, USA. Available at www.medscape.come/viewarticle/523616_2
- Kwee A, Smink M, van der Laar R, *et al*, 2007. Outcome of subsequent delivery after a previous early preterm cesarean section. *Journal of Maternal-Fetal and Neonatal Medicine*, 20(1): 33-37

56 NIH Consensus Development Conference: Vaginal Birth After Cesarean: New Insights, Bethesda, Maryland, March 8-10, 2010.

57 Grobman W. 2010. Rates and prediction of successful vaginal birth after cesarean. NIH Consensus Development Conference: Vaginal Birth After Cesarean: New Insights, Bethesda, Maryland, March 8-10, 2010.

58 NIH Consensus Development Conference: Vaginal Birth After Cesarean: New Insights, Bethesda, Maryland, March 8-10, 2010. Final Statement. See: http://consensus.nih.gov/2010/images/vbac/vbac_statement.pdf

59
- Blackwell SC, Hassan SS, Wolfe HM, 2000. Vaginal birth after caesarean in the diabetic gravida. *J Reprod Med*, 45(12): 987-990
- Guise JM, Denman MA, Emeis C. et al. 2010. Evidence-based Practice Center Presentation I: Trial of Labor, Vaginal Delivery Rates, and Relevant Factors, NIH Consensus Development Conference: Vaginal Birth After Cesarean: New Insights, Bethesda, Maryland, March 8-10, 2010.

60 Guise JM, Eden K, Emeis C, *et al*, 2010. Evidence-based practice center presentation I: Trial of labor, vaginal delivery rates and relevant factors. NIH Consensus Development Conference: Vaginal Birth After Cesarean: New Insights, Bethesda, Maryland, March 8-10, 2010.

61 Guise JM, Eden K, Emeis C, *et al*, 2010. Evidence-based practice center presentation I: Trial of labor, vaginal delivery rates and relevant factors. NIH Consensus Development Conference: Vaginal Birth After Cesarean: New Insights, Bethesda, Maryland, March 8-10, 2010.

62 NIH Consensus Development Conference: Vaginal Birth After Cesarean: New Insights, Bethesda, Maryland, March 8-10, 2010.

63 NIH Consensus Development Conference: Vaginal Birth After Cesarean: New Insights, Bethesda, Maryland, March 8-10, 2010.

64
- Goodall PT, Ahn JT, Chapa JB, *et al*, 2005. Obesity as a risk factor for failed trial of labor in patients with previous caesarean delivery. *American Journal of Obstetrics and Gynecology*, 192(5): 1423-1426
- Juhasz G, Gyamfi C, Gyamfi P, *et al*, 2005. Effect of body mass index and excessive weight gain on success of vaginal birth after cesarean delivery. *Obstet Gynecol*, 106(4): 741-746
- Lydon-Rochelle MT, Cahill AG, Spong CY, 2010. Birth after prior cesarean delivery: short-term maternal outcomes. NIH Consensus Development Conference: Vaginal Birth After Cesarean: New Insights, Bethesda, Maryland, March 8-10, 2010.

65
- Shipp TD, Zelop C, Repke JT, *et al*, 2002. The association of maternal age and symptomatic uterine rupture during a trial of labor after prior caesarean delivery. *Obstet Gynecol*, 99: 585-588
- Kaczmarczyk M, Sparén P, Terry P, *et al*, 2007. Risk factors for uterine rupture and neonatal consequences of uterine rupture: a population-based study of successive pregnancies in Sweden. *BJOG*, 114(10): 1208-1214
- Bujold E, Blackwell SC, Gauthier RJ, 2004. Cervical ripening with transcervical foley catheter and the risk of uterine rupture. *Obstet Gynecol*, 103(1): 18-23

66 Bujold E, Hammoud AO, Hendler I, *et al*, 2004. Trial-of-labor in patients with a previous cesarean section: does maternal age influence the outcome? *Am J Obstet Gynecol*, 190(4): 1113-1118

67 Ravasia DJ, Brain PH, Pollard JK, 1999. Incidence of uterine rupture among women with müllerian duct anomalies who attempts vaginal birth after caesarean delivery. *Am J Obstet Gynecol,* 181(4): 877-881.

68 Kaczmarczyk M, Sparén P, Terry P, *et al,* 2007. Risk factors for uterine rupture and neonatal consequences of uterine rupture: a population-based study of successive pregnancies in Sweden. *BJOG,* 114(10): 1208-1214.

69 Marpeau L, 2000. Faut-il laisser accoucher les sièges par voie basse? In: [unattributed] *Mise à jour en gynécologie obstétrique.* Paris, Collège National des Gynécologues et Obstétriciens Français, pp 127-144, published by Vigot Diffusion. Quoted by Vercoustre L, Roman H, 2006. Essai de travail en cas de césarienne antérieure – revue de la littérature. *J Gynecol Obstet Biol Reprod,* 35: 35-45.

70 • De Meeus JB, Ellia F, Magnin G, 1998. External cephalic version after previous caesarean section: a series of 38 cases. *Eur J Obstet Gynecol Reprod Biol,* 81: 65-68
• Flamm BL, Fried, MW. Lonky NM, 1991. External cephalic version after previous caesarean section. *Am J Obstet Gynecol,* 165: 370-372. Quoted by Vercoustre L, Roman H, 2006. Essai de travail en cas de césarienne antérieure – revue de la littérature. *J Gynecol Obstet Biol Reprod,* 35: 35-45

71 Quiñones JN, Stamilio D, Paré E. Et al. 2005. The effect of prematurity on vaginal birth after cesarean delivery: success and maternal morbidity, *Obstet & Gynecol,* 105(3): 519-524.

72 Quiñones JN, Stamilio D, Paré E. Et al. 2005. The effect of prematurity on vaginal birth after cesarean delivery: success and maternal morbidity, *Obstet & Gynecol,* 105(3): 519-524.

73 • Ford AA, Bateman BT, Simpson LL, 2006. Vaginal birth after caesarean delivery in twin gestations: a large, nationwide sample of deliveries. *American Journal of Obstetrics and Gynecology,* 195(4): 1138-1142
9 studies quoted by Vercoustre L, Roman H, 2006. Essai de travail en cas de césarienne antérieure – Revue de la littérature. *J. Gynecol Obstet Biol Reprod,* 35: 35-45, as follows:
• Strong TH, Phelan JP, Ahn MO, Sarno AP. Vaginal birth after cesarean section in the twin gestation. *Am J Obstet Gynecol* 1989; *161*: 29.
• Miller DA, Mullin P, Hou D, Paul RH. Vaginal birth after cesarean section in twin gestation. *Am J Obstet Gynecol* 1996; *175*: 194-8.
• Odeh M, Tarazova L, Wolfson M, Oettinger M. Evidence that women with a history of cesarean section can deliver twins safely. *Acta Obstet Gynecol* 1997; 76:663-6.
• Aboulfalah A, Abbassi H, el Karroumi M, Himmi A, el Mansouri A. Twin delivery after cesarean section: is a trial of labor warranted? *J Gynecol Obstet Biol Reprod* 1999; 28: 820-4.
• Wax JR, Philput C, Mather J, Steinfeld JD, Ingardia CJ. Twin vaginal birth after cesarean. *Conn Med* 2000; 64: 205-8.
• Myles T. Vaginal birth of twins after previous cesarean section. *J Maternal Fetal Med* 2001; 10: 171-4.
• Delaney T, Young DC. Trial of labour compared to elective caesarean in twin gestations with a previous caesarean delivery. *J Obstet Gynaecol Can* 2003; *25*: 289-92.
• Sansregret A, Bujold E, Gauthier RJ. Twin delivery after a previous caesarean: a twelve-year experience. *J Obstet Gynaecol Can* 2003; 25: 294-8.
• Coutty N, Deruelle P, Delahousse G, Le Goueff F, Subtil D. Vaginal birth after caesarean delivery in twin gestation: is trial of labor allowed? *Gynecol Obstet Fertil* 2004; 32: 855-9.

74 • NIH Consensus Development Conference: Vaginal Birth After Cesarean: New Insights, Bethesda, Maryland, March 8-10, 2010.
• American College of Obstetricians and Gynecologists, August 2010, Vaginal birth after previous cesarean delivery. Practice Bulletin No 115 – Clinical Management Guidelines for Obstetrician-Gynecologists. See http://www.ourbodiesourblog.org/wp-content/uploads/2010/07/ACOG_guidelines_vbac_2010.pdf

Notes and references   271

75   Srinivas SK, Stamilio DM, Stevens EJ, *et al*, 2006. Safety and success of vaginal birth after cesarean delivery in patients with preeclampsia. *American Journal of Perinatology*, 23(3): 145-152.

76   Srinivas SK, Stamilio DM, Stevens EJ, *et al*, 2006. Safety and success of vaginal birth after cesarean delivery in patients with preeclampsia. *American Journal of Perinatology*, 23(3): 145-152.

77
- Lieberman E, 2001. Risk factors for uterine rupture during a trial of labor after a cesarean section. *Clin Obstet & Gynecol*, 44: 609-621
- Goyet M, Bujold E, 2006. Society for Maternal-Fetal Medicine, Jan 30-Feb 4, 2006. Miami Beach. Florida. Quoted in *Medscape OB/Gyn & Women's Health* 2006 11(1)
- Kaczmarczyk M, Sparén P, Terry P, *et al*, 2007. Risk factors for uterine rupture and neonatal consequences of uterine rupture: a population-based study of successive pregnancies in Sweden. *BJOG*, 114(10): 1208-1214
- Elkousy MA, Sammel M, Stevens E, *et al*, 2003. The effect of birth weight on vaginal birth after caesarean delivery success rates. *American Journal of Obstetrics and Gynecology*, 188 (3): 824-830
- Parry S, Severs CP, Schdev HM, *et al*, 2000. Ultrasonographic prediction of fetal macrosomia. Association with caesarean delivery. *J Reprod Med*, 45(1):17-22
- Vercoustre L, Roman H, 2006. Essai de travail en cas de césarienne antérieure – revue de la littérature. *J Gynecol Obstet Biol Reprod*, 35: 35-45, quoting Lao TT, Chin RKH, Leung BFH, 1987. Is X-ray pelvimetry useful in a trial of labour after caesarean section? *European Journal of Obstetrics, Gynecology and Reproductive Biology*, 24(4): 277-283

78
- Sacks DA, Chen W, 2000. Estimating fetal weight in the management of macrosomia. Obstet Gynecol Surv 55(4): 229-239
- Lao TT, Chin RKH, Leung BFH, 1987. Is X-ray pelvimetry useful in a trial-of-labor after caesarean section? *EJOG* 24(4): 277-283

79
- Coassolo KM, Stamilio DM, Paré E, *et al*, 2005. Safety and efficacy of vaginal birth after cesarean attempts at or beyond 40 weeks of gestation. *Obstetrics & Gynecology*, 106 (4):700-706
- Lieberman E, 2001. Risk factors for uterine rupture during a trial of labor after a cesarean section. *Clin Obstet & Gynecol*, 44: 609-621
- Zelop CM, Shipp TD, Cohen A, *et al*, 2001. Trial of labor after 40 weeks' gestation in women with prior caesarean. *Obstet Gynecol*, 97(3): 391-393
- Goyet M, Gauthier RJ, 2001. Should we allow a trial of labor after a previous caesarean for dystocia in the second stage of labor? *Obstet Gynecol*, 98(4): 652-655
- Lieberman E, Ernst EK, Rooks JP, *et al*, 2004. Results of a national study of vaginal birth after cesarean in birth centers. *Obstet Gynecol*, 104(5 Part 1): 933-942
- Kaczmarczyk M, Sparén P, Terry P, *et al*, 2007. Risk factors for uterine rupture and neonatal consequences of uterine rupture: a population-based study of successive pregnancies in Sweden. *BJOG*, 114(10): 1208-1214

80   Coassolo KM, Stamilio DM, Paré E, *et al*, 2005. Safety and efficacy of vaginal birth after cesarean attempts at or beyond 40 weeks of gestation. *Obstetrics & Gynecology*, 106(4): 700-706.

81
- Jastrow N, Chaillet N, Roberge S et al, 2010, Sonographic lower uterine segment thickness and risk of uterine scar defect – a systematic review, *JOGC*, 32(4):321-327 .
- NIH Consensus Development Conference: Vaginal Birth After Cesarean: New Insights, Bethesda, Maryland, March 8-10, 2010

82
- Grobman W, 2010. Rates and prediction of successful vaginal birth after cesarean. NIH Consensus Development Conference: Vaginal Birth After Cesarean: New Insights, Bethesda, Maryland, March 8-10, 2010.
- Guise JM, Denman MA, Emeis C, *et al*, 2010. Agency for Healthcare Research and Quality – Evidence Report/Technology Assessment No 191, *Vaginal Birth After Cesarean: New Insights*, Publication no 10-E001.

83   NIH Consensus Development Conference: Vaginal Birth After Cesarean: New Insights, Bethesda, Maryland, March 8-10, 2010. Note: Usually, for this book this reference relates to the systematic review of scientific studies that was done for the Conference : Guise JM, Denman MA, Emeis C, et al, 2010. Agency for Healthcare Research and Quality – Evidence Report/Technology Assessment No 191, Vaginal Birth After Cesarean: New Insights, Publication no 10-E001.

84   Lieberman E, Ernst EK, Rooks JP, *et al*, 2004. Results of a national study of vaginal birth after cesarean in birth centers. *Obstet Gynecol*, 104(5 Part 1): 933-942.

85   • Lieberman E, Ernst EK, Rooks JP, *et al*, 2004. Results of a national study of vaginal birth after cesarean in birth centers. *Obstet Gynecol*, 104(5 Part 1): 933-942
    • David M, Gross MM, Wiemer A, *et al*, 2009. Prior cesarean section—an acceptable risk for vaginal delivery at free-standing midwife-led birth centers? Results of the analysis of vaginal birth after cesarean section (VBAC) in German birth centers. *EJOG* 142(2): 106-110

86   Lieberman E, Ernst EK, Rooks JP, *et al*, 2004. Results of a national study of vaginal birth after cesarean in birth centers. *Obstet Gynecol*, 104(5 Part 1): 933-942.

87   • Guise JM, Denman MA, Emeis C, et al, 2010. Agency for Healthcare Research and Quality – Evidence Report/Technology Assessment No 191, Vaginal Birth After Cesarean: New Insights, Publication no 10-E001.
    • Goyet M, Gauthier RJ, 2001. Should we allow a trial of labor after a previous caesarean for dystocia in the second stage of labor? *Obstet Gynecol*, 98(4): 652-655

88   Grobman WA, Gilbert S, Landon MB, *et al*. 2007. Outcomes of induction of labor after one prior caesarean *Obstet Gynecol* 109(2 Pt1):262-269.

89   • Landon MB, Hauth JC, Leveno KJ, *et al* (National Institute of Child Health and Human Development Maternal-Fetal Medicine Units Network), 2004. Maternal and perinatal outcomes associated with a trial of labor after prior caesarean delivery. *NEJM* 351: 2581-2589.
    • Guise JM, Denman MA, Emeis C, *et al*, 2010. Agency for Healthcare Research and Quality – Evidence Report/Technology Assessment No 191, *Vaginal Birth After Cesarean: New Insights*, Publication no 10-E001.

90   Bujold E, Blackwell SC, Hendler I, *et al*, 2004. Modified Bishop's score and induction of labor in patients with a previous caesarean delivery. *Am J Obstet Gynecol*, 191(5): 1644-1648.

91   Guise JM, Denman MA, Emeis C, *et al*, 2010. Agency for Healthcare Research and Quality – Evidence Report/Technology Assessment No 191, *Vaginal Birth After Cesarean: New Insights*, Publication no 10-E001.

92   Latendresse G, Murphy PA, Fullerton JT, 2005. A description of the management and outcomes of vaginal birth after caesarean birth in the homebirth setting. *J Midwifery Women's Health*, 50(5): 386-391.

93   Latendresse G, Murphy PA, Fullerton JT, 2005. A description of the management and outcomes of vaginal birth after caesarean birth in the homebirth setting. *J Midwifery Women's Health*, 50(5): 386-391.

94   Grobman WA, 2010. Rates and prediction of successful vaginal birth after cesarean. NIH Consensus Development Conference: Vaginal Birth After Cesarean: New Insights, Bethesda, Maryland, March 8-10, 2010.

95   Lydon-Rochelle M, Holt VL, Easterling TR, *et al*, 2001. Risk of uterine rupture during labor among women with a prior cesarean delivery. *NEJM*, 345: 3-8.

96   • Goyet M, Bujold E, 2006. Society for Maternal-Fetal Medicine, Jan 30 - Feb 4, 2006, Miami Beach, Florida, USA. Quoted in *Medscape OB/Gyn & Women's Health* 2006 11(1)
    • Goyet M, Gauthier RJ, 2001. Should we allow a trial of labor after a previous caesarean for dystocia in the second stage of labor. *Obstet Gynecol*, 98(4): 652-655

Notes and references 273

97   See the Chapter 2 (on risk) and also the following: British Columbia Perinatal Health Program, 2008. *Caesarean birth task force report.* Vancouver, Canada. February 2008.

98   Macones G, Peipert J, Nelson D, *et al,* 2005. Maternal complications with vaginal birth after cesarean delivery: a multicenter study. *Am J Obstet Gynecol,* 193(5): 1656-1662.

99   Lydon-Rochelle M, Hold VL, Easterling TR, *et al,* 2001. Risk of uterine rupture during labor among women with a prior caesarean delivery. *NEJM* 345:3-8.

100   NIH Consensus Development Conference: Vaginal Birth After Cesarean: New Insights, Bethesda, Maryland, March 8-10, 2010.

101   • Guise JM, Denman MA, Emeis C, et al, 2010. Agency for Healthcare Research and Quality – Evidence Report/Technology Assessment No 191, Vaginal Birth After Cesarean: New Insights, Publication no 10-E001.
      • Goyet, M, Bujold E, 2006. Society for Maternal-Fetal Medicine, Jan 30 - Feb 4, 2006, Miami Beach, Florida, USA, quoted in Medscape *OB/Gyn & Women's Health* 2006 11(1)

102   Walmsley K, Hobbs L, 1994. Vaginal birth after lower segment caesarean section. *Modern Midwife,* 4(4): 20-21.

103   Grobman WA, 2010. Rates and prediction of successful vaginal birth after cesarean. NIH Consensus Development Conference: Vaginal Birth After Cesarean: New Insights, Bethesda, Maryland, March 8-10, 2010.

104   Guise JM, Denman MA, Emeis C, *et al,* 2010. Agency for Healthcare Research and Quality – Evidence Report/Technology Assessment No 191, *Vaginal Birth After Cesarean: New Insights,* Publication no 10-E001.

105   Guise JM, Eden K, Emeis C, *et al,* 2010. Agency for Healthcare Research and Quality – Evidence Report/Technology Assessment No 191, *Vaginal Birth After Cesarean: New Insights,* Publication no 10-E001.

106   • Brill Y, Windrim R, 2003. Vaginal birth after caesarean section: review of antenatal predictors of success. *J Obste Gynaecol Can,* 25(4): 275-286. 246
      • Martin JN, 1988. Vaginal birth after caesarean section. *Obs & Gyn Clinics in North America,* 15(4):729

107   Martin JN, 1988, Vaginal birth after caesarean section: review of antenatal predictors of success, J Obste Gynaecol Can, 2594): 275-286

108   Dr Schiffin, quoted in: Batisti-Richards L, 1987. *The VBAC Experience.* Bergin & Garvey, p103.

109   • Stratton B, 2006. 50 ways to protest a VBAC denial. *Midwifery Today,* No 78. See www.midwiferytoday.com/articles/50ways_vbac.asp
      • Stratton B, 2004. Confronting an anti-VBAC hospital. *Clarion* 19(4):1
      • Sundaramurthy, A, 2004. Fighting for a hospital VBAC. *Clarion* 19(4): 9-11

110   See Middlesex Superior Court CA No 88-6450, Mass 1992, USA. See http://www.mass.gov/courts/courtsandjudges/courts/middsupmain.html and the www.advocatesforpregnantwomen.org

111   Federal Public Prosecutor supports Parto do Princípio and sponsors hearing on c-section abuse, 30 September, 2007. See www.partodoprincipio.com.br

112   For more information on Vermont and New Hampshire's project see: Birth choices after a cesarean section. Oct 3, 2002. Also see the Northern New England Perinatal Quality Improvement Network at www. nnepqin.org

113   See http://goliath.ecnext.com/coms2/gi_0199-2840899/Mother-friendly-hospital-designated-Bulletins.html

Chapter 4—Consider the emotional aftermath

1 Oblasser C, Ebner U, Wesp G. 2008. *Der Kaiserschnitt hat kein Gesicht*. Salzburg: Edition Riendenburg.

2 Baldwin R, Palmarini T, 1986, *Pregnant Feelings*. Berkeley, CA, USA: Celestial Arts.

3 Amfousse L, 1988. Personal communication with the author.

4 Grégoire L, Saint-Amant S (eds), 2004. *Au cœur de la naissance – Témoignages et réflexions sur l'accouchement*. Montreal, Canada: Éditions Remue-ménage.

5 National Consensus Conference on Aspects of Cesarean Birth, McMaster University, 1985.

6 Chaillet N, 2005. Exploratory study on women's satisfaction after a caesarean. Unpublished data.

7 Norwood C, 1984, *How to Avoid a Cesarean Section*. New York: Simon et Schuster, p 31.

8 Faúndes A, De Pádua KS, Duarte, Osis MF, *et al*, 2004. Opinião de mulheres e médicos brasileiros sobre a preferência pela via de parto. *RevSaúde Pública*, 38(4): 488-494.

9 Selo-Ojeme D, Abulhassan N, Mandal R, *et al*, 2008. Preferred and actual delivery mode after a caesarean in London, UK. *Int J. Gynaecol Obste*, online, April 24.

10 *Sunday Morning*, Radio-Canada, March 9, 1986 (interview).

11 Klein M and the Medical Sub-Committee (ed: Yves Lefèvre), 1987. Controversies in Obstetrical Management and Maternal Care. Direction des communications, Ministère de la Santé et des Services Sociaux, Quebec, Canada.

12 Panuthos C. The psychological effects of cesaeran deliveries. *Mothering*. Winter 1983, No.26, p 61.

13 Shearer E. *Cesarean prevention and VBAC*. Conference organised by Edmonton VRAC Association and Edmonton Childbirth Education Association, Edmonton, June 1987.

14 • Schneider G, 1981. Management of normal labour and delivery in the case room a critical appraisal. *CMA Journal*, 125: 350-352
   • Oakley A, 1983. Social consequences of obstetric technology: the importance of measuring 'soft' outcomes. *Birth*, 10(2): 99-109
   • Humenick SS, 1981. Mastery: the key to childbirth satisfaction - a review. *Birth and the Family Journal*, 8(2): 79-90

15 Klein M, and the Medical Sub-Committee, 1987 (ed: Yves Lefèvre). Controversies in Obstetrical Management and Maternal Care. Direction des Communications, Ministère de la Santé et des Services Sociaux, Quebec, Canada.

16 Fillipi V, 2007. Subsequent mental health impairment in women with severe obstetric complications. *Lancet*, 370:1329-1337. Quoted at www.orgyn.com/en/authfiles/printfiles/print_495993995.asp Oct 13, 2007.

17 National Institutes of Health, 1981. *Cesarean Childbirth*. Public Health Service, US Department of Health and Human Services, 1981.

18 Fenwick J, Gamble J, Mawson J, 2003. Women's experiences of Caesarean section and vaginal birth after caesarean: a birthrites initiative. *International Journal of Nursing Practice*, 9(1): 10.

19 Chit Ying L, Levy VA, Shan CO, *et al*, 2001. A qualitative study of the perceptions of Hong Kong Chinese women during caesarean section under regional anaesthesia. *Midwifery*, 17: 115-122.

20 Cohen N, Estner L, 1983. *Silent Knife: Cesarean Prevention and VBAC*. South Hadley: Bergin and Garvey.

21 National Institute of Health, 1980. *Cesarean Childbirth*. Statement online, Sep 22-24; 3(6): 1-30.

22 *ICEA News*, January 23, 1984.

23 Baptisti-Richards L, 1987. *The Vaginal Birth After Cesarean Experience – Birth Stories by Parents and Professionals*. Westport, CT, USA: Bergin and Garvey.

24 Panuthos C, 1983. The psychological effects of cesarean deliveries. *Mothering*, 26: 62.

25 See http://www.childbirthconnection.org/article.asp?ck=10166#psychological

26 Swain JE, Tasgin E, Mayes LC, *et al.* 2008. Maternal brain response to own baby-cry is affected by cesarean section delivery. *J Child Pscyhol Psychiatry*, 49(10):1042-1052.

27 Affonso DA (ed), 1981 (1st ed). *Impact of Cesarean Childbirth*. Philadelphia: FA Davis.

28 Marut JS, Mercer RT, 1979. Comparison of primiparas' perceptions of vaginal and cesarean births. *Nursing Research*, 28: 260-266.

29 National Institute of Health. *Cesarean Childbirth*, p 458. NIH Consensus Statement 1980 Sep 22-24;3(6):1-30.See: http://consensus.nih.gov/1980/1980Cesarean027html.htm

30 Harrisson M, 1982. *A Woman in Residence*. New York: Penguin Books, p80.

31 • *Pre and Perinatal Psychology Journal*, Psychology Association of North America Human Sciences Press, New York. See www.birthpsychology.com/Journal/
    • Verny T, Kelly J, 1981. *The Secret Life of the Unborn Child*. New York: Dell.

32 Authors like David Chamberlain, PhD, who is a pioneer in birth psychology, and one of the founders of the Association for Pre- and Perinatal Psychology and Health (APPPAH).

33 Verdult R, 2009. Caesarean birth: psychological aspects in adults. *Journal of Prenatal and Perinatal Psychology and Medicine*, 21(1/2):17-28.

34 • Bailham D, Joseph S, 2003. Post-traumatic stress following childbirth: a review of the emerging literature and directions for research and practice. *Psychology, Health and Medicine*, 8(2): 159-168
    • Ryding EL, Awijma K, Wijma B, 1998. Experiences of emergency caesarean section: a phenomenological study of 53 women. *Birth*, 25(4): 246-251

35 Nicholls K, Ayers S, 2007. Childbirth-related post-traumatic stress disorder in couples: a qualitative study. *British Journal of Health Psychology*, 12(4): 491-509.

36 Ayers S, 2007. Thoughts and emotions during traumatic birth: a qualitative study. *Birth*, 34 (3): 253-263.

37 Jukelevics N, 2004. Once a cesarean, always a cesarean: the sorry state of birth choices in America. *Mothering*, 123: 46-55.

38 Korte D, Scaer R, 1984. *A Good Birth, A Safe Birth*. New York: Bantam Books.

39 Deming M, Comello N, 1988. Grieving and healing. *The Cesarean Prevention Clarion*, 5 (3,4).

Chapter 5—Create a supportive environment

1 Da Motta CCL, Rinne C, Naziri D, 2006. The influence of emotional support during childbirth: a clinical study. *Journal of Prenatal and Perinatal Psychology and Health*, 20(4): 325-341.

2 The more detailed version of this document intended for health professionals is available at http://www.rcog.uk/files/rcog-corp/uploaded-files/GT45BirthAfterPreviousCeasarean.pdf

3 Balwin R, Palmarini T, 1986. *Pregnant Feelings*. Berkeley: Celestial Arts, p 4.

4 Panuthos C, 1983. The psychological effects of cesarean deliveries. *Mothering*, 26: 64.

5 • Saisto T, Halmesmaki E, 2003. Fear of childbirth: a neglected dilemma. *Acta Obstetrica and Gynecological Scandinavia*, 82: 201-208
    • Zar M, Wijma K, Wijma B, 2001. Pre and postpartum fear of childbirth in nulliparous and parous women. *Scandinavian Journal of Behaviour Therapy*, 30(2): 75-81

6 Consult the web site www.bonapace.com. This method is taught in Canada.

7   See http://www.activebirthcentre.com/pb/classesandteachers.shtml for more information

8   Coalition for Improving Maternity Services (CIMS), 2007. Evidence basis for the ten steps of mother-friendly care. *Journal of Perinatal Education*, 16(1): Supplement. Winter 2007. Available at http://www.motherfriendly.org/products.php. Available at http://www.motherfriendly.org/products.php

9   See http://www.wordfromhomenetworkmarketing.com/maxwell-maltz-quotes.html

10 These three women worked in the field of psychotherapy and wrote books on mental health. Further details are as follows:
    - Labonté created 'L'approche globale du corps', writing among other books *Se Guérir Autrement, C'est Possible.* Montreal, Éditions de l'Homme, 2001.
    - Gayle Peterson is a senior therapist and international expert who wrote, among other books, *An Easier Childbirth: Birthing Normally.* Berkeley, CA : Shadow and Light Publications, 1993.
    - Claudia Panuthos directs a childbirth counselling centre and wrote (with Catherine Romeo) *Ended Beginnings: Healing Childbearing Losses.* South Hadley, MA, USA: Bergin & Garvey, 1984 and *Transformation Through Birth—A Woman's Guide.* South Hadley, MA, USA: Bergin & Garvey, 1984.

11 NIH Consensus Development Conference: Vaginal Birth After Cesarean: New Insights, Bethesda, Maryland, March 8-10, 2010.

12 These statistics can be found at the following websites:
    - http://www.statistics.gov.uk/pdfdir/ipm0909.pdf
    - http://www.statistics.gov.uk/StatBase/ssdataset.asp?vlnk=7412&Pos=&ColRank=2&Rank=480

13 World Health Organization, 1985. Appropriate technology for birth. *Lancet*, Aug 24.

14 Johnson KC, Daviss BA, 2005. Outcomes of planned home births with certified professional midwives: large prospective study in North America. *British Medical Journal*, 330(7505): 1416-1427.

15 Althabe F, Belizan JF, 2006. Caesarean section: the paradox. *Lancet*, 36: 1472-1473.

16 Rooks JP, Weatherby NL, Ernst EKM, 1989. Outcomes of care in birth centers: The National Birth Center Study. *NEJM*, 321(26): 1804-1811

17 Anonymous. Cesarean section – why does the national US cesarean section rate keep going up? Dec 2007. www.childbirthconnection.org/article.asp ?ck=10456

18 Coalition for Improving Maternity Services, Grassroots Advocates Committee. Birth Survey Project, 2007. See www.thebirthsurvey.com

19 Latendresse G, Murphy PA, Fullerton JT, 2005. A description of the management and outcomes of vaginal birth after caesarean birth in the homebirth setting. *J Midwifery Women's Health*, 50(5): 386-391.

20 Coalition for Improving Maternity Services (CIMS), 2007. Evidence basis for the ten steps of mother-friendly care. *Journal of Perinatal Education*, 16(1): Supplement. Winter 2007. Available at http://www.motherfriendly.org/products.php

21 Fisher C, Hauck Y, Fenwick J, 2006. How social context impacts on women's fears of childbirth: a Western Australian example. *Social Science and Medicine*, 63: 64-75.

22 Jukelevics N, 2004. Once a cesarean, always a cesarean: the sorry state of birth choices in America. *Mothering*, 123: 46-55.

23 Fédération des infirmières et infirmiers du Québec, Canada, 1987. Femmes et maternité, féconder de nouveaux choix – donner naissance à de nouvelles ressources. See http://catalogue.cdeacf.ca/Record.htm?idlist=1&record=19108548124919267209

24 Hodnett ED, Gates S, Hofmeyr GJ, Sakala C, 2003. Continuous support for women during childbirth. The Cochrane Library. *Cochrane Database Syst Rev* 2003;(3):CD003766. See http://www.ncbi.nlm.nih.gov/pubmed/12917986

Notes and references 277

25   Klaus MH, Obertson MO, (eds), 1982. *Birth, Interaction and Attachment – Exploring the Foundation for Modern Perinatal Care*. Skillman, NJ, USA: Johnson & Johnson Baby.

26   Hodnett ED, Gates S, Hofmeyr GJ, Sakala C, 2007 (revised). Continuous Support for Women During Childbirth. The Cochrane Library. 2007. Issue 3 See http://www.childbirthconnection.org/pdfs/continuous_support.pdf

27   • Hodnett ED, Gates S, Hofmeyr GJ, Sakala C, 2005. Continuous support for women during childbirth - Cochrane Review. *The Cochrane Library*, Issue 2, Chichester, UK: John Wiley.
      • Yogev S, 2004. Support in labour: a literature review. *MIDIRS Midwifery Digest*, 14(4): 486-492

28   • Rosen P, 2004. Supporting women in labor: analysis of different types of caregivers. *Journal of Midwifery and Women's Health*, 49(1): 24-31
      • Brüggemann OM, Parpinelli MA, Duarte Osis JF, 2005. Evidências sobre o suporte durante o trabalho de parto/parto: uma revisão da literatura. *Cad. Saúde Publica*. Rio de Janeiro, 21(5):1316-1327

29   Simkin P, Klaus P, 2004. *When Survivors Give Birth: Understanding and Healing the Effects of Early Sexual Abuse on Childbearing Women*, Seattle, WA, USA: Classic Day Publishing.

30   • Rosen P, 2004. Supporting women in labor: analysis of different types of caregivers. *Journal of Midwifery and Women's Health*, 49(1): 24-31
      • Yogev S, 2004. Support in labour: a literature review. *MIDIRS Midwifery Digest*, 14(4): 486-492
      • Wolman WL, Chalmers B, Hofmeyr GJ, *et al*, 1993. Postpartum depression and companionship in the clinical birth environment: a randomized, controlled study. *Am.J. Obstet Gynecol*, 168(5): 1388-1393

31   Yogev S, 2004. Support in labour: a literature review. *MIDIRS Midwifery Digest*, 14(4): 486-49.

32   Simkin P, Klaus P, 2004. *When Survivors Give Birth: Understanding and Healing the Effects of Early Sexual Abuse on Childbearing Women*, Seattle, WA, USA: Classic Day Publishing.

33   • Hodnett D, Gates S, Hofmeyr GJ, *et al*, 2007. Continuous support for women during childbirth. *The Cochrane Library*, Issue 3
      • Campbell DA, Lake MF, Falk M, *et al*, 2006. A randomized control trial of continuous support in labor by a lay doula. *JOGNN*, 35(4): 456-464.

34   • Yogev S, 2004. Support in labour: a literature review, *MIDIRS Midwifery Digest*, 14(4): 486-492
      • Pascali-Bonaro D, Kroeger M, 2004. Continuous female companionship during childbirth: a crucial resource in times of stress or calm. *Journal of Midwifery and Women's Health*, 49(4): Suppl. 1: 19-27— quoting Hofmeyr GJ, Nikodem VC, Wolman WL, *et al*, 1991. Companionship to modify the clinical birth environment: effects on progress and perceptions of labour and breastfeeding. *British Journal of Obstetrics and Gynaecology*, 98(8): 756-764.

35   Hodnett E. 2002. Caregiver support for women during childbirth. Cochrane Database Systematic Reviews. Issue 1—CD000199. See http://www.ncbi.nlm.nih.gov/pubmed/11869571

36   Hofmeyr GJ, Nikodem VC, Wolman WL, *et al*, 1991. Companionship to modify the clinical birth environment: effects on progress and perceptions of labour, and breastfeeding. *British Journal of Obstetrics and Gynaecology*, 98(8): 756-764.

37   Yogev S. 2004. Support in labour: a literature review. *MIDIRS Midwifery Digest*, 14(4): 486-492.

38   Vadeboncoeur H, 2004. *La naissance au Québec à l'aube du troisième millénaire: de quelle humanization parle-t-on?* Doctoral thesis, Sciences humaines appliquées, Université de Montreal, Canada.

39 Kennell JH, McGrath SK, 1993. Labor support by a doula for middle income couples. The effect on caesarean rates. *Pediatric Res*, 33: 12A. Quoted by Klaus MH, Kennell JH, Klaus PH, 2002. *The Doula Book*, Cambridge, MA: Perseus. Chapter 8, Note 5.

40 Lacharité C, Mailhot L, Boilard H, *et al*, 2001. L'accompagnement à la naissance – une forme de soutien efficace pour promouvoir l'adaptation parentale des pères et des mères lors de la période postnatale. Actes du 6e Symposium québécois de recherche sur la famille. In Lacharité C, Pronovost G, (eds), 2002. *Comprendre la famille*. Quebec, Canada: Presses Universitaires du Québec.

41 Pepleau H, 1972. A working definition of anxiety. Presentation to the Association of Hawaïan Nurses, University of Hawaï. Quoted by Affonso D, 1981. *Impact of Cesarean Childbirth*. Philadelphia, PA, USA: Davis.

42 National Institutes of Health, 1981. *Cesarean Childbirth*. Public Health Service, US Department of Health and Human Services, p 424.

43 *The Personnel and Guidance Journal*, June 1984, p 619-623. Now published as the *Journal of Counseling and Development*. See http://www.counseling.org/Publications/Journals.aspx for more information.

44 • Davidson K, Jacoby S, Brown MS. Prenatal perineal massage: preventing lacerations during delivery. *J Obstet Gynecol Neonatal Nurs*, 2000 Sep-Oct; 29(5): 474-9
   • Shipman MK, Boniface DR, Tefft ME, McCloghry F. Antenatal perineal massage and subsequent perineal outcomes: a randomised controlled trial. *Br J Obstet Gynaecol*, 1997 Jul; 104(7): 787-91.

45 Simkin P, 2007. Birth plans: after 25 years, women still want to be heard. *Birth* 34(1): 49-50.

Chapter 6—Make wise decisions during labour

1 What is suggested in this chapter is almost entirely evidence-based, i.e. based on the results of scientific studies. See www.childbirthconnection.org/article.asp?ck=10375 (2006). Also see Notes 2 and 3 below, and Jukelevics N. 2004. Once a cesarean always a cesarean: The sorry state of birth choices in America. *Mothering*, No.123:46-55.

2 WHO, 1996. *Care in Normal Birth: A Practical Guide*. Department of Reproductive Health and Research. WHO/FRH/MSM/96.24. Available at: http://www.who.int/reproductivehealth/publications/maternal_perinatal_health/MSM_96_24_/en/index.html

3 For a list of healthy birth practices, see http://www.lamaze.org/ChildbirthProfessionals/ResourcesforProfessionals/CarePracticePapers/tabid/90/Default.aspx

4 This systematic review was published in the *Journal of Perinatal Education* in March 2007. It looked at practices which were the focus of the Mother-Friendly Initiative. You can find out more about this initiative at www.motherfriendly.org

5 Singata M, Tranmer J, Gyte GML, 2010. Restricting oral fluid and food intake during labour. *Cochrane Database of Systematic Reviews*. Issue 1, Art. No CD003930. DOI: 10.1002/14651858.

6 • Department of Health and Social security, 1979. *Report on confidential enquiries into maternal deaths in England and Wales 1973-1975*. London: HMSO
   • Pritchard JA, MacDonald PC, 1976. *Williams Obstetrics* (15th edition). New York: Appleton-Century Crofts.

7 • Scheepers H, Essed GG, Brouns F, 1998. Aspects of food and fluid intake during labour. Policies of midwives and obstetricians in The Netherlands. *European Journal of Obstetrics, Gynecology, and Reproductive Biology*, 7(1): 37-40
   • Schuitemaker N, van Roosmalen J, Dekker G, *et al*, 1997. Maternal mortality after cesarean section in The Netherlands. *Acta Obstetricia and Gynecologica Scandinavica*, 76(4): 332-334. Quoted in CIMS, 2007 (Goer H. et al).

Notes and references

8   Coalition for Improving Maternity Services (CIMS), 2007. Evidence basis for the ten steps of mother-friendly care. *Journal of Perinatal Education*, 16(1): Supplement. Winter 2007. Available at http:/www.motherfriendly.org/products.php

9   Cluett ER, Burns E, 2009. Immersion in water in labour and birth. *Cochrane Database of Systematic Reviews*, Issue 2. Art. No.: CD000111. DOI: 10.1002/14651858.CD000111.pub3.

10   Royal College of Obstetricians and Gynaecologists & Royal College of Midwives, 2006. Joint Statement No 1: Immersion in water during labour and birth. See http://www.rcog.org.uk/womens-health/clinical-guidance/immersion-water-during-labour-and-birth

11   See Sarah Buckley's website—www.sarahjbuckley.com. She is a GP and the author of several books on childbirth.

12   Michel SC, Rake A, Treiber K *et al.* 2002. MR obstetric pelvimetry: effect of birthing position on pelvic bony dimensions. *Am. J Roentgenol* 179(4):1063-1067.

13   Nasir A, Korejo R, Noorani KJ. 2007. Childbirth in squatting position. *J Pak Med Assoc* 57(1): 19-22.

14   Coalition for Improving Maternity Services (CIMS), 2007. Evidence basis for the ten steps of mother-friendly care. *Journal of Perinatal Education*, 16(1): Supplement. Winter 2007. Available at http:/www.motherfriendly.org/products.php

15   Choquet J, 2007. Primum non nocere: impact des interventions obstétricales sur l'allaitement. Journée Programme Périnatalité Petite Enfance. CSSS de la Pommeraie, Cowansville. Note: This was a presentation at a conference.

16   For more on fetal positioning, see Jean Sutton and Pauline Scott's book: *Understanding and Teaching Optimal Fœtal Positioning*, 1996. New Zealand: Birth Concepts.

17   Cheng YW, Hopkins LM, Caughey AB, 2004. How long is too long: Does a prolonged second stage of labor in nulliparous women affect maternal and neonatal outcomes? *Am J Obstet Gynecol* 191(3): 933-938.

18   Yildirim G, Beji NK, 2008. Effects of pushing techniques in birth on mother and fetus: a randomized study. *Birth,* 35(1): 31-32.

19   Verheijen EC, Raven JH, Hofmeyr GJ. Fundal pressure during the *second stage of labour*. *Cochrane Database of Systematic Reviews* 2009, Issue 4. Art. No. CD006067. DOI: 10.1002/14651858.CD006067.pub2

20   Rice Simpson K, 2004, *Fundal Pressure During the Second Stage of Labour*, 1st May, Statewide Perinatal Care Program, Department of Pediatrics, 200 Hawkins Dr., Iowa City, Iowa

21   Simpson KR, Knox E, 2001. Fundal pressure during second stage of labor. *MCN,* 26(2), March-April.

22   Interviews carried out for the French edition of this book.

23   Royal College of Obstetricians and Gynaecologists, 2007, *Birth After Previous Caesarean Birth*, Green-top Guideline No 45, Feb 2007.

24   Leung AS, Leung EK, Paul RH. Uterine rupture after previous cesarean delivery: Maternal and fetal consequences. *Am J Obstet Gynecol* 1993;169:945-50.

25   American College of Obstetricians and Gynecologists, 2010. Vaginal birth after previous cesarean delivery. Practice Bulletin 115.

26   Klein M and the Medical Sub-committee (ed:Yves Lefèvre), 1986,*Controversies in Obstetrics and Maternity Care*, Comité régional d'humanisation des soins en périnatalité, CSSSRMM, p 28.

27   Coalition for Improving Maternity Services (CIMS), 2007. Evidence basis for the ten steps of mother-friendly care. *Journal of Perinatal Education*, 16(1): Supplement. Winter 2007. Available at http:/www.motherfriendly.org/products.php

28 Choquet J. 2007. *Primum Non Nocere*. Presentation given on November 29, at the Brome-Missisquoi-Perkins Hospital, Quebec, Canada.

29 Coalition for Improving Maternity Services (CIMS), 2007. Evidence basis for the ten steps of mother-friendly care. *Journal of Perinatal Education*, 16(1): Supplement. Winter 2007. Available at http:/www.motherfriendly.org/products.php

30 Alfirevic Z, Devane D, Gyte GML, 2006, "Coninuous cardiotocography (CTG) as a form of electronic fetal monitoring (EFM) for fetal assessment during labour", *Cochrane Database of Systematic Reviews*. Issue 3.

31 Task Force on Predictors of Fetal Distress, March 2004, quoted by Anderson G, 1994, Canadian Task Force on the Periodic Health Examination. Canadian *Guide to Clinical Preventive Health Care*, Ottawa, Health Canada. 1994: 158-165. Reproduced under: Intrapartum Electronic Fetal Monitoring. See www.ctfphc.org/Full_Text_printable/Ch15full.htm

32 Bergstrom L, Roberts J, Skillman L, *et al*, 1992. 'You'll feel me touching you, sweetie': vaginal examinations during the second stage of labor. *Birth*, 19(1), 10-18.

33 NICE Clinical Guideline 55. Intrapartum care, p 25, 1.6.7.

34 Vadeboncoeur H, 2004, *La naissance au Québec à l'aube du 3e millénaire: de quelle humanisation parle-t-on?* Doctoral thesis. Sciences humaines appliquées, Université de Montréal.

35 Odent M, 1988. Personal communication with the author.

36 Coalition for Improving Maternity Services (CIMS), 2007. Evidence basis for the ten steps of mother-friendly care. *Journal of Perinatal Education*, 16(1): Supplement. Winter 2007. Available at http:/www.motherfriendly.org/products.php

37 Coalition for Improving Maternity Services (CIMS), 2007. Evidence basis for the ten steps of mother-friendly care. *Journal of Perinatal Education*, 16(1): Supplement. Winter 2007. Available at http:/www.motherfriendly.org/products.php

38 Vadeboncoeur H, 2004, *La naissance au Québec à l'aube du 3e millénaire: de quelle humanisation parle-t-on?* Doctoral thesis. Sciences humaines appliquées, Université de Montréal.

39 Harrison M. 1983. *A Woman in Residence*. New York: Penguin.

40 Vadeboncoeur H. 1989. *Une autre césarienne ? Non merci*. Montréal: Éditions Québec-Amérique.

41 Conversation with Dr. Bujold, 2008.

42 Jukelevics N, 2004. Once a cesarean, always a cesarean: the sorry state of birth choices in America. *Mothering*, 123: 46-55.

43 This diagram is inspired by a diagram in Brody Howard and JR Thompson JR, 1981. The Maxim in strategy in modern obstetrics, *Journal of Family Practice*, No 12:979.

44 Tracy SK, Sullivan E, Wang YA, *et al*, 2007. Birth outcomes associated with interventions in labour amongst low risk women: a population based study. *Women and Birth*, 20(2): 41-48.

45 • Dyer C, 1998. Trusts face damages after forcing women to have caesareans. *BMJ* 1998;316:1477, May 16
    • Dyer C, 1997. Appeal court rules against compulsory caesarean sections. *BMJ* 1997;314:993, April 5

46 WHO, 1996. *Care in Normal Birth: A Practical Guide*. Department of Reproductive Health and Research. WHO/FRH/MSM/96.24. Available at: http://www.who.int/reproductivehealth/publications/maternal_perinatal_health/MSM_96_24_/en/index.html

47 The Maternity Care Working Party, UK, 2007. Normal Birth Consensus Statement. See http://www.nctpregnancyandbabycare.com/about-us/what-we-do/maternity-services-user-involvement/making-normal-birth-a-reality

48 Gerbelli C, 2001. La péridurale. Université du Québec à Trois-Rivières, Canada. See www.ecofamille.com/1-11596-Laperidurale.php

49 • Torvaldson S, Roberts CL, Simpson JM, Thompson JF, Ellwood DA. Intrapartum epidural analgesia and breastfeeding: a prospective cohort study. *Int Breastfeeding J.* 1:1-24, 2006
   • Jordan S, Emery S, Bradshaw C, Watkins A, Friswell W. The impact of intrapartum analgesia on infant feeding. *BJOG*, 112: 927-934, 2005
   • Choquet J, 2007. Primum non nocere, impact des interventions obstétricales sur l'allaitement. Journée Programme de Périnatalité Petite Enfance. Cowansville, CSSS de la Pommeraie. Note: This was a presentation at a conference.
   • Forster DA, McLachlan, 2007. Breastfeeding initiation and birth setting practices: a review of the literature, *J Midwifery Women's Health*. 2007; 52(3): 273-280.
   • Anim-Somuah M, Smyth RMD, Howell CJ, 2005. Epidural versus non-epidural or no analgesia in labour. *Cochrane Database of Systematic Reviews*, Issue 4. Art. No: CD000331. DOI: 10.1002/14651858.CD000331.pub2

50 Hacker N, Moore JG, Gambone J, 2004 (4th ed). *Essentials of Obstetrics and Gynecology*. Vol. 1. Philadelphia: Elsevier.

51 Templeton SK, 2009. Mothers face crackdown on epidural births. *Sunday Times*. March 1. Available at http://www.timesonline.co.uk/tol/news/uk/article5822051.ece

52 See http://www.ic/nhs.uk/webfiles/publications/maternityeng2005/ NHSMaternityStatistics260506_PDF.pdf and http://www.ic.nhs.uk/statistics-and-data-collections/hospital-care/maternity/nhs-maternity-statistics-2008-09

53 Coalition for Improving Maternity Services (CIMS), 2007. Evidence basis for the ten steps of mother-friendly care. *Journal of Perinatal Education*, 16(1): Supplement. Winter 2007. Available at http://www.motherfriendly.org/products.php

54 • Klein MC, 2006. Does epidural analgesia increase rate of caesarean section? *Canadian Family Physician*, 52: 419-421
   • Klein MC, 2006. L'analgésie péridurale accroît-elle les taux de césariennes? *Le Médecin de famille canadien*. See http://www.cfpc.ca/cfp/2006/Apr/Vol52-apreditorials-2_fr.asp

55 Kotaska AJ, Klein MC, Liston RM, 2006. Epidural analgesia associated with low-dose oxytocin augmentation increases cesarean births: a critical look at the external validity of randomized trials. *American Journal of Obstetrics and Gynecology*, 194: 809-814.

56 Baumgardner DJ, Muehl P, 2003. Effect of labor epidural anesthesia on breast-feeding of healthy full-term newborns delivered vaginally. *Journal of the American Board of Family Practice*, 16(1): 7-13.

57 Riordan J, Gross A, Angeron J, *et al*, 2000. The effect of labor pain relief medication on neonatal suckling and breastfeeding duration. *Journal of Human Lactation*, 16(1):7-12.

58 Ransjö-Ardvison AB, Matthiesen AS, Lilja G, *et al*, 2001. Maternal analgesia during labor disturbs newborn behavior: effects on breastfeeding, temperature and crying. *Birth*, 28(1): 5-12.

59 Kiehl EM, Anderson GC, Wilson ME, *et al*, 1996. Social status, mother-infant time together, and breastfeeding duration. *J Hum Lact*,12(3): 201-206.

60 Choquet J, 2007. *Primum non nocere, impact des interventions obstétricales sur l'allaitement*. Journée Programme de Périnatalité Petite Enfance. Cowansville: CSSS de la Pommeraie. Note: This was a presentation at a conference.

61 Walsh D, 2009. Pain and epidural use in normal childbirth. *Evidence-based Midwifery* 7(3).

62 Klein MC, Gauthier RJ, Robbins, JM *et al*, 1994. Relationship of episiotomy to perineal trauma and morbidity, sexual dysfunction, and pelvic floor relaxation. *Am J Obstet Gynecol*. 171(3): 591-598.

Chapter 7—Remember the reasons for birthing normally...

1   National Health Service Information Centre, 2008, UK.

2   Centers for Disease Control and Prevention's National Center for Health Statistics (NCHS), 2010.

3   United States Department of Health and Human Services. Benefits of Breastfeeding. See http://www.bcphp.ca/sites/bcrcp/files/Publications/CBTF_REPORT.pdf

4   Kitzinger S, 1984. Unpublished document, International Childbirth Education Association conference, St-Louis, Missouri.

5   This is what Sheila Kitzinger wrote in her introduction to *Birth Reborn* by Michel Odent (Birth Works, 1994).

6   Newton N *et al*, 1966. Parturient mice: effect of environment on labor. *Science*, 151: 1560-1561.

7   If you read French, you can read this interview in the October edition of *Periscoop* at http://www.aspq.org/view_page.php?type=theme&id=aucun&article=2556

8   British Columbia Perinatal Health Program, 2008. *Caesarean Birth Task Force Report 2008*. Available at http://www.bcphp.ca/sites/bcrcp/files/Publications/CBTF_REPORT.pdf

9   Panuthos C, 1984. *Transformation Through Birth – A Woman's Guide*. South Hadley, MA : Bergin & Garvey, p6

10   Schmid V. 2011. *Birth Pain: Explaining Sensations, Exploring Possibilities*. Chester le Street: Fresh Heart Publishing

11   Jordan B, Davis-Floyd R, 1993. *Birth in Four Cultures: A Crosscultural Investigation of Childbirth in Yucatan, Holland, Sweden and the United States*. Prospect Heights: Waveland Press.

12   De Koninck M, 1988. Femmes, enfantement et changement social: le cas de la césarienne, doctoral thesis. Université Laval, Quebec, Canada.

13   Simkin P, 1992. Just another day in a woman's life? Nature and consistency of women's long term memories of their first birth experience. *Birth*, 19:64-81.

14   Halldorsdottir S, Karlsdottir SI, 1996. Empowerment or discouragement: women's experience of caring and uncaring encounters during childbirth. Health *Care for Women International*, 17(4)361-379.

15   • Menage J, 1993. Post-traumatic disorder in women who have undergone obstetric and/or gynaecological procedures: a consecutive series of 30 cases of PTSD. *Journal of Reproductive et Infant Psychology*. 11(4): 221-228
       • Ayers SM, Pickering AD, 2001. Do women get posttraumatic stress disorder as a result of childbirth? A prospective study of incidence. *Birth*, 28(2): 111-118
       • Soet JE, Brack GA, Dilorio C, 2003. Prevalence and predictors of women's experience of psychological trauma during childbirth. *Birth*, 30(1): 36-46.

16   Bailham D, Joseph S, 2003. Post-traumatic stress following childbirth: a review of the emerging literature and directions for research and practice. *Psychology Health and Medicine*, 8 (2): 159-168.

17   Soderquist J, Wijma K, Wijma B. Traumatic stress after childbirth: the role of obstetric variables. *J Psychosom Obstet Gynaecol*, 2002; 23:31.

18   • Simkin P, 1991. Just another day in a woman's life? Women's long-term perceptions of their first birth experience, Part I. *Birth*, 18(4):203-210
       • Simkin P, 1992. Just another day in a woman's life? Nature and consistency of women's long term memories of their first birth experience. *Birth*, 19:64-81

19   Peterson G, 1996. Childbirth, the ordinary miracle: effects of devaluation of childbirth on women's self-esteem and family relationships. *Pre and Perinatal Psychology Journal*, 11(2): 101-109.

20   Oakley A, Rajan L, 1990. Obstetric technology and maternal emotional well-being: a further research note. *Journal of Reproductive and Infant Psychology,* 8(1):45-55.

21   Littlewood J, McHugh N, 1997. *Maternal Distress and Postnatal Depression,* Basingstoke: MacMillanPress.

22   Rocheleau L, 2001. Étude exploratoire des attentes et des besoins des femmes en périnatalité. Unpublished Master's dissertation. Montréal: Université du Québec à Montréal, Canada.

23   Johnson LH, 1997. *Childbirth as a Developmental Milestone.* Doctoral thesis, Psychoanalysis and Women's Studies, The Union Graduate School, Cincinnati, Ohio, USA.

24   Bizieau S, 1996. Que peut apporter le respect de la physiologie de l'accouchement? Évaluation des pratiques médicales autour de la naissance. Actes du colloque Naissance et Société, June 7, 1996, *Cahiers de l'Université de Perpignan,* No 22.

25   I explored the idea of birth as a transformative and fulfilling event, and as an event which can promote personal growth in a literature review I carried out in 2004 on the multiple dimensions of childbirth, for the Association pour la Santé Publique du Québec, Canada. This review is: *La naissance en 2004: qu'est-ce que l'humanisation?* L'Association pour la Santé Publique du Québec. Unpublished document.

26   Stadlmayr W, Bitzer J, Hosli I, *et al,* 2001. Birth as a multidimensional experience: comparison of the English and German-language versions of Salmon's Item List. *Journal of Psychosomatics Obstetrics and Gynecology,* 22: 205-214.

27   Rocheleau L, 2001. *Étude exploratoire des attentes et des besoins des femmes en périnatalité.* Unpublished Master's dissertation, Montréal, Université du Québec à Montréal, Canada.

28   Vadeboncoeur H, 2004. La naissance en 2004: Qu'est-ce que l'humanisation? Literature review done for L'Association pour la Santé Publique du Québec. Unpublished document.

29   Misago C, Kendall C, Freitas P *et al,* 2001. From 'culture of dehumanization of childbirth' to 'childbirth as a transformative experience: changes in five municipalities in north-east Brazil. *International Journal of Obstetrics and Gynecology,* 75 (1): S67-S72.

30   Green JM, Coupland VA, Kitzinger J, 1990. Expectations, experiences and psychological outcomes of childbirth: a prospective study of 825 women. *Birth,* 17(1):15-24.

31   Stadlmayr W, Bitzer J, Hosli I, *et al,* 2001. Birth as a multidimensional experience: comparison of the English and German-language versions of Salmon's Item List. *Journal of Psychosomatics Obstetrics and Gynecology,* 22: 205-214.

32   Callister LC, 2004. Making meaning: women's birth narratives. *JOGNN: Journal of Obstetric, Gynecologic and Neonatal Nursing,* 33(4): 508-518.

33   DeVries R, Salvesen HB, Wiegers TA, *et al,* 2001. What (and why) do women want? The desires of women and the design of maternity care. In *Birth By Design – Pregnancy, Maternity Care, and Midwifery in North America and Europe,* DeVries R *et al* (eds). New York: Routledge, pp 243-265.

34   Lemay C, 1999. *Anthropology of Homebirth: Voice of Women and Midwives.* Manilla: International Confederation of Midwives, Philippines.

35   Klassen PE, 2001. Sacred maternities and postbiomedical bodies: religion and nature in contemporary home birth. *Signs,* 26(3): 775-809.

36   Viisaiven K, 2001. Negotiating control and meaning: home birth as a self-constructed choice in Finland. *Social Science and Medicine,* 52(7):1109-1121, p 1114.

37   Baldwin R, Palmarini T, 1986. *Pregnant Feelings.* Berkeley: Celestial Arts, p 2.

38   Aria B, Dunham C, 1991. *Mamatoto: A Celebration of Birth.* London: Virago, p 98.

Glossary

adhesions a frequent consequence of any surgery because scarring takes place. After a caesarean adhesions can develop between the uterus and the surrounding organs or affect the abdominal wall, sometimes to the point of causing intestinal obstruction. They can cause pain after the operation (sometimes persistent pain) and pain in future pregnancies, since the expansion of the uterus pulls, stretches or breaks any adhesions. With any subsequent caesarean, surgery becomes more complicated as the surgeon has to deal with scarring and adhesions from the previous operation(s) and this increases the length of the operation too.

adrenaline (also called 'epinephrine') the hormone which is sometimes called the 'fight-or-flight' hormone because it is produced spontaneously by the body in times of great stress. Strangely enough, although stressful situations generally prevent a good labour and birth, adrenaline is naturally produced as part of a 'fetus ejection reflex'.

alternative therapies: a variety of therapeutic or preventive health care practices, such as osteopathy, homeopathy, naturopathy, chiropractic, self-hypnosis or biofeedback

amniotic fluid the clear, odourless, sterile fluid in which your baby floats when he or she is in your womb. As well as nourishing your little one, it also protects him or her from bumps and—oddly enough—is also the place where your little one wees! The fluid is replaced every three hours (by natural processes) which is one reason why it seems important to drink plenty of water.

amniotomy breaking the woman's waters, i.e. the membranes which keep them in, so they flow out. This is sometimes done so as to speed up labour, but it is clearly an intervention.

anaesthesia (general) the use of intravenously-administered drugs to induce loss of consciousness, during which patients are not arousable, even by painful stimulation. Since patients often cannot continue to breathe on their own while anaesthetised, other drugs are used to sustain breathing. A local anaesthetic or a regional anaesthetic (e.g. an epidural) blocks off pain in a specific part of the body and does not result in loss of consciousness

analgesia the use of drugs (familiarly known as 'painkillers') to relieve pain

analgesics drugs which aim to be mild to moderate painkillers e.g. paracetamol and co-dydramol.

anterior the 'front' of a woman's body. Your little one is said to be in an 'anterior' position (or 'anterior presentation', or 'anterior lie') when his or her back is against your front (stomach). This contrasts with a 'posterior' position in which the fetal back lies against the woman's back. An anterior position is more favourable for a smooth labour and birth.

Apgar score a score out of 10 given to newborns to indicate health. See page 16.

augmentation (or acceleration) stimulation or acceleration of labour, usually by the administration of drugs intravenously (e.g. Pitocin) or by performing an amniotomy, known as ARM

biofeedback the process of becoming aware of various physiological functions with instruments which provide information on the activity of those systems. The aim in doing this is to be able to manipulate physiological functions at will so as to improve health or performance. It is reportedly possible control brainwaves, muscle tone, skin conductance, heart rate and pain perception. Along with physiological changes achieved, subjects also report experiencing changes in thoughts, emotions and behaviour.

biomedical model an approach to birth which treats this event as essentially a medical one, centering on its 'management', on interventions and technology. This approach has also been labelled 'technocratic' (by Robbie Davis Floyd), 'industrialised' (by Michel Odent) and 'medicalised' (by various writers).

birth canal an unhelpful term which supposedly describes the route your little one travels when he or she is born. Of course, the term is unhelpful because the word 'canal' suggests a hard, straight, man-made passageway, while the reality is a soft, womanly, curvaceous route.

birthframe a term coined in this book to refer to an account by a woman, man, child or professional which describes any aspect of a pregnancy or birthing experience or experiences

birthing ball another name for a large inflated gym ball, which some women find helpful during labour

birth centre (also 'birthing centre') a small unit run by midwives which specialises in birth and which aims to create a private and comfortable environment for birthing women. In some places birth centres are located outside hospitals and in others they are parts of hospitals. In both cases, they are run by midwives, not consultants.

birthing pool a pool (similar to a paddling pool) which may be inflated or assembled (or a permanent fixture) and used at home or in hospital. Birthing pools usually have pumps and heaters which allow water to be put in and heated to an ideal temperature. They are available for hire.

blood pressure the force exerted by circulating blood on the walls of blood vessels— one of the main so-called 'vital signs'. It is important to check blood pressure during pregnancy because although it must be high *enough* to ensure that your little one gets enough oxygen (through the placenta), it must also not rise too high, because high blood pressure is one of the symptoms of pre-eclampsia, which *may* (in a few rare cases) be a prelude to the life-threatening condition eclampsia.

bonding a process involving the development of a close, loving relationship, which is said to occur between mother (or father) and newborn babies after the baby's birth

bradycardia an abnormally slow or unsteady heart rhythm

breaking the waters – see 'amniotomy'

breech when a fetus is in a position where it will be born buttocks first, or feet first. 'Complete breech' means that the baby's hips and knees are flexed so that the baby is sitting cross-legged, with feet beside the bottom. Also see 'frank breech', 'footling breech', and 'kneeling breech', if relevant.

brow presentation when the fetal head is not well 'flexed', i.e. not well tucked into his or her chest. This usually necessitates a caesarean section. Also see 'flexed position'.

Caesar caesarean section

caesarean abdominal surgery carried out under regional or general anaesthesia, which involves extracting the baby from the mother's uterus through an abdominal incision. A caesarean is said to be primary when it's the first one the woman has; a repeat caesarean is a subsequent one; an elective caesarean is a planned caesarean; an emergency caesarean is one which is carried out during labour, either because it's a real emergency (cord prolapse, placenta praevia, etc) or because a medical decision has been taken to perform one (for failure to progress, failed instrumental birth, etc); a caesarean on demand is one which is carried out for no medical reason.

cardiotocograph [CTG] a graph produced by an electronic fetal monitor

care guide a term coined in this book to replace the commonly used term 'birth plan'. Like a birth plan, it is a document which details a woman's wishes for her labour and birth.

castor oil vegetable oil which is sometimes used to stimulate contractions; it sometimes works because it stimulates the intestines, which also means that the uterus becomes stimulated.

catheter a thin, flexible tube which is inserted into the bladder in order to drain off urine

cephalic in a head-down position in the womb (i.e. not breech), , which is an ideal position for the birth

cephalo-pelvic disproportion the situation where a woman's pelvis is supposedly too small (or inappropriately shaped) for the fetal head to pass through. In the past it was frequently given as the reason for an emergency caesarean, but it is now largely discredited in most cases. However, it may still be an issue if a woman has suffered (or is suffering from) scoliosis, kyphosis or rickets. A scan is also often suggested for women with diabetes because this condition often results in an overly large baby.

cervix the muscle at the base of the womb. When you go into labour, this muscle will first soften, then shorten and finally open out (like a blossoming flower)—'dilate' in medical jargon—so as to enable your fully-grown baby to leave your womb and enter the world. While you are pregnant, he or she is being kept safe and sound in your womb as a result of this very effective muscle's work.

coccyx see 'tailbone'

Cochrane Library a website which periodically publishes reviews of scientific studies carried out by the Cochrane Collaboration. This is an international network of people helping caregivers, policy makers, patients, etc make informed decisions about human health. The Cochrane systematic reviews are highly respected evaluations of medical research. Also see 'systematic review' and 'meta-analysis'.

commanded pushing when a midwife or doctor instructs a woman to push at certain moments, perhaps according to what they are observing on a monitor, or based on their view of what is happening. (For example, the woman may be asked to hold her breath while a caregiver counts the seconds, or she may be asked to push with all her might.) It contrasts with 'spontaneous pushing', where a woman pushes spontaneously, based on her intuitive view of timing or her instinctive knowledge of how to give birth.

compression (of the umbilical cord) when the umbilical cord becomes pressed (perhaps during the birth), which may mean the fetus is deprived of oxygen. This is obviously dangerous for the growing baby.

consultant a senior medical expert, typically an obstetrician, working from a hospital in the UK, Australia or Ireland

contractions an unhelpful term to describe the flexing of the uterine muscles when a woman goes into labour and gives birth. The word is unhelpful because it suggests a narrowing and 'drawing in', when in fact an expansion and 'drawing out' is occurring.

contraction stress test [CST] (also called a 'stress test' or 'oxytocin challenge test') a pre-labour procedure which aims to check how well the placenta is functioning and therefore whether a fetus will be able to cope with the reduced levels of oxygen that normally occur during labour contractions. First synotcinon (artificial oxytocin) is injected intravenously, then the pregnant woman is connected up to an electronic fetal monitor. Also see 'EFM'.

convenience factor a non-medical reason for doing (or not doing) something. In this book it's mentioned as one of the reasons to explain the rising caesarean rate.

convulsions when a person's body shakes rapidly and uncontrollably, which occurs if muscles contract and relax repeatedly. Convulsions are a symptom of the life-threatening condition eclampsia so are a sign of an emergency treatment.

cord umbilical cord

cord prolapse when the umbilical cord drops down out of the woman's body before the baby is born—a dangerous eventuality because it is likely to lead to cord compression, which can mean the baby is deprived of oxygen and therefore at risk

correlation this means that researchers find a link between two factors, e.g. smoking and birth weight—i.e. a research project may show a clear link (a 'correlation') between the amount a pregnant woman smokes and the subsequent birth weight of her baby

crown when your little one has travelled down the so-called 'birth canal' and his or her head ('crown') stays visible at the vaginal opening, without slipping back in. This occurs just before the birth.

c-section caesarean section

deep transverse arrest see 'transverse arrest'

dehiscence a rupture or 'bursting open' of some part of the body; this may happen with an abdominal wall after surgery, for example. Uterine rupture is a form of dehiscence.

dilated open; fully dilated' means a cervix has opened to 10cm

dilation the process by which the cervix opens up (to 10cm) so as to allow a baby to be born. Midwives and doctors usually measure the extent of dilation using their fingers.

doula a mother figure a woman can rely on before, during or after giving birth. Normally, doulas follow some kind of formal training before gaining work experience – and they are often experienced mothers themselves. They usually meet their pregnant clients a few times during the woman's pregnancy, then they offer support throughout the whole of the labour and birth, as well as postnatally. Some doulas work within organisations and some are autonomous, while others are employed by a company. See Useful contacts for more information.

dystocia a vague term used to refer to an abnormal or difficult labour or birth. It is often the reason given for an emergency caesarean, being expressed as 'failure to progress', although what exactly constitutes a slow labour, or one which is not progressing sufficiently fast, is widely disputed.

eclampsia a serious complication of pregnancy, characterised by convulsions, which may occur before, during or after labour. It usually occurs after the onset of pre-eclampsia, although sometimes no symptoms of pre-eclampsia are found. When it occurs before labour has begun, the fetus needs to be delivered immediately and the mother also requires treatment.

ectopic pregnancy a pregnancy in which the egg fails to travel down to the womb after being fertilised in the fallopian tubes

edema see 'oedema'

EFM [electronic fetal monitoring] monitoring which involves connecting a woman up to an electronic fetal monitor. It is carried out either intermittently or continuously throughout labour, or during the third trimester, in which case it is called the 'non-stress test'. Two disc-shaped transducers are usually laid on the woman's abdomen in order to measure both the fetal heart rate and uterine contractions (if any). For obvious reasons, this monitoring restricts a woman's movement and gives her a feeling of being observed.

electronic fetal monitoring (also 'external fetal monitoring') see 'EFM'

emergency caesarean a caesarean which is unplanned, which is felt to be necessary during labour; also called an 'in-labour caesarean'

endorphins the body's natural painkillers, i.e. feel-good hormones which are produced spontaneously during an undisturbed natural labour

enema a procedure in which liquids are introduced into the rectum and colon via the anus with a view to stimulating the expulsion of faeces (poo)

engaged a fetus is considered to be 'engaged' when his or her head drops down into the pelvis, ready for the birth

epidural anaesthesia produced by injecting a local anaesthetic into the epidural space of the lumbar or sacral region of the spine. This causes regional anaesthesia from the abdomen or pelvis downward and it is often used to control pain during childbirth. Drugs used in an epidural include narcotics.

episiotomy a cut made through the perineum (with a pair of scissors) so as to enlarge the vaginal opening, performed under local anaesthetic and sutured closed after the birth. Rarely performed now in the UK (although this is worth checking), but it is still a routine procedure in many countries of the world. It is a necessary and life-saving procedure if the baby's shoulder gets stuck or in the case of a breech birth which is not going well. Of course, it is also necessary if forceps are used.

external cephalic version [ECV] a manual attempt (by an obstetrician) to turn a fetus who is in the breech position at or after 37 weeks' gestation. It only has a 50% success rate and may result in distress to the fetus if he or she becomes entangled in the umbilical cord. This procedure should only be performed where facilities for an emergency caesarean are immediately available.

external version see 'external cephalic version'

faeces poo (excrement)

failure to progress the situation when one or more caregivers decide, during a particular woman's labour, that her labour is not moving forward. The assessment of labour in this respect is extremely subjective and is widely disputed in the medical literature

fascia a layer of flexible, fibrous connective tissue (which can withstand stretching), which is found round muscles, blood vessels and nerves—e.g. in the perineum

fetal distress a situation in which the life of an unborn baby appears to be threatened

fetal movement counting the counting of fetal movements a woman may be asked to do when she is overdue; she is usually asked to record these on a 'kick chart'. This is one way of monitoring that her little one is literally still 'alive and kicking'.

fetal scalp electrode [FSE] a device which is screwed into the fetal scalp while it is still in the birthing canal; it connects up with a monitor, which monitors the fetal heart rate. A version which uses a sensor rather than a clip is now also available.

fetal scalp monitor a monitoring machine which provides care providers with information about fetal heart activity, using an electrode which is screwed into the fetal scalp. Monitoring of this type can only take place when the woman's cervix is at least 1-2cm dilated and after the membranes have ruptured, either spontaneously or after an amniotomy.

fetal stethoscope (also 'fetoscope' and 'Pinard') a stethoscope shaped like a listening trumpet, which is put on a pregnant woman's abdomen so as to listen to the fetal heartbeat. This type of stethoscope has the advantage that it does not involve the use of ultrasound, unlike the Doppler Sonicaid. See page 195.

fetoscope see 'fetal stethoscope'

fetus (also 'foetus') a word used to describe the baby growing in your womb from the end of Week 8 of your pregnancy, by which time all the major systems and organs will have developed

fetus ejection reflex (also called a 'fetal ejection reflex') a sudden and compelling rush of energy which automatically makes birth simple, active and intuitive

first stage the stage of labour/birth in which the cervix opens so as to allow the baby to emerge in the second stage

first trimester the first three months of pregnancy

first-degree tear see 'tear'

flexed position when the fetus is curled up and his or her head is tucked into the chest

footling breech birth when one or two feet are born first. This occurs rarely at term, but is relatively common in premature births.

forceps a handheld, hinged instrument made from high-grade carbon steel, used to grasp and apply pressure. In a forceps birth, when a woman's cervix is fully dilated and her bladder has been emptied (perhaps with a catheter) the woman is placed in the lithotomy position, a mild anaesthetic is administered (if an epidural is not already in place) and the two sections of the forceps are individually inserted and locked into position around the baby's head. The fetal head is then rotated to bring the baby to an occiput anterior position (if this is not already the case), an episiotomy is performed, and the baby is pulled out.

forewaters the amniotic fluid which is in front of the fetal head when the baby is engaged. When these waters break the gush is usually dramatic and unmistakable as a leak of amniotic fluid. Also see 'hindwaters'.

frank breech when a baby's bottom is born first, and his or her legs are flexed at the hip and extended at the knees (with feet near the ears). 65-70% of breech babies are born in the frank breech position.

gentle gymnastics a movement approach developed by the French woman, Thérèse Bertherat, who called her system 'anti-gymnastique' (anti-gymnastics). Very gentle movements are performed in a conscious manner so as to become conscious of tensions within the body and learn how to release them.

gestate grow (fetus)

gestation the period when a baby is growing inside its mother

gestational diabetes diabetes which occurs for the first time during pregnancy

GP [general practitioner] a doctor in the UK, Australia or Ireland

haemoglobin [Hb] the iron-containing oxygen-transporting metalloprotein in the red blood cells of the blood

haemoglobin concentration what is tested for in a blood count, in order to check whether or not a woman is suffering from anaemia

haemorrhage excessive bleeding, which is life-threatening

haemorrhoids (also known as 'piles') enlarged and swollen blood vessels in or around the lower rectum or anus. They are very common in pregnancy, especially when the woman experiences constipation, which again underlines the importance of a good diet with plenty of water and roughage.

head down position with the baby's head facing downwards in the womb, which is an ideal position for the birth

heparin lock a small tube connected to a catheter which is inserted into a vein in the arm. It allows easy access for IV transfusions.

high blood pressure see 'pre-eclampsia'

hindwater leak see 'hindwaters'

hindwaters the amniotic fluid which is behind the fetal head when the baby is engaged. When these waters break there is usually intermittent trickling which is difficult to distinguish from the odd leak of urine (common at the end of pregnancy), or from thin vaginal discharge. Also see 'forewaters'.

hormone a natural chemical messenger which travels in the blood and carries a signal from one cell (or group of cells) to another. Their production and orchestration are crucial to successful birth, but highly susceptible to influence through disturbance.

hypertension high blood pressure. This is potentially dangerous in pregnancy if associated with high levels of protein in the urine. Also see 'pre-eclampsia'.

hysterectomy the surgical removal of a woman's womb

iatrogenic problem caused by the diagnosis, manner or treatment of a doctor

ICU [intensive care unit]

incision the medical word for 'cut'

incontinence the inability to control the flow of urine (wee), faeces (poo) or flatus (farts), which may result after some pregnancies or births, either vaginal or caesarean (because of the pressure during pregnancy on the pelvic floor)

independent midwife a midwife who works independently of the National Health Service (the NHS) in the UK

induced see 'induction'

induction any procedure which triggers the beginning of a woman's labour. Approaches used range from amniotomy to the use of cod liver oil and the use of drugs administered through an IV drip.

informed choice in terms of health, a choice is only considered 'informed' when the person who is making it has been given adequate information about a particular situation, including information about benefits and risks of all options which might be chosen. Information must be provided in a form which is understandable to the person involved (in terms of his or her ability to understand and communicate). The person should also benefit from nonjudgmental advice and support regarding the choices he or she wants to make. Also see 'informed consent' and 'informed refusal'.

informed consent a legal procedure used to ensure that a patient or client knows all of the risks and benefits involved in an intervention. It includes informing him of her about the nature of the intervention, possible alternatives and the potential risks and benefits of the intervention.

informed refusal after the information has been provided—see 'informed choice' and 'informed consent' above—this is an outcome in which the person receiving the information decides to refuse an intervention or course of treatment.

in-labour caesarean a caesarean operation which is deemed necessary while the woman is in labour

instrumental delivery when a baby is pulled out of a woman's vagina with the help of either ventouse (a vacuum extractor) or forceps (i.e. tongs, similar to salad tongs)

internal (or internal examination) an internal vaginal examination performed by a care giver to check cervical dilation

intervention any action taken or attempt at communication

interventionist having a preference for intervention

intestinal obstruction partial or complete blockage of the bowel which means that intestinal contents are unable to pass through

intrapartum during labour and birth

invasive officially this term refers to any medical procedure which penetrates or breaks the skin or a body cavity, i.e. which involves making an incision into the body or the removal of biological tissue. In this book the definition is extended to mean any procedure which penetrates a body cavity, like a vaginal examination, or the insertion of an internal monitor.

Kegel muscles the muscles which form the 'pelvic floor', which support the pelvic organs, including the vagina, bladder and rectum. For obvious reasons, maintaining use of these muscles is important so as to avoid incontinence.

Kegels term used to describe the exercises you can do so as to strengthen the muscles of your pelvic floor, originally devised by Dr Arnol Kegel

lithotomy position a common position used for surgical procedures involving the pelvis and lower abdomen. In this position the patient lies on her back with her knees bent and kept spread apart and above her hips through the use of stirrups. Of course, a woman giving birth is not a patient because she is not ill—she is simply a woman—and this position is not suitable for birth.

lithotomy stirrups U-shaped devices which hold a patient's legs up while she is in the lithotomy position undergoing surgery. See 'lithotomy position'.

litigation the process of taking a case to court so as to obtain compensation and/or a conviction

LMP [last menstrual period] the first day of your last period, which is used to calculate the day your baby is due to be born

LOA [left occiput anterior] the term used to describe your little one's position when the back of his or her head (the occiput) is pointing down and facing towards the left side of your body, with his or her back round to the front of your body. This is the best position for your baby to be in when you go into labour.

LOP [left occiput posterior] the term used to describe the fetal position when the back of the fetal head (the occiput) is pointing downwards and faces the left side of a mother's body, when the fetal back is round to the back of the woman's body, parallel to her spine. If the baby is still in this position when the woman goes into labour, she is said to have a 'posterior' labour.

lower uterine segment the lower part of the uterine cavity, as opposed to the upper uterine segment (the main portion of the body of the uterus). The type of uterine incision carried out in the lower part of the uterine cavity is less prone to rupture, and is called a low transverse incision (i.e. a horizontal cut, below the bikini line).

malpresentation the abnormal presentation of a fetus in its mother's womb, i.e. any presentation which is not a head-down position

medicalisation within the field of sociology, medicalisation is understood as the process by which social phenomena are defined and treated as medical conditions by doctors and other health professionals. Childbirth became medicalised in the 19th century. Saying that birth is 'medicalised' means that giving birth is increasingly seen as belonging to the medical domain.

meta-analysis within the field of statistics this word is used to refer to an analysis of the results of several studies with related research hypotheses. Meta-analyses are often, but not always, an important part of a systematic review of a given area of medical research.

Misoprostol a synthetic prostaglandin, used to help the cervix efface, so that it is more likely to dilate during labour. Other prostaglandins exist, which perform the same function. Misoprostol was not branded for use during pregnancy or labour and it may have detrimental effects.

morbidity illness in any particular case

mortality death in any particular case

mucous plug a mass of capillaries and mucous which fill the 'os', the small hole in the cervix, so as to keep infection out of your womb. It comes away as the cervix begins to open up at the beginning of labour, so noticing some stringy jelly (which may be streaked with blood) is a sign that your labour will begin within the next week or even day.

non-stress test [NST] electronic fetal monitoring which is carried out in the third trimester to check the fetal heartbeat

obstetrics the *surgical* medical speciality which relates to anything to do with the care of women (and her babies) during pregnancy and birth, and afterwards. Most obstetricians are also qualified gynaecologists. Note that a midwife is the *non-surgical* speciality which deals with women having babies, which explains why they have to refer women to an obstetrician in cases where, for example, a caesarean is necessary.

occipito-posterior position see 'posterior'

oedema a build-up of excess fluid within body tissues, which causes swelling. This is common in pregnancy and is nothing to worry about unless it is also accompanied by high blood pressure or high amounts of protein in the urine.

osteopathy osteopathy or osteopathic medicine is an approach which was first developed by Andrew Taylow Still, an American physician. It focuses on the role of the musculoskeletal system in health and disease. Practitioners can be found in many countries in Europe and beyond.

overdue a woman who is still pregnant (without having given birth yet) beyond her due date, which is generally calculated as being 40 weeks (or 280 days) after the first day of her last menstrual period

oxytocin a hormone produced naturally during orgasm, birth and while breastfeeding. During labour this hormone causes contractions, which make your cervix dilate and the baby move down and be born. During breastfeeding it is the hormone which enables your milk to be released into the milk ducts in your breasts. Note that synthetic oxytocin is often simply called 'oxytocin' by caregivers who are setting up a drip, even though the real name of the artificial hormone is 'syntocinon' (or 'pitocin' in the USA). (The synthetic version of the hormone is often used to induce or augment labour.) The artificial hormone does not have the same properties as naturally-produced oxytocin and it does not travel round the body in the same way, or result in the same behavioural changes (i.e. loving behaviour), which are associated with the natural hormone. The synthetic hormone also interferes with the production of the natural hormone and its use to stimulate or augment contractions often results in contractions which are too strong to be tolerated without recourse to strong pharmacological pain relief. As detailed on pages 44-45, the use of synthetic oxytocin during a VBAC labour may also increase the risk of uterine rupture.

oxytocin drip an IV drip which administers an artifical oxytocic, i.e. oxytocin

pelvo-cephalic disproportion see 'cephalo-pelvic disproportion'

perinatal morbidity this refers to the incidence or prevalence of disease or disability around the time of a baby's birth and, in this book, complications which aren't lethal

perinatal mortality this refers to the number of babies who die in the perinatal period (i.e. before and soon after birth)

perinatal outcome this relates to the baby's health—or otherwise—around the time of a baby's birth and refers to disease, disability and death

perineal massage the practice of massaging the perineum, i.e. the area of muscle around the vagina, during pregnancy. The idea is to try and prevent tearing during the second stage of labour. Research has suggested it can reduce second or third degree tears by 5% to 7%.

perineum the part of the body below the abdomen between the legs, which includes the anus and vagina and is the outlet to the abdomen. This part of the body has plenty of nerve endings (so is sensitive during labour and sex) and it consists of superficial and deep fascias and muscles. (Also see 'fascia'.) If the perineum is 'intact' after birth it means there has been no tearing.

physiological processes the natural processes the body will normally go through when no interventions of any kind are used and no 'pain relief' is attempted

Pinard stethoscope (sometimes simply called a 'Pinard') a fetal stethoscope shaped like a trumpet, which does not involve the use of ultrasound; named after the French obstetrician Adolphe Pinard (1844-1934)

pitocin synthetic oxytocin, known in the UK as syntocinon. Also see 'synoticinon'.

placenta an organ which develops during the first trimester of pregnancy from the same sperm and egg cells that form your little one. Its function is to transfer nutrients, oxygen, antibodies, and hormones from your own blood to your little one, and to transfer waste back out to your own organs (which will then process it).

placenta abruptio when a woman's placenta prematurely comes away from the uterine wall, suddenly depriving the fetus of oxygen. If symptoms indicate this may have occurred (i.e. bleeding with severe abdominal pain) the mother risks bleeding to death, so must go straight to A&E for emergency care.

placenta accreta the abnormal adherence of part of the placenta to the myometrium (the muscle of the uterus), when the placenta grows into the myometrium. This condition, which threatens the mother's health, is a complication of caesareans and may necessitate manual removal of the placenta after the birth, which in turn means the increased risk of parts being left behind and consequent infection. (The most effective treatment for placenta accreta is actually considered to be hysterectomy, i.e. removal of the womb.) Placenta accreta is serious complication and the risk of it occurring increases as each additional caesarean is performed.

placenta praevia when the placenta lies in the lower part of the uterus and covers part or all of the cervix. If it is only partially covered (Type I or II) a vaginal birth is possible. If the cervix is completely covered (Type III or IV) a caesarean section is necessary because the baby could not otherwise get out of the womb. If you are told you have placenta praevia at or before 20 weeks, the placenta may still work its way higher up as your womb stretches to accommodate your growing baby.

posterior the 'back' of a woman's body. A fetus is said to be in a 'posterior' position (or 'occipito-posterior position') when its back is against the woman's back. This contrasts with an 'anterior' position in which your little one's back lies against your front. An anterior position is more favourable for a smooth labour and birth. Also see 'posterior labour'.

posterior labour a labour which occurs when the fetus is in a posterior position (i.e. its back lies against the mother's back). This generally results in a more painful labour because there are no painfree breaks between contractions. If the woman is conscious and moving about as she wishes it is very possible that the fetus will turn to an anterior position in time for the actual birth.

postmature birth a birth which occurs after 42 weeks of pregnancy (or 43 weeks, according to some definitions). If the placenta is really no longer functioning properly and the baby is truly postmature (i.e. if it is not just a case of the due date having been incorrectly calculated), the newborn baby is likely to be thin and underweight, with slender limbs, dry wrinkled skin and longer hair and nails than usual in a newborn.

postmaturity the condition of a baby born after 42 weeks of gestation or 294 days after the LMP

postpartum haemorrhage [PPH] excessive (life-threatening) bleeding which occurs after a woman has given birth. Whether or not this is occurring is usually assessed *visually*, i.e. in rather a subjective, non-scientific manner, by care givers, but it is certainly something to be taken very seriously if bleeding is ongoing and does not stop with treatment (which is usually an injection of syntometrine).

post-traumatic stress disorder an anxiety disorder which can develop after a person experiences a terrifying event or ordeal in which grave physical harm occurred or was threatened. People with PTSD usually have persistent frightening thoughts and memories of their ordeal (i.e. flashbacks) and they may feel emotionally numb, especially with people they were once close to. Sleep problems are possible, feelings of detachment and numbness and people with PTSD are usually easily startled.

PPH see 'postpartum haemorrhage'

pre-eclampsia (also 'toxaemia' or 'pre-eclamptic toxaemia') a medical condition in which high blood pressure (140/90 or more) occurs at the same time as high levels of protein in the urine (300mg or more per day). It is potentially dangerous for both mother and baby, which explains why it is routinely checked for during antenatal appointments. It's worth knowing that it is much more common in first pregnancies than in subsequent ones. It may also occur immediately postpartum or 6-8 weeks after the birth. Eclampsia—the rare development which occurs in 1 in 2,000 pregnancies—is a much more dangerous progression of this condition.

primigravida a woman in her first pregnancy

prolonged pregnancy a pregnancy which extends beyond 42 weeks. Somewhere between 4-14% of women are thought to experience longer pregnancies.

prostaglandins hormones (often administered in the form of pessaries to induce labour) which may have many actions. They may cause constriction or dilatation of muscles, they may sensitise spinal neurons to pain, affect cell growth and even affect the production of other hormones, amongst other things.

protocols a medical protocol is a set of predetermined criteria which define nursing, midwifery or medical interventions and describe situations in which the caregivers make judgments about a course of action so that effective management can be provided for common problems. In obstetrics, not all protocols are evidence-based (i.e. based on scientific research)—some protocols may be traditional or local ways of doing things.

randomised control trial the type of scientific experiment considered the most reliable within the field of medicine. Randomised control trials involve the random selection of subjects who are allocated different interventions (or not, in the case of the 'control group') in order to test these particular interventions.

ring of fire a burning sensation experienced by women as their baby's head presses against the entrance to the vagina, just moments before baby is born

risk a word which has at least two meanings: 1. the possibility of suffering harm or loss, or facing danger, and 2. a factor, thing, element, or course of action (or inaction) involving uncertain dangers or hazards

ROA [right occiput anterior] the term used to describe the fetal position when the back of the fetal head (the occiput) is pointing downwards and towards the right side of a mother's body, when the fetal back is round to the front of the woman's body. According to optimal fetal positioning experts Jean Sutton and Pauline Scott, a fetus lying in this position just before labour begins will often drop round to a posterior position for labour... so it is not an ideal position for your little one.

ROP [right occiput posterior] the term used to describe the fetal position when the back of the fetal head (the occiput) is pointing downwards and faces the right side of a mother's body, when the fetal back is round to the back of the woman's body, parallel to her spine. If the baby is still in this position when the woman goes into labour, she is said to have a 'posterior' labour, which is not ideal.

rotation the word used to describe the movement (turning round) of a fetus in the birth canal so as to pass through the pelvis

scan see 'ultrasound scan'

second stage the stage of birth when the baby is born

second trimester the second three months of pregnancy

second-degree tear see 'tear'

section (also c-section) caesarean section

self-hypnosis a heightened state of focused concentration (i.e. trance), with the willingness to follow instructions (suggestibility), which may occur spontaneously (e.g. when watching a film). Specific approaches to self-hypnosis have been developed for pregnant women because research has shown that it can be beneficial for labour.

semi-squat a position in which the woman is upright, with her knees slightly bent. Of course, during the second stage of labour women may want to be supported in this position, or hang from something suspended from the ceiling.

serosa (uterine) a thin layer of tissue that covers the uterus (i.e. the fundus and the posterior body of the uterus). A true uterine rupture also involves rupture of the serosa.

SGA [small for gestational age] where a fetus appears to be smaller than he or she should be, considering his or her age

shiatsu a manipulative therapy developed in Asia, which incorporates techniques from traditional Japanese massage, acupressure and stretching, focusing on acupuncture meridians (which, in turn, are important lines within acupuncture)

shoulder dystocia a term used to describe the situation where a baby's right shoulder cannot be born or where it can only be born with significant expert manipulation

show a discharge of a jelly-like substance, which may be smeared with blood. Also see 'mucous plug'.

single-layer suturing technique see page 47

small-for-dates (or 'small-for-gestational-age') see 'SGA'

Sonicaid (also 'Doptone', 'Doppler machine' or 'carotid Doppler machine') a device which uses low-frequency ultrasound waves to measure frequencies which are translated into sounds. [See 'ultrasound' too.] It is used to listen to the fetal heartbeat but other sounds will also be heard, e.g. that of blood through the placenta.

sonogram a diagnostic medical image created using ultrasound echo (sonographic) equipment. Women are often given or sold one of these images after having an ultrasound scan.

stage one see 'first stage'

stage three see 'third stage'

stage two see 'second stage'

stress incontinence accidental leaks of urine (or faeces) after coughing, sneezing or laughing. Urinary stress incontinence is fairly common in late pregnancy, unfortunately!

stripping of the membranes see 'sweeping'

supine position when a woman is lying on her back. Also see 'lithotomy position' and 'tailbone'.

suppositories solid medications inserted into a woman's anus, perhaps as an enema, or to induce labour

sweeping when a pregnant woman's amniotic membranes are loosened or broken so as to induce or accelerate labour. In the USA this same procedure is called 'stripping of the membranes'.

syntocinon a synthetic form of oxytocin, sometimes used in a drip to induce or speed up contractions during labour

syntometrine see 'ergometrine'

systematic review a review of the academic literature which deals with a specific question. A systematic review is meant to identify, appraise, select and synthesise all high quality research evidence which is relevant to that particular question. Also see 'metaanalysis' and 'Cochrane Library'

tailbone (the 'coccyx') the final segment of the human vetebral column, made up of two or three solid bones with rudimentary joints. During birth if the woman is lying down the pressure of the baby passing through the 'birth canal' can make one of these joints break, which can cause considerable pain subsequently. If, on the other hand, the woman is in a forward, leaning-forward position the angles and internal dimensions of the abdomen change dramatically. As the baby passes through the pelvis both the sacrum and coccyx (tailbone) are lifted out of the way, meaning no damage occurs.

tearing damage to a woman's vagina and possibly also other body parts, categorised into four degrees. In a 1st degree tear, there is superficial damage but no tearing of muscles. When 2nd degree tearing occurs, both vaginal walls and muscles may be torn, but the anal sphincter remains intact. In the case of a 3rd degree tear, the tearing extends to the anal sphincter, but the rectum is still intact. A 4th degree tear involves tearing right up to and including the rectum. Tearing is less likely when a woman is completely conscious and if it occurs at all it is less severe and heals more effectively when there is no episiotomy. Tears can be treated fairly easily in the UK, unlike in other parts of the world, where women may become socially ostracised as a result of unrepaired tears.

thickness of the uterine scar research began into this in the mid 1990s—i.e. the thickness of the scar, where the caesarean was carried out, was measured with the idea of determining if a thin scar leads to more uterine ruptures, or not. Research results have been contradictory, because different measuring techniques were used.

third stage the stage of birth where the placenta comes out

third trimester the third three months of pregnancy

third-degree tear see 'tear'

transition the end of the first stage of labour, when the cervix dilates from 7 to 10cm. Symptoms of transition may be extreme and may include longer, stronger contractions, trembling, shaky legs, vomiting, irritability, backache, shiveriness or sweatiness, as well as despair or extreme grumpiness!

transverse arrest when the fetus gets stuck as it is descending the so-called birth canal. This may occur as a result of commanded pushing when the fetus is in a posterior position during the second stage of labour. Also see 'commanded pushing'.

transverse lie when a fetus lies horizontally across its mother's womb. It is common until 27 weeks of pregnancy, by which time the (larger) fetus should have settled into a head-down or breech position, ready for the birth. If the fetus is still lying transverse during labour, a caesarean must be performed.

trimester one of the three periods of pregnancy, lasting approx. three months

ultrasound acoustic energy with a frequency above human hearing. Also see 'ultrasound scan' and the photo caption above

Glossary 297

ultrasound scan a process in which images are produced using ultrasound (see 'ultrasound' entry above) so as to date and assess a developing pregnancy

umbilical cord the flexible cord which connects your little one to you (inside your womb), which contains umbilical arteries and a vein. It is along this cord that nutrients, oxygen, antibodies and hormones from your own blood pass to your little one, and that waste transfers back to you.

uterine to do with the womb

uterine rupture a separation of the uterine incision (all its layers at the site of the scar, including the membrane). If this occurs, a caesarean has to be carried out quickly so that the baby can be born safely and the woman's uterus repaired.

uterus see 'womb'

vacuum extraction / ventouse (also 'ventouse delivery') the use of a device, called a vacuum extractor, to pull out a baby. A traction cup is attached to the fetal head, negative pressure is applied and traction is made on a chain passed through a suction tube. Vacuum extraction is an alternative to forceps and does not require an episiotomy.

vacuum extractor (also 'ventouse') see 'vacuum extraction'

vagina the passageway which leads from a woman's womb out of her body. It is commonly thought to include the vulva or female genitals generally, but strictly speaking it only includes the internal tubular passageway.

vaginal exam a check carried out by a midwife to ascertain how dilated a woman's cervix is

VBAC [vaginal birth after caesarean] when a woman who has previously had one or more caesareans has a vaginal birth for a subsequent child

VBAC rates meaning the number of VBACs arranged which actually occur (i.e. as vaginal births), it should be noted that there is more than one way of calculating rates. Some countries or hospitals take the number of women who completed a VBAC and divide this by the number of women who had a previous caesarean. For instance, if 10 women had a VBAC on a total of 40 women who previously gave birth by caesarean, the VBAC rate is said to be 25% (i.e. a quarter). Other countries or hospitals divide the number of VBACs by the total number of births, which gives a much lower VBAC rate. With this system, if the total number of births is 100 and 10 out of 100 women completed a VBAC, the VBAC rate is calculated as being 10 %.

vena cava the main vein running down a mother's back, which takes blood from the placenta and therefore also from the fetus. It is easily compressed by the heavy uterus when the mother is lying on her back.

ventouse vacuum extractor. See 'vacuum extraction'.

version see 'external cephalic version'

vertex position where your little one's presenting part is the occiput of the flexed head, i.e. not the feet (breech)

vulva a woman's exterior genitalia (genitals)

water birth a birth in which the woman labours in water (preferably after reaching more than 5cm dilation) and possibly also gives birth under water

waters the amniotic fluid around your baby when he or she is in your womb. Also see 'amniotic fluid'.

waters breaking also known as SROM (spontaneous rupturing of the membranes), this is when the amniotic membranes break, thereby releasing amniotic fluid – in a continuous flow, a gush, or in dribbles.

womb (also 'uterus') the 'bag' of muscle which holds your growing baby and which gradually expands to create a huge bump!

Index

ACOG (American College of Obstetricians and Gynecologists) 12, 22, 23, **25, 26**, 27, 44, 47-51, **84-95**, 99, 100, 117, 196, 197, 203

accomplishment, sense of 172, **226-228**

adhesions 46, 55, 64

admission to hospital 196

advantages of:

caesareans 52, 53

having a doula **171, 172, 173**

vaginal birth for the baby 96, 191, 218

VBAC 51, 72—also see Chapters 3 and 7, Birthframe 26 (on p 239) and most of the other birthframes

AIMS (Association for Improvement in the Maternity Services) 13, 98, 167, 220

allergies 52, 57, 64, 72

amniocentesis 41, 58, 59

amnioscope 199

amniotomy 45, 59, 78, 171, **189, 199, 201**, 210—also see Birthframes 4, 5, 7, 14, 27 (on pp 33, 35, 70, 177, 242)

anaesthesia 53, 54, 63, 64, 77, 191, 194, 206, 207, 209—also see 'epidurals'

analgesia 77, 194, 201, 203, 223

antenatal appointments 19, 76, 100

antenatal classes 19, 76, 121, 153, 154

anxiety 38, 62, 121, 172, 173, 198

Apgar score 52, 172, 198, 226

approaches:

alternative therapies 202

bio-medical 232

Mother-Baby 14, 19, 21, 55, 72, 73, 122, 170, 171, 172

natural 224

ARM (artificial rupture of the membranes)—see 'amniotomy'

asthma 52, 57, 64, 72, 88, 300

attachment—see 'bonding'

augmentation (or acceleration) of labour 41, 44, 45, 54, 59, 93, 94, 99, 158, 189, 192, 201, 202, 203

autonomy 119

Baby-Friendly Hospital Initiative 19, 20, 21, 100

baths during labour, benefits of **192**, 208

also see Birthframes 4, 6, 9, 13, 14, 17, 21, 22, 25, 27 (on pp 33, 66, 104, 140, 177, 182, 216, 233, 237, 236, 242)

bikini line incision—see 'low transverse incision'

biomedical model of childbirth 156, 220

birth attendants (fathers, partners, other companions) 73, 152, 161, 175, 188, 192, 232—also see Birthframes 2, 21 (on pp 4, 216)

birth centres 41, 92, 166, 176, 202, 211

birth environment 151, 153, 174
birthing balls 190, 211, 285
birth plans—see 'care guides'
birthing stool 191
birth weight 57, 66, 90, 189
bleeding 40, 46, 47, 99—also see 'haemorrhage'
blood clots 53, 54
bonding 52, 61, 72, 73, 102, 113, 171, **172**
Brabant, Isabelle 12, 115
bradycardia 40—also see 'fetal heartbeat'
breastfeeding:
    factors negatively affecting 54, 55, 64, 119, 122, **206**, **207**, 211
    initiation 72—also see Birthframe 6 (on p 66)
    difficulties sucking—see Birthframe 3 (on p 31)
    duration 207
breech babies 9, 46, 77, 78, 79, 80, 89, 209
breech babies in past caesarean 82, 84
breech position—see 'presentation'
Bujold, Emmanuel 42, 45, 86, 97, 201
caesareans:
    delay from decision to operation (in the case of uterine rupture) 197
    due dates and caesareans 56, 57
    elective 12, 15, 24, 26, 30, 39, 41, 42, 53, 56, 57, 60, 82, 196—also
        see Birthframes 9, 12, 24 (on pp 104, 135, 235)
    emergency 22, 23, 25, 39, 41, 49, 55, 59, 63, 75, 91, 95, 113, 114,
        121, 166, 168, 191, 197
    how to avoid having another one **189**
    indications for 77, 78
    more than one previous caesarean **86**, 99—also see Birthframes 24, 26
        (on pp 235, 239)
    on demand 11, 12, 53, 62, 72, 76
    previous 15, 22, 23, 25, 39, 41, 42, 44, 51, 53, **76**, 77, 78, 83, **84**, 90,
        91, 94, 95, 100, 112, 128, 151, 153, 167, 196, 202, 209—also
        see Birthframe 22 (on p 233)
    primary 85
    rates **8**, **9**, **10**, 14-16, 18-21, 23, **27-29**, **53-56**
    reasons to choose 74-76, 96, 97
    repeat caesareans 11, 15, **24-26**, 30, 39, 41-43, **48**, 48, 50, 51, 53,
        54, 56, 59, 60, 64, 71, 74, 75, 76, 95, 96, 97, 98, 99, 100, 166,
        203—also see Birthframes 15, 18 (on pp 179, 212), and
        'caesareans, elective'
    risks of 52-58—also see 'risks of caesareans'
    trivialisation of 9, 11
    unnecessary **77**, 169
    also see all birthframes

cardiac arrest 64
care guides (birth plans) 175
catecholamines 55, 60
cephalo-pelvic disproportion 23, 81, 85, 151, 286, 292—also see 'pelvimetry'
        and 'ultrasound' and Birthframes 6, 12 (on pp 66, 135)
cephalic (external) version **78**, **90**—also see Birthframe 27 (on p 242)
cervical dilation **92**, 161, **162**, 190, 202, 209
cervix, soft 22, 43, 45, 63, **81**, 91, **92**, **93**, 95, 160, **189**
      also see Birthframes 4, 5, 12, 13, 14, 15, 17, 21, 23, 24, 26 (on   pp
        33, 35, 135, 140, 177, 179, 182, 216, 233, 234, 235, 239)
Chaillet, Nils 252
Changing Childbirth 20
Childbirth Connection 54, 57, 60, 121, 165, 220
choice of:
      birth centre **164**
      doctor or consultant 164, **167**, **168**, 169, 170
      doula—see 'doula'
      hospital 83, 99, **164**
      midwife 164, **167**, **168**, 169, 170
choices (decisions) 1, 12, 19, 22, 25, 29, 38, 58, 60, 71, 74, 77, 83, 86, 97,
        101, 168, 164, 165, 167, 206—also see 'choice' and
        Birthframes 9, 17, 27 (on pp 104, 182, 242)
circumstances linked with the circumstances of your VBAC:
      being induced in any way 94
      being induced when the cervix is favourable (i.e. soft) 92
      being less than 4cm dilated at admission 92
      experiencing failure to progress during the active phase of labour   93
      experiencing labour progressing well 95
      having a baby with its head engaged and descended lower 94
      having an epidural 95
      having a soft cervix at the beginning of labour 93
      having a VBAC at home 93
      having a VBAC in a birth centre 92
      having a VBAC in a country where midwives are the main
      caregivers 92
      having a VBAC in a low volume hospital 92
      having a VBAC in a rural hospital, or in a private hospital 91
      having movements restricted during labour 94
      having non-reassuring fetal heart traces 95
      having synthetic oxytocin in a drip to induce labour 93
      having the length of labour limited in advance 94
circumstances linked with your personal characteristics or situation:
      being asthmatic 88
      being diabetic (type 1 diabetes) 88

being healthy before the pregnancy 87
being obese or having a high BMI 88
being over 30 years old 89
being short 89
being single 87
being white 87
expecting a boy 87
have high blood pressure 88
having an unusually shaped uterus (bicornate, etc) 89
having less than 12 years schooling 88
circumstances linked with your present pregnancy:
expecting a 'big' baby (expected to be over 4kg at birth) 90
expecting twins 90
giving birth at or beyond 40 weeks 91
having a baby who is presenting breech 89
having an external cephalic version (to turn a breech baby) 89
having a premature baby 90
having a thin uterine scar 91
having hypertension or pre-eclampsia 90
circumstances linked with your previous caesarean:
classical uterine incision (i.e. vertical in the upper part of uterus) 87
incomplete cervical dilation previously achieved 85
low vertical uterine incision or unknown type of incision 85
more than one previous caesarean 86
past caesarean with premature baby 86
previous uterine rupture 87
previous vaginal birth (before caesarean, or a past VBAC) 85
prior surgery to the uterus 84
reason for past caesarean: breech presentation 84
reason for past caesarean: cephalo-pelvic disproportion 85
reason for past caesarean: failure to progress 84
reason for past caesarean: fetal distress 84
single layer technique, single level suture for uterine incision 86
classical incision (i.e. vertical in upper part of uterus) 15, 42, 46, 63, 85, 87
also see Birthframe 25 (on p 236)
Cochrane Library 172, 191, 198, 207
commanded pushing—see 'second stage'
complications (maternal, fetal, surgical)—see 'risks of caesareans', 'risks of
VBAC'
complications, long term **55**, **57**, 64, 122
complications, short term 52, **53-55**, 56, 57
compresses 192, 209—also see Birthframe 5 (on p 35)
conferences—see 'consensus conferences'

confidence 19, 38, 74, 96, 119, 151, 156, 158, 169, 173, 188, 204, 224, 226, 227, 228—also see Birthframes 5, 6, 9, 10, 14, 17, 20, 26 (on pp 35, 66, 104, 130, 177, **182**, 214, 239)

congenital malformations 64

consensus conferences 22, 24, 26, 28, 30, 39, 41, 44, 63, 83, 115, 119, 122, 164, 197

consent 49, 199, 205—also see 'informed choice' and Birthframes 21, 26 (on pp 216, 239)

consent form 99

consultants 8, 11, 12, 14, 17, 18, 20, 24, 27, **28**, 29, 30, 42, 45, 48, 49, **50, 51, 58**, 71, 76, 77, 96, **97**, 100, 102, 114, 115, 117, 152, 167, 175, 201, 202, 221, 224, 230—also see Birthframes **4**, 9, 11, 13, **16, 18**, 24 (on pp **33**, 104, 133, 140, **181, 212**, 235)

contact:
    father-baby 73
    first or early contact **72, 73**, 74, 102, 113, 121, 180
    mother-baby 14, 21, 119, 132, 203
    skin-to-skin **72**, 73, 180
    also see 'bonding'

contractions 11, 13, 15, 45, 60, 61, 64, 81, 93, 99, 155, 156, 158, **160**, 161, 167, 170, 173, 190, 191, 192, 193, 198, 201, 203, 207, 208, 222, 224, 225, 231—also see Birthframes 1, 2, 3, **4**, 5, **6, 8, 9**, 10, 11, 12, **13**, 14, **17**, 18, 21, 22, 24, 25, 26, 27 (on pp 2, 4, 31, **33**, 35, **66, 103, 104**, 130, 133, 135, **140**, 177, **182**, 212, 216, 233, 235, 236, 239, 242)

contraindications 42, 84, 85, 89, 93, 94, 152

cord compression 41—also see 'cord prolapse'

cord prolapse 59, 78, 200

culture 18, 224, 228, 232—also see Birthframes 9, 15 (on pp 104, 179)

Cytotec 44—also see 'prostaglandins'

Dauphin, Francine 59

Davis-Floyd, Robbie 13

death, intra-uterine 57—also see 'risks of VBAC'

decisions (women's) 1, 7, 11, 12, 22, 25, 29, 39, 58, 61, 62, 65, **71**, 73, **74, 75**, 76, 77, 83, 96, 97, 100, **102**, 112, 116, 119, 151, 174, 175, 176, 196, 202, 206, 209, 229, 230—also see Birthframes 14, 15, 17, 19, 20, 21, 23, 24, 25, 26, 27 (on pp 177, 179, 182, 213, 214, 216, 234, 235, 236, 239, 242)

dehiscence 40-41, 83, 93, 287—also see 'uterine rupture'

De Koninck, Maria 13, 75, 225

depression xv, 54, 64, 118, 119, 121, 123-124, 128, 171, 172, 218, 226, 246—also see Birthframes 1, 12, 18, 20, 26 (on pp 2, 135, 212, 214, 239)

dilation—see 'cervical dilation'

doctors—see 'GPs'

Doppler—see 'Sonicaid'

doulas x, 17, 38, 45, 73, 96, 116, 153, 164, 167, **170-173**, 176, 190, 192, 199, 223, 246, 287—also see Birthframes 4, 5, 10, 11, 14, 15, 18, 20, 24, 25, 26, 27 (on pp 33, 35, 130, 133, 177, 179, 212, 214, 235, 236, 239, 242)

drinking during labour 81, 191, 197, 211

drips—see 'syntocinon'

drugs for pain relief 201, 203, 208, 223

due dates 56, 57, 61, 99, 166—also see Birthframes 1, 2, 4, 6, 10, 12, 13, 14, 18, 19, 21, 22, 24, 25, 26, 27 (on pp 2, 4, 33, 66, 130, 135, 140, 177, 212, 213, 216, 233, 235, 236, 239, 242)

dystocia—see 'failure to progress'

eating during labour 81, 191, 197, 211

EFM (electronic fetal monitoring), continuous or intermittent 23, 50, 77, 79, 81, 96, 100, 117, 170, 171, 189, 198, 200, 210, 211, 285, 286, 287, 288, 292—also see Birthframes 3, 4, 7, 10, 19, 24, 25 (on pp 31, 33, 70, 130, 213, 235, 236)

electronic fetal monitoring—see 'EFM'

embolisms 54, 64

emergency caesareans—see 'caesareans'

emotions 1, 73, 113, 114, 116, 120, **125, 126, 127**, 128, 163, 192, 222, 223, 225

empowerment 172, 225, 232, 233

endorphins 60, 206, **222-224**, 288

Enkin, Murray 59, 191, 196, 201, 202, 248

epidurals 13, 18, 20, 22, 40, 54, 55, 59, 74, 95, 113, 114, 173, 189, 190, 194, 203, 206-208, 210-211, 284, 289—also see Birthframes 1, 3, 4, 6, 9, 11, 12, 14, 17, 18, 19, 23, 26, 27 (on pp 2, 31, 33, 66, 104, 133, 135, 177, 182, 212, 213, 234, 239, 242)

episiotomy 18, 21, 114, 190, 194, 206, 208-209, 211, 226, 288, 289, 296, 297—also see Birthframes (on pp 6, 32, 103, 134, 178, 212, 213, 240)

external cephalic version 78, 79—also see Birthframe 27 (on p 242)

external version—see 'external cephalic version'

failure to progress 77, 78, 81, **84, 93**, 99, 151, 155, 156, 202—also see Birthframes 9, 11 (on pp 104, 133)

family, in labour and birth 13, **120**, 154, 169, 224, 225, 226—also see Birthframes 10, 12, 13, 17, 21 (on pp 130, 135, 140, 182, 216)

family, in pregnancy—see Birthframe 13 (on p 140)

fear of childbirth 18, 28

fear 9, 12, **18**, 22, 23, 27, 30, 38, 42, 58, 75, 76, 96, 119, 121, 124, 153, 154, 168, 173, 190, 192, 221, 222, 223, 226, 229

fear of litigation—see 'litigation, fear of'

fertility problems 55, 64
fetal descent 40, 192, 263
fetal distress 41, 59, 77, 78, **79**, **84**, 170, 190, 193, 194, 198, 199, 200,
        201, 207—also see Birthframes 23, 27 (on pp 234, 242)
fetal heartbeat, fetal heart rhythms 40, 45, 50, 63, 79, 95, 99, 189, 190, **198**,
        211—also see Birthframes 3, 5, 23, 27 (on pp 31, 35, 234, 242)
fever 54, 206, 207, 211
Flamm, Bruce 40, 45
forceps 15, 20, 45, 60, 64, 82, 114, 121, 128, 158, 164, 190, 193, 194,
        198, 203, 206, 226, 288, 289, 291, 297—also see Birthframes
        1, 2, 4, 6, 12, 14, 19 (on pp 2, 4, 33, 66, 135, 177, 213)
friend, support from (during labour) 171, 173, 189, 221—also see Birthframes
        5, 17, 19, 21 (on pp 35, 182, 213, 216)
friendship 155
genital herpes 78
gestation 46, 56, 61, 90, 91, 210
gestational diabetes 14, 117—also see Birthframes 6, 27 (on pp 66, 242)
GPs 11, 14, 17, 18, 19, 29, 50, 96, 102, 115, 118, 152, 167, 168, 204, 222,
        289—also see Birthframes 4, 8, 17, 25, 27 (on pp 33, 103, 182,
        236, 242)
guidelines 15, 20, 23, 24, 26, 28, 30, 42, **44**, 45, 47, **48**, 49, 50, 57, **63**, **84-
        95**, 99, 100, 152, 164, **194**, 196, 197, 199, 203, 204
guilt 20, 119, 121, 127, 210—also see Birthframe 21 (on p 216)
haemorrhage 40, 41, 54, 59, 63, 78, 206, 288, 290, 293, 294
head, fetal 39, 56, 73, 78, 81, 160, 161, 190, 199, 209—also see Birthframes
        1, 5, 6, 7, 9, 10, 11, 12, 13, 17, 19, 21, 25, 26, 27 (on pp 2, 35,
        66, 70, 104, 130, 133, 135, 140, 182, 213, 216, 236, 239,
        242)
head, engagement 189, 193, 210—also see Birthframes 4, 6, 8, 9 (on pp 33,
        66, 103, 104)
head, presentation of 22, 80, 81, 94
head rotation 20, 206—also see Birthframe 20 (on p 214)
headaches 206, 211, 223—also see Birthframes 14, 15 (on pp 177, 179)
healing **126**, **128**, 129
health, baby's 14, 39, 114, 118, 119, 124, 155, 226
health, maternal 14, 27, 39, 75, 78, 155, 156, 165, 175, 218, 226
        also see Birthframe 15 (on p 179)
heparin lock 197, 290
herpes—see 'genital herpes'
home birth 13, 17, 51, 227, 228, 229—also see Birthframes 5, 17, 18, 21, 25
        (on pp 35, 182, 212, 216, 236)
hormones 22, 55, 60, 61, 64, 190, 201, 222, 224—also see Birthframe 13 (on
        p 140)

hospitals 8, 9, 11, 13, 15, 17, 19, 20, 22, 23, **24**, 25, 26, 27, 28, 30, 41, 42, 44, 47, 48, 49, 50, 51, 53, 54, 55, 56, 62, 63, 72, 73, 74, 75, 82, 83, **91**, **92**, 96, 97, 99, 100, 101, 114, 115, 116, 117, 125, 151, 152, 153, **164**, **165**, 166, 167, 169, 170, 171, 172, 175, 176, 189, 190, 193, 196, 197, 198, 202, 203, 204, 205, 207, 210, 211, 218, 220, 221, 222, 223, 227, 229, 230, 231—also see Birthframes 1, 2, 3, 4, 5, 6, 7, 8, 9, 10, 11, 12, 13, 14, 15, 16, 17, 18, 19, 20, 21, 22, 24, 25, 26, 27 (on pp 2, 4, 31, 33, 35, 66, 70, 103, 104, 130, 133, 135, 140, 177, 179, 181, 182, 212, 213, 214, 216, 233, 235, 236, 239, 242)
humanisation of birth 13, 19, 72, 165, 227
hydration—see 'drinking during labour'
hypertension 56, 78, 90, 290
hypnosis 123, 158
hypotension 206, 211
hysterectomy 40, 44, 55, 63, 64, 166, 290
identity (sense of self) 118, 227, 228
impact—see 'reactions to caesarean'
    of a VBAC on the mother, father, couple, baby 228, 231, 232
    also see Birthframes 1, 10 (on pp 2, 130) and most of the other birthframes too
incision 15, 22, 25, 26, 39, 40, 42, 43, 46-47, 49, 51, 54, 55, 62, 63, 84, 85, 86-95, 290, 292—also see Birthframes 2, 14, 25 (on pp 4, 177, 236)
incision, type 26, 42, 43, **46**, **47**, 63, **85**
incision, risks associated with 22, 39, 40, 42, 47, 55, 62, 63
indications for a caesarean (absolute, relative)—see 'caesarean, indications for'
induction of labour 18, 21, 22, 41, 42, **43**, **44**, 45, 46, 51, 54, 59, 62, 63, 78, 93, **94**, 95, 99, 158, 166, 176, 189, 202, 204, 206, 210—also see Birthframes 13, 15, 27 (on pp 140, 179, 242)
infant/neonatal mortality 14, 15, **16**, 52, 56, 64, 92, 165, 203
infection 199, 207, 209—also see Birthframes 2, 15 (on pp 4, 179)
infection related to caesaeans 46, 52, 53, **54**, 64
infertility—see 'fertility problems'
information (obtaining it, becoming well-informed) 16, 17, **19**, 20, 21, 22, 25, 26, 63, 74, 76, 77, 84, 96, 98, 99, 116, 121, 126, 165, 174, 175, 199, 201, 211—also see Birthframes 3, 10, 14, 15, 26 (on pp 31, 130, 177, 179, 239)
informed choices or decisions 19, 26, 28, 38, 49, 102
instrumental delivery—see 'forceps' and 'ventouse, vacuum delivery'
integrity 119, 120, 226
intensive care 52, 53, **56**, 61, 64, 100, 198—also see Birthframes 2, 10 (on pp 4, 130)
internal examinations—see 'vaginal examinations'

306 birthing normally after a caesarean or two

International Mother-Baby Childbirth Initiative **19-21**, 83
interval (between caesarean and VBAC) 99, 167
interventions, during labour 3, 14, **18**, 19, 21, 27, 38, 43, 45, 51, 52, 54, **58**,
59, 62, 64, 99, 127, 128, 153, 165, 166, 172, 194, 199, 201,
202-204, 205, 206, 207, 208, 211, 220, **221**, 222, 223, 226,
230, 232—also see 'amniotomy', 'anaesthesia', 'augmentation or
acceleration of labour', 'caesarean', 'EFM', 'epidural',
'episiotomy', 'external version', 'forceps', 'induction', 'manual
exploration of the uterus', 'pelvimetry', 'Pitocin', 'prostaglandins',
'routines', Syntocinon', 'vaginal examinations' and Birthframes 2,
6, 9, 15, 20, 25, 26, 27 (on pp 4, 66, 104, 179, 214, 236, 239,
242)
interventions, neonatal 73, 209
intestinal, serious problems 55, **64**
intimacy 73, 172, 192, 222, 226—also see Birthframes 6, 10, 17 (on pp 66,
130, 182)
IVs—see 'drips' and 'syntocinon'
Jimenez, Vania 18, 22
Johnson, Lucy 226
Jones, Ricardo Herbert 220, 223
Jukelevics, Nicette 12, 123, 169
Kegel exercises 209, 291—also see Birthframe 14 (on p 177)
Kitzinger, Sheila 19, 98, 118, 220-221, 225, 228
Klaus, Marshall 171
Klein, Michael 14, 38, 118, 207, 254
labour:
active phase 79, **81**, 93, 99, 189, 192, 198, 199, 207—also see
Birthframes 17, 18, 21 (on pp 182, 212, 216)
benefits for the baby **60, 61,** 62
latent phase 45, **81**, 198, 199—also see Birthframes 18, 26 (on pp 212,
239)
lesions—see 'nervous system'
litigation 23, 27, **29**, 30, **49**, 50, 204
litigation, fear of 23, 27, 28, **29**, 30, 49, 50, 204
low birth weight 57
low transverse incision (bikini-line incision) 22, 25, 26, 39, 42, **46**—also see
'incision, type'
Lydon-Rochelle 44
Making Normal Birth A Reality 20
manual exploration of the uterus 40
massage 45, 157, 161, 173, 175, 192, 209, 223—also see Birthframes 6, 11,
14, 24, 26 (on pp 66, 133, 177, 235, 239)
massage chairs 191

maternal mortality 14, 15, **52**, **53**, 64, 92, 203—also see Birthframe 9 (on
    p 104)
medical associations 13, 30, 39, 46, 48, 50, 63, 100
medicalisation of childbirth 38, 204, 226, 229—also see Birthframe 17 (on
    p 182)
medico-legal considerations—see 'litigation'
membranes (spontaneous rupture of, waters breaking or rupturing) 59, 92,
    199—also see Birthframes 1, 2, 4, 5, 6, 7, 10, 12, 13, 17, 18, 21,
    22, 27 (on pp 2, 4, 33, 35, 66, 70, 130, 135, 140, 182, 212,
    216, 233, 242)
midwives:
    antenatal classes with 514—also see Birthframe 20 (on p 214)
    associations 48, 51, 98, 204, 220
    collaboration with physicians 222
    during labour 32, 45, **51**, 82, **92**, 98, 164, 168, 173, 175, 201, 220,
        228—also see Birthframes 10, 12, 13, 17, 21, 24, 25 (on pp
        130, 135, 140, 182, 216, 235, 236)
    influence of, on women 102, 104, 117
    influence on place of birth 166, 167, 168
    shortage of   30, 152
Misoprostol 18, 44, 63, 94, 291—also see 'syntometrine'
mobility during labour 190, 197, 211
monitoring—see 'EFM', 'Sonicaid' and 'Pinard'
mother-baby dyad 19—also see 'International MotherBaby Childbirth Initiative'
Mother-Friendly Childbirth Initiative 21, 83, 100
mourning, previous birth(s) 123, **113**-128—also see 'healing'
narcotics 206
neonatal mortality—see 'infant/neonatal mortality
nervous system (lesions) 57, 64
newborns 54, 56, 61, 62, 64, 73, 119, 197, 198, 203, 206, 215—also see
    Birthframe 3 (on p 31)
NICE (National Institute for Clinical Excellence) 15, 20, 23, 39, 44, 48, 79, 83,
    84, 91, 93, 94, 100, 152, 199
NIH Consensus Development Conference—VBAC: New Insights 24-26, 28, 30,
    41, 44, 63, 83, 164, 197
non-reassuring fetal heart rate tracing 95, 99, 201
obstetric interventions—see 'interventions'
obstetricians—see 'consultants'
Odent, Michel 13, 199, 220, 221-222, 223
official policies or recommendations 22, 48, 97, 204
overdue—41, 78, **91**—also see Birthframes 11, 18, 23 (on pp 133, 212, 234)
oxygen deprivation (lack of oxygen) 42, 63, 77, 78, 79, 199, 207
oxytocin, natural 55, 72, 192, 222-223, 292—also see Birthframe 13 (on
    p 140)

oxytocin, synthetic 11, 42, 44, 63, 93, 94, 99, 158, 190, 192, 201, 207, 286, 288, 293, 295—also see Birthframes 1, 5, 22 (on pp 1, 35, 233)

pain:

after caesarean 53-55, 64, **116**, 120, 130, 152, 209, 239

during sexual intercourse—55, 120

emotional 70, 115, 116, 120, 123-126, 152—also see Birthframes 9, 10, 17 (on pp 104, 130, 182)

in labour, of contractions 13, 15, 20, 21, 75, 81, 120, 170, 172, 173, 189, 190, 191, 192, 193, 199, 201, 203, 207, **208**, 222, **223**, **224**, 225, 230, 232—also see Birthframes 3, 6, 9, 12, 13, 14, 17, 21, 25, 26, 27 (on pp 31, 66, 104, 135, 140, 177, 182, 216, 236, **239**, 242)

pelvic 64

intestinal—see 'adhesions'

pelvic 64—see 'adhesions'

preparation for 156, 158—also see Chapter 5

relief—see 'drugs for pain relief' and 'pain, preparation for'

what helps to alleviate it 61, 68, 69, 171, 173, 178, **191-194**, 208, 209, 236—also see Birthframes 6, 14, 25 (on pp 66, 177, 236)

what increases it 201, 207, 208—also see 'amniotomy', 'oxytocin, artificial', 'position, lithotomy', 'position, supine'

Paling Perspective scale 59

pelvic pain—see 'pain, pelvic'

pelvimetry 90—also see Birthframe 18 (on p 212)

perinatal mortality 59, 165, 198, 221

perineal massage 175, 209—also see Birthframe 11 (on p 133)

Peterson, Gayle 75, 225

pulmonary hypertension, persistent 56

physiological pushing—see 'second stage'

Pinard 79, 210, 289, 293—also see Birthframe 13 (on p 140)

pitocin 59, 99, 284, 293—also see 'oxytocin, artificial' and 'syntocinon'

placenta abruptio (placental abruption) 293, 166

placenta accreta 55, 166

placenta praevia 22, 46, 55, 78, 293, 296—also see Birthframe 7 (on p 70)

pneumonia 54

positions:

for labour and birth: 41, 50, 79, 99, 150, 178, **191**, 209—also see Birthframes 4, 20, 26, 27 (on pp 33, 214, 239, 242)

lithotomy 189

on all fours 191

side lying 209

squatting—see Birthframe (19 on p 213)

supine 50, 198, 200

upright (or vertical) 81, 185, 191, **193**, 209

postmaturity—see 'pregnancy, prolonged'

postnatal recovery 74, 113, 120—also see Birthframes5, 22, 23 (on pp 35, 233, 234)

postpartum haemorrhage—see 'haemorrhage'

post-traumatic stress disorder 14, 98, 121, 123, 124, 128, 225

power—see 'empowerment'

PPH—see 'haemorrhage'

pre-eclampsia 78, 90, 285, 287, 290, 294—also see Birthframe 15 (on p 179)

pregnancy, ectopic 55, 58, 59

pregnancy, prolonged (after 42 weeks) 41, 78, **91**—also see Birthframes 11, 18, 23 (on pp 133, 212, 234)

prematurity 18, 46, 53, 57, 58, 86, 92—also see Birthframes 2, 8 (on pp 4, 103)

preparation:

    finding a supportive caregiver **167-169**—also see 'doula'

    for VBAC generally xiv-xv, 18, 19, 22, 76, 103, 114, 125, **151-157**, **175**—also see Chapters 5 and 6 and Birthframes 5, 7, 10, 11, 12, 13, 22, 26, 27 (on pp 35, 70, 130, 133, 135, 140, 233, 239, 242)

    mental **158**, 159, 160, 161, 162

    physical **155-157**

    place of birth (choice of) **164-166**

presentation (position of the baby) **80**, 81, 157—also see the Glossary, for each position, as follows:

    anterior 80

    cephalic (i.e. head down or vertex) 80

    breech 77, 78, **79**, **80**, 84—also see Birthframe 13 (on p 140)

    brow—see Birthframe 1 (on p 2)

    face—see Birthframes 5, 16, 25 (on pp 35, 181, 236)

    posterior **191**, 194—also see Birthframes 4, 21 (on pp 33, 216)

prolactin 55

prostaglandins 11, 22, 42, 43-45, 54, 60, 63, 94, 95, 201, 291, 294—also mentioned in Birthframe 2 (on p 4)

protocols (in hospitals or birth centres) 24, 63, **83**, 96, 100, **164**, **189**, 198, **202**

psychological impact of:

    caesareans 113, **119**—also see Chapter 4

    VBACs—see 'psychological growth'

psychological growth **226**, **227**, 232

PTSD—see 'post-traumatic stress disorder'

pulmonary hypertension 56

pushing—see 'second stage'

questions (having) 83, 102, 114, 115, 166, 168, 175—also see 'useful questions' and Birthframes 1, 4, 5, 9, 10, 11, 13, 15, 16, 23, 27 (on pp 2, 33, 35, 104, 130, 133, 140, 179, 181, 234, 242)

rates of caesareans—see 'caesarean, rates'
rates of VBACs—see 'VBAC, rates'
reactions to caesareans of:
>   babies 121
>   fathers 120, 121
>   mothers 113, 114, **115**, **116**, **117**, **118**, **119**, **121**, **123**, 128
>   other people around 117, 119
>   also see 'post-traumatic stress disorder' and 'depression'
refusal to arrange a VBAC
>   hospital's or consultant's or midwife's **97**, 100, 152, 153
>   woman's 96, 97
>   also see Birthframe 26 (on p 239) and other birthframes
respiratory distress—see 'respiratory problems'
respiratory problems affecting the baby
>   benefits of labour to prevent 60
>   effects of caesareans 52, **56**, **57**, 60, 61, 65, 100, 166
restrictions for VBAC 95, 96
>   in medical guidelines 23, 24, 25, 27, 44, 50, 51, 52, 196, 197, 203
rights (patient rights, human rights) 71, 98, 151, 210
respect 164, 174, 210, 220, 226—also see Birthframes 10, 17, 22, 26 (on pp
>   130, 182, 233, 239)
risks of caesareans 12, 13, 14, 19, 20, 25, 26, 38, **53-58**, 59, **60**, **64**—also
>   see 'complications, short term' and 'complications, long term'
risks of VBAC 17, 20, 22, 25, 26, 38, **39-47**, **49**, **50**, **51**, 59, 60, **62**, **63**—also
>   see 'uterine rupture' and Birthframe 4 (on p 33)
risk, level of—see 'risks of VBAC'
rite of passage 117, 221, 225, 232—also see Birthframe 17 (on p 182)
routines:
>   affecting the baby right after the birth **73**
>   during labour 19, 96, **189**, 199, 202, 204, 206, 208
RCOG (Royal College of Obstetricians and Gynaecologists) 20, 23, 41, 42, 45,
>   48, 50, 57, **83-95**, 152, 192, 196, 204
safety 14, 23, 26, 39, 75, 83, 84-95, 97, 101, 120, 161, 220—also see
>   Birthframes 13, 25 (on pp 140, 236)
scans 90, 189, 210, 286, 295, 296—also see 'ultrasound' and Birthframes 6,
>   8, 10, 12, 14, 17, 19, 26 (on pp 66, 103, 130, 135, 177, 182,
>   213, 239)
scar, emotional scar of a caesarean—see Chapter 4
scar, uterine—see 'incision'
second stage (the pushing phase of labour)
>   commanded (or directed) pushing **193**, 194
>   spontaneous (or physiological) pushing **193**, 194
secondary effects of caesareans—see 'risks of caesareans'
separation of the incision—see 'uterine rupture'

Index   311

separation, mother-baby 55, **72**, 208, 221, 226—also see Birthframes 6, 11
　　　　(on pp 66, 133)
septicaemia 54—also see 'infection'
sex:
　　　　impact of a caesarean or a VBAC and 82, 120, 124
　　　　pain from adhesions and 55, 56, 120
　　　　also see Birthframes 10, 13 (on pp 130, 140)
situations—see 'circumstances'
slowing down of labour— see 'failure to progress'
social factors 13, 71, 76, 117, 173, 219, 224, 230
SOGC (Society of Obstetricians and Gynaecologists of Canada) x, 20, 44, 49,
　　　　100, 197, **84-95**
Sonicaid 50, 79, 198, 210, 289, 295—also see Birthframes 4, 9 (on pp 33,
　　　　104)
spontaneous labour 41, 44, 61, 62, 64, 71, 93, 94, 99, 155, 204
spontaneous pushing—see 'second stage'
spontaneous vaginal delivery 60, 158, 171—also see Birthframes 17, 21 (on
　　　　pp 182, 216)
station—see 'fetal descent'
statistics—see 'caesarean, rates'
stitches—see 'sutures' and 'suturing techniques'
success (for VBAC) **84-95**
support—see 'doulas'
surfactant 57, 60
surveys:
　　　　Listening to Mothers 12, 201
　　　　Mother Friendly Childbirth Initiative 21
　　　　Transparency in Maternity Care 165
　　　　WHO on maternal and perinatal health 8
sutures (single-layer, two-layer) 43, **47, 63, 86, 167**
suturing techniques (double or single layer) 43, **47**, 63, **86**, 167
syntocinon 22, **44, 45**, 54, 59, 64, **93, 99**, 118, 158, 192, **201**, 202, **203**,
　　　　207—also see Birthframes 1, 2, 4, 5, 6, 14, 23, 25 (on pp 2, 4,
　　　　33, 35, 66, 177, 234, 236)
syntometrine 288, 293, 294, 295
Szejer, Myriam 62
tearing 171, **176**, 191, **193**, 207, 208, 209—also see 'episiotomy' and
　　　　Birthframes 5, 12, 13 (on pp 35, 135, 140)
technology 13, 22, 101, 154, 224, **226**
transformation xiv-xv, 120, **227, 228, 229**, 232—also see 'psychological
　　　　development'
transverse lie 78, 80, 296—also see Birthframe 10 (on pp 130)
twins 9, 14, 23, 26, 78, 90, 117, 247—also see Birthframe 19 (on p 213)

ultrasound 40, 79, 198, 283, 289, 295, 296—also see 'scans' and Birthframe
13 (on p 140)
useful questions:
frequently asked about VBAC labour and birth **196**
of the NIH Consensus Development Conference on VBAC 24, 26
to ask the caregiver **153, 169, 176**
to ask the hospital or birth centre **164** (before labour), **205** (during
labour)
to ask yourself (to deal with feeling guilty) **127**
uterine incision—see 'incision'
uterine rupture 30, **39, 40, 41, 42, 43, 44, 45, 46, 47,** 49, 50, 56, 58, **59, 63,**
83, 84, 85, 86, 87, 90, 93, 94, 95, 100, 152, 166, 196, 197,
201, 202, 207, 210—also see 'risk of VBACs' and Birthframes 3,
5, 6, 9, 11, 15, 27 (on pp 31, 35, 66, **104,** 133, 179, 242)
level of risk, **41,** 42, 46, 47, 53, 58, **59,** 60, 63, **99,** 102
signs of **40**
uterine segment, thickness 40, 41, 63, 167—also see Birthframe 4 (on p 33)
vaginal birth, factilitating factors **190-196**
vaginal birth, why give birth vaginally? **224-229**
vaginal examinations **199,** 222
VBAC (vaginal birth after caesarean):
preparation—see 'preparation for VBAC'
rates of **16,** 17, 18, 23, 26, 27, 30, 56, 96, **99,** 152
risks of—see 'risks of VBAC'
benefits of, for the baby—see 'labour, benefits for the baby'
ventouse, vacuum delivery 20, 45, 60, 64, 121, 158, 164, 171, 190, 193,
194, 198, 206, 291, 297—also see Birthframes 3, 6 (on pp 31,
66)
visualisation 158-163—also see Birthframes 6, 9, 11, 12, 13, 14, 17, 22, 27
(on pp 66, 104, 133, 135, 140, 177, 182, 233, 242)
Wagner, Marsden 51
warm water **192,** 208, 211—also see Birthframes 6, 9, 13, 14, 17, 21, 22, 27
(on pp 66, 104, 140, 177, 182, 216, 233, 242)
women's satisfaction 54, 98, 114, 116, **172, 173,** 227—also see Birthframe
10 (on p 130)
WHO (World Health Organization) 19, 20, 51, 56, 78, 165, 190, 218, 220

Right: Artwork by the author's sister, Rachel Vadeboncoeur—
a piece in stained glass called 'Intuition'

Intuition... 313

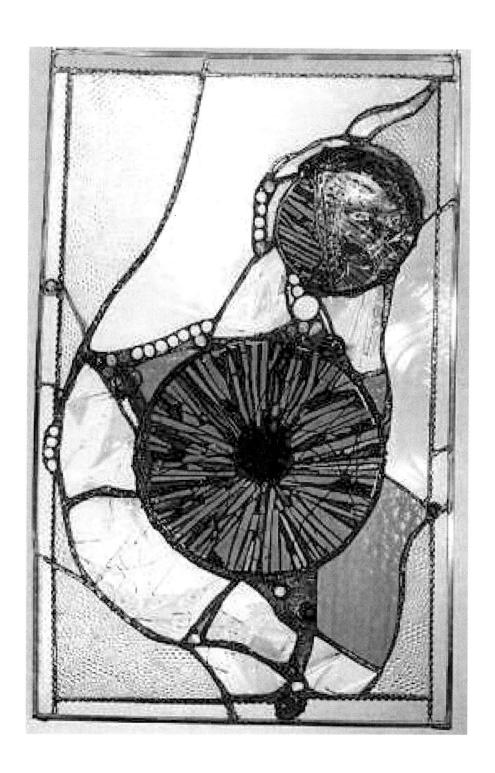

About the author

Many years after having children, Hélène Vadeboncoeur discovered that ever since her maternal great-great-grandmother gave birth in Ivy Bridge (England), most of the women she knew, as well as her direct ancestors, had had some serious problems while giving birth. Her own mother had had to fight in order to *not* be put asleep while having her first baby. Pondering these issues and considering her own experiences, in her early 40s Hélène decided to become a childbirth researcher.

Before having children Hélène had worked in the field of education, teaching children with learning disabilities. After having her own children, her priorities changed and she started working as a freelance researcher and consultant, mostly in the field of childbirth. One of her first contracts was to write a long article on VBAC for the Quebec women's magazine *Naissance-Renaissance, L'Une à L'Autre* [meaning 'Birth-Rebirth, Woman to Woman']. This article won her a prize from a Canadian association of specialised journalists and Hélène later expanded the original article into a book on VBAC, addressing women directly. It was, and still is, the only book ever published in French on VBAC and was the basis for a second edition and also for this book, which has been adapted for Britain.

All along, Hélène has been preoccupied by the lack of informed choice women seem to have when facing childbirth. In an attempt to explore reasons and options, when Hélène was in her early 40s she decided to go back to university to learn more about evidence-based obstetrics, which was at that time a relatively new preoccupation in the field of birth.

While studying for an MSc in Public Health, Hélène worked for five years for the Quebec Ministry of Health and Social Services and part of her work involved setting up out-of-hospital birthing centres. For her dissertation, Hélène did a comparative study on what had led two Canadian provinces to take very different approaches to the legalisation of midwifery. (Quebec had chosen to run pilot projects, while Ontario had chosen to legalise midwifery immediately.) Hélène then did a PhD in Applied Social Sciences at the University of Montreal and this time, she focused on the 'humanisation' of childbirth, doing an ethnographic study in a progressive hospital. (In case you don't know, ethnography is the study of people and cultures and usually involves research techniques such as participant observation, interviews and questionnaires.) While she was doing her PhD, Hélène also taught on the new university midwifery training programme in Quebec and she taught a course on research at the University of Montreal. Over that period, she also went on several overseas trips to find out more about birth practices around the world. As part of this research, she spent some time at the University of Sheffield, at the research centre of the School of Nursing and Midwifery, and she visited a few other British and Brazilian centres, often making presentations on her visits. She also visited several progressive obstetric wards and birthing centres, and exchanged information with many fellow researchers.

About the author

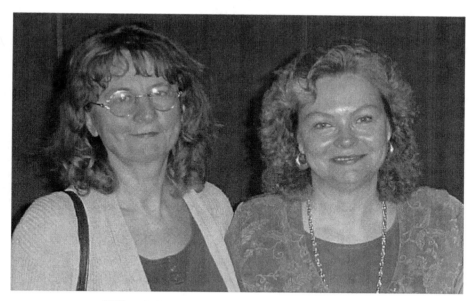

Hélène (left) with Robbie Davis-Floyd at a conference

Hélène eventually concluded that although in the last few decades some positive changes have occurred—for example midwifery has been legalised in some places where it was previously illegal, birth centres have been set up, and many obstetric wards have been renovated—the approach in many hospitals still seems to be based on the biomedical model of birth. In other words, she feels that birth is still seen as an event, which needs to be medically managed and decisions are too often only made by caregivers while in fact—in her view—it should really be seen as a multidimensional and physiological event with the birthing woman well informed and at the centre of the decision-making process.

Hélène's current work includes teaching doulas and participation in research projects, some of which are being carried out on an international level. In recent years, she has continued to coordinate studies at an innovative new centre in Montreal, which is providing health and social services to vulnerable pregnant immigrants who are also new mothers and she acts as a consultant to a local grassroots VBAC organisation. She is on the Board of Directors of the International MotherBaby Childbirth Organization (the IMBCO), is involved in the Quebec public health association, and also sits on several scientific committees for birth conferences. She is regularly interviewed by the media about caesareans and VBAC and often speaks at childbirth conferences around the world. Her published work includes many articles for scientific journals, in both French and English.

In case you're wondering where Hélène lives, it's in a beautiful spot by a lake in Canada. She loves to swim in the summer and skate, snowshoe or cross-country ski in the winter. It's an inspiring setting for her work on birth.

Photo © Regroupement Les Sages-Femmes du Québec, Canada

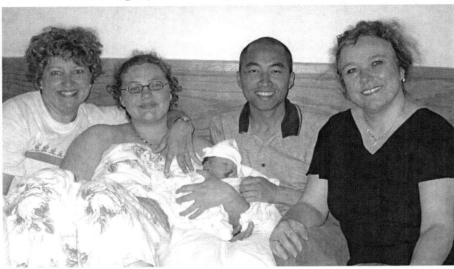

A happy family after a normal birth

A few words of thanks:

Here's an email the author received after the French edition was published...

I would like to thank you for the birth I experienced. I vaginally birthed a little boy on 9 November 2006, after having a caesarean on 21 April 2004. My consultant did not support my decision to have a VBAC. But after reading your book, I had arguments to put to him and, above all, confidence in myself, so that it was possible to refuse another caesarean. I had to hold firm in my decision and keep on insisting on it right up until the very last minute, but I did succeed and it was an extraordinary experience.

The birth went superbly well, without any complications. Afterwards, I felt so proud of being able to stand up and take care of my baby. Your book was just what I needed. I certainly do not have the impression that this VBAC took place in the normal course of events... In the hospital where I gave birth I felt like an alien from outer space when I said I didn't want to have another caesarean. When I arrived at the labour ward all kinds of conditions were imposed on my labour, none of which had been discussed with my consultant. But even then, I was prepared, thanks to having read your book. Without it, I would never have given birth normally.

Marie-Claude, 20 August 2007
[Read her birth story inside the book.]

Soo Downe

Professor of Midwifery Studies at the University of Central Lancashire:

The need to reduce caesarean section rates is well recognised by many authorities across the world. While it is essential to avoid unnecessary surgical birth for first-time mothers, it is also important to increase rates of VBAC for women who would like this option. To date, efforts to support this increase by the use of clinical guidelines alone have been variably successful.

This book is important because it combines a heart, head and hands approach. The use of good quality, well presented evidence, rich personal stories, and accounts of professional views speaks directly to the definition given by David Sackett and colleagues that evidence based medicine is a combination of best evidence, patients' values and clinical expertise.

This book therefore promises to be useful for many people—for individual women (and their partners) certainly, but also for maternity care staff and services committed to improving maternity care overall.

> This book is important because it combines a heart, head and hands approach

Also available from Fresh Heart:

Books for you:

- *Birth: Countdown to Optimal: Information and Inspiration for Pregnant Women* by Sylvie Donna
- *Birth Pain: Power to Transform!* by Verena Schmid
- *Birth Your Way: Choosing to Give Birth at Home or in a Birth Centre* by Sheila Kitzinger

Books for your partner, friends and relatives:

- *Surprising, Inspiring Birth: Accounts of Birth to Inform, Amuse and Reassure* by various authors

Books for your caregivers:

- *Promoting Normal Birth: Research, Reflections & Guidelines* by various authors (an international collaboration)
- *Optimal Birth: What, Why & How* by Sylvie Donna
- *Birth Pain: Explaining Sensations, Exploring Possibilities* by Verena Schmid
- *Welcoming Baby* by Debby Gould

See the Fresh Heart website for more information and prices.

All books can be bought online (paying by PayPal), or from any other online store (e.g. Amazon), or they can be ordered through your local bookshop.

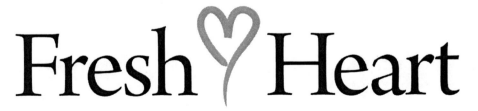

www.freshheartpublishing.co.uk

An invitation to share your own story...

At Fresh Heart we're interested in hearing about your own experiences so as to inform future editions of this book, but you may also want to have your own story published. If so, you can be named or anonymous and your account might be used either on the website or in a book, with your permission, of course.

To contact us to tell us about your experiences or for any other reason, simply click on 'Contact us' at the website below. If you're not online, write to us at:

My Story
Fresh Heart Publishing
PO Box 225
Chester le Street
DH3 9BQ
UK

LaVergne, TN USA
02 November 2010

203107LV00004B/1/P